Essentials of Nutrition and Diet Therapy

Essentials of Nutrition and Diet Therapy

Editor: Caleb Robbins

Callisto Reference

www.callistoreference.com

Callisto Reference,
118-35 Queens Blvd., Suite 400,
Forest Hills, NY 11375, USA

Visit us on the World Wide Web at:
www.callistoreference.com

ISBN: 978-1-64116-631-7 (Hardback)

Cataloging-in-Publication Data

Essentials of nutrition and diet therapy / edited by Caleb Robbins.
p. cm.
Includes bibliographical references and index.
ISBN 978-1-64116-631-7
1. Nutrition. 2. Diet therapy. 3. Food. 4. Dietetics. I. Robbins, Caleb.

RA784 .E87 2021
613.2--dc23

Table of Contents

Preface

The main aim of this book is to educate learners and enhance their research focus by presenting diverse topics covering this vast field. This is an advanced book which compiles significant studies by distinguished experts in the area of analysis. This book addresses successive solutions to the challenges arising in the area of application, along with it; the book provides scope for future developments.

The branch of science which interprets the interaction of nutrients present in food with respect to maintenance, health, disease and growth of organisms is known as nutrition. It studies various biological processes such as absorption, assimilation, biosynthesis and excretion. Some of the different nutrients studied under this field are carbohydrates, fats, proteins, vitamins and minerals. Diet therapy is a domain of dietetics which is concerned with the usage of foods for therapeutic purposes. It generally involves the alteration of the dietary lifestyle of a person in order to promote optimum health. Some of the therapies which fall under diet therapy are full liquid diet, clear liquid diet, pureed diet, renal diet and high fiber diet. This book provides comprehensive insights into the field of nutrition and diet therapy. It strives to provide a fair idea about this discipline and to help develop a better understanding of the latest advances within this field. Scientists and students actively engaged in this field will find this book full of crucial and unexplored concepts.

It was a great honour to edit this book, though there were challenges, as it involved a lot of communication and networking between me and the editorial team. However, the end result was this all-inclusive book covering diverse themes in the field.

Finally, it is important to acknowledge the efforts of the contributors for their excellent chapters, through which a wide variety of issues have been addressed. I would also like to thank my colleagues for their valuable feedback during the making of this book

Editor

Dietary flavonoid intake in older adults: how many days of dietary assessment are required and what is the impact of seasonality?

Katherine Kent[1*], Karen E. Charlton[2,3], Simone Lee[1], Jonathon Mond[1], Joanna Russell[4], Paul Mitchell[5] and Victoria M. Flood[6,7]

Abstract

Background: Within- and between-person variation in nutrient intake is well established, but little is known about variability in dietary flavonoid intake, including the effect of seasonality.

Methods: Within- and between-individual variability of flavonoid intake, and intake of flavonoid subclasses was examined in older adults ($n = 79$; mean age 70.1 y (range: 60y-80y)), using three separate 4-day weighed food records (WFR) collected approximately 4 months apart. The effects of seasonality were also examined. Mixed-effects linear regression models were used to estimate within- and between-individual variance components for flavonoids and subclasses. The number of days of dietary assessment required for a high level of hypothetical accuracy was calculated from variance ratios.

Results: Within- and between-individual variability was high for flavonoid intake, and intake of flavonoid subclasses, with variance ratios > 1. It was calculated that six days of WFR data are required for total flavonoid intake, and between 6 and 10 days was required for flavonoid subclasses. There was no effect of seasonality for total flavonoid intake or intake of flavonoid subclasses, with the exception that flavan-3-ol and flavanone intakes which were relatively low in summer, and in summer and winter, respectively.

Conclusion: While the effects of seasonality on total flavonoid intake may be small, within- and between-individual variation associated with flavonoid intake assessment appears to be substantial across 12 days of WFR data in older adults. It is recommended that a minimum of 6 days of weighed food records are collected to minimise the impact of within- and between-individual variability on total flavonoid intake assessments in this population.

Keywords: Flavonoids, Within-individual variation, Between-individual variation, Variance ratio, Dietary assessment, Seasonality

Introduction

Flavonoids are a large group of naturally occurring plant-based compounds that are commonly consumed through a diet rich in fruit, vegetables, tea, wine and soy-based foods [1]. Habitual consumption of dietary flavonoids has been consistently linked with improvements in chronic conditions associated with ageing, certain cancers [2], cardiovascular [3] and neurodegenerative diseases [4–9]. Flavonoids are divided into six major classes: anthocyanins, flavan-3-ols, flavanones, flavones, flavonols and isoflavones [10].

Precise estimation of nutrient intake is essential for establishing a relationship between diet and disease. Flavonoids are abundant, wide-spanning and diverse in the human diet, and their quantity in foods is heavily influenced by a food's growth and processing conditions [11]. For these reasons, estimations of dietary flavonoid intake need to take into account their complexity and

* Correspondence: Katherine.Kent@utas.edu.au
[1]Centre for Rural Health, Faculty of Health, University of Tasmania, Locked Bag 1322, Launceston, TAS 7250, Australia

variability. There are substantial variations in population estimates of dietary flavonoid intake [12–17], which may lead to inconsistent associations with health outcomes. A recent review reported a wide range for mean total flavonoid intakes of between 209 to 1017 mg/d (mean 435 mg/d) in Australian, European, and US adult populations [12]. This variability may relate to true differences in dietary patterns, such as differences in the food supply and cultural eating patterns between countries [18, 19]. However, it may also reflect well-known limitations associated with the assessment methods typically used to assess flavonoid and subclass intake [12], described below.

To determine the flavonoid composition of a diet, dietary intake data needs to be cross-referenced with a flavonoid-specific food composition database (FCDB). The dietary assessment method most commonly applied in the literature to determine flavonoid intakes is retrospective analysis of FFQs that aren't developed or validated to measure flavonoid intakes specifically [20, 21]. This method, while useful when analysing large existing datasets has limitations for the accurate assessment of flavonoid intakes and can lead to inaccurate results, as often within the FFQs, foods which are nutritionally similar are grouped together (to make the FFQs shorter -i.e., green and red grapes), but these food items often possess very different flavonoid profiles. In addition to the well-known limitations of dietary assessment methods in general [22], in the case of flavonoids, there are additional methodological issues relating to the choice of FCDBs used to assign flavonoid content information to dietary data. These issues relate to the completeness and appropriateness of the flavonoid FCDB [12], which is in turn related to availability of analytical food data [23]. In Australia, for example, very little analytical food data exists for the flavonoid composition of foods, meaning that there are no Australian-specific flavonoid FCDBs to use. Additionally, flavonoid FCDBs are unable to account for inherent variability of the flavonoid composition of foods [11], which may fluctuate according to cultivar type, season, and/or processing and preparation methods [24]. Lastly, one recent study demonstrated significant variations in estimates of flavonoid intake when two different flavonoid FCDBs were applied to the same dietary data [25]. A comparison of the anthocyanin content of fruits and vegetables demonstrated marked variability in anthocyanin content values yielded by three different food composition database sources, namely the USDA tables, Phenol-Explorer and an Australian- specific flavonoid subclass (anthocyanin) database [23].

Differences in reported flavonoid intakes may be also be attributed to bias associated with different dietary assessment methodologies, leading to further errors in estimation of intake. For example, a Food Frequency Questionnaire (FFQ) and a 24 h diet recall would produce fundamentally different estimates of flavonoid intake, given the inherent differences in the recall and reporting periods of each tool. When assessing flavonoid intake, the majority of studies have applied a FFQ [26–28] to capture habitual intake, while fewer studies have utilised either single [29, 30] or multiple 24 h recalls [31], diet history methods [32] and food records [33]. The use of FFQs to determine flavonoid intake has limitations, as often a retrospective secondary analysis of flavonoid intake is conducted [34] from a FFQ tool that has not specifically been designed to assess flavonoid intake. Often, these tools group food items which are nutritionally similar but which possess very different flavonoid profiles. This is especially relevant for assessing fruits and vegetables [23]. Until recently [35–38], there has been a lack of validated dietary tools for estimating flavonoids and flavonoid subclasses, which is a major limitation to progress in establishment of dietary recommendations.

The known variability associated with estimating dietary flavonoid intake is often attributed to the aforementioned limitations of dietary assessment methodologies, with no consideration of the potential influence of within-individual variation (the inherent day-to-day fluctuation) in flavonoid intake. However, within-individual variation could be significantly contributing to the reported differences in population-based estimates of dietary flavonoid intake. There is substantial within- and between-individual variation for all dietary components, and it is generally well established that macronutrients show smaller variation than micro-nutrients [39]. Research has established that the number of days of dietary assessment required for accurate estimation of macronutrients intake is a 7-d recording period. However, the majority micronutrients require a longer time period (but less than 1 month) [40]. It has previously been hypothesised that 'antioxidant' dietary components would require more days of dietary assessment than macronutrients, but one study has shown that total flavonoid intakes would require 8 days of dietary assessment, but 10 days would be needed for energy assessment in the same population.

Despite this preliminary analysis, the number of days of dietary data needed to precisely assess flavonoid intakes is currently unclear, with only the one study addressing this issue to date in younger adults and only in relation to total flavonoid and isoflavone intake [40]. The inherent differences in eating patterns between younger and older adults, underpins the different major dietary sources of flavonoids in these groups, where the contributions of wine and tea to total flavonoid intake increases with age [41], and given these differences, a focused investigation on the variability in flavonoid intake for older adults is warranted. Information on within- and between-individual variation in flavonoid and subclass intake can be used to calculate the number of days of dietary assessment that are required to precisely estimate intakes of these food components.

Also of potential relevance when considering variability in flavonoid intake assessment, is the potential influence of seasonality. The influence of season on dietary consumption patterns has been established [42]. Seasonality has been shown to influence nutrient [43] and antioxidant [44] intakes, and may influence food availability [45]. However, the effect of seasonality on dietary flavonoid intake has not yet been adequately investigated. Given that fruits and vegetables are major sources of dietary flavonoids, the effect of seasonality on flavonoid intake could be significant.

The primary aims of the current research were: (1) to assess the between and within-individual variability of dietary flavonoid intake; and (2) to calculate the number of days required to assess usual intake of flavonoids and flavonoid subclasses within a defined level of accuracy using 12 days of weighed food record (WFR) data. A secondary aim of the research was to determine if seasonality impacted on total flavonoid or flavonoid subclass intake in this population.

Methods

Study population

The Blue Mountains Eye Study (BMES) is a longitudinal, population-based study of chronic health outcomes in residents aged 49 years and over in a defined area (the Blue Mountains, population of approximately 80,000 in 2016) west of Sydney, Australia [46]. All procedures of the Blue Mountains Eye Study were approved by the Human Research Ethics Committees of the University of Sydney and the Western Sydney Area Health Service, and were conducted adhering to the tenets of the Declaration of Helsinki. Written, informed consent was obtained from all study participants and de-identified data was provided to the research team. The dietary assessment methods utilised in this study have been described in detail elsewhere [46]. Briefly, twelve days of WFRs, comprising three separate 4-day WFRs were collected approximately 4 months apart in 1994 in a randomly selected sub-sample of the BMES cohort ($n = 79$). The WFR data were collected in the sub-sample for the purpose of validating a FFQ administered in the full population group [47], and the sample size was selected based on validation for energy intake (for full details please see [47]). The sub-sample comprised 45 females (57%) and 34 males with a mean age of 70.1 years (age range: 60y to 80y) and a mean body mass index (BMI, kg/m^2) of 21.3 (± 3.3) [47].

Flavonoid and subclass assessment

The 12 days of WFR data were selected to provide a comprehensive assessment of flavonoid intake, and given a previous study [40] showing that 8 days of dietary data are needed to calculate flavonoid intakes precisely, this data was likely to be robust enough for the proposed analysis. A strength of this dataset is that it is collected for 4-day periods over three separate time points, which allows for the analysis of within-individual variation in flavonoid intake. The dietary data were collected to reflect intake over a 12-month period, thereby spanning the different seasons [47–49]. WFR data was provided to the research team in a Microsoft Access (2010) database, which was developed for the purpose of storing and managing the large BMES data set. The dietary data comprising the WFRs were cross-referenced with the USDA Database for the Flavonoid Content of Selected Foods (Release 3.1) [24] to assign each food reported a total flavonoid value and a value for each flavonoid subclass: flavonols, flavan-3-ols, anthocyanins, flavones, flavanones. Isoflavone intake was not assessed as isoflavone consumption in Australia is very low (14) (isoflavones are largely provided by soy foods) and the isoflavone content of foods is not reported in the USDA flavonoid database. The content data was assigned based on the most similar and appropriate food/beverage available in the reference USDA flavonoid database. The USDA Database was chosen as our reference database as internationally it is one of the most comprehensive and commonly applied flavonoid FCDBs, despite containing limited information pertaining to some cooked foods. Additionally, the flavonoid content values may not have accurately reflected that of Australian-specific produce. However, the use of the USDA database to determine the flavonoid intakes is justified in this study given the lack of Australian-specific data for total flavonoid intakes [23].

After flavonoid-contents were assigned to the WFR data, the dietary data was linked with the population characteristics stored in the Excel Access (2010) database, using the query tool. The linked data table was then exported to SPSS version 23.0 (IBM Corporation, Somers, NY, USA) for statistical analysis. The mean and range of flavonoid intake per 4-day food record and intake of flavonoids and flavonoid subclasses per person per day have been reported previously, in addition to the major sources of flavonoids and flavonoid subclasses [17].

Statistical analysis

Data analysis was performed using SPSS version 23.0 (IBM Corporation, Somers, NY, USA). Analysis indicated that the distributions of total flavonoid and all subclass intakes showed departure from normality.

Calculation of number of days required for assessing usual nutrient intakes

Untransformed data for flavonoid and subclass intake were used in the analysis for within- and between-individual variation, in line with previous research [50, 51], for three reasons. First, the data (estimates of the relative contributions of variance for each dietary variable) were not substantially affected by log transformation. Second, transforming data would have introduced further error associated with transformation/back transformations, and previous research indicated that transformation did not improve the assumption of homoscedasticity across variables [52]. Third, untransformed data was presented in a meaningful unit (mg), and transforming data would have created difficulty with interpretation the results [53].

For total flavonoids and each subclass, median intake, mean intake, standard deviation (SD), and the within- and between-person variations were calculated using a mixed-effects regression model with a restricted likelihood estimator [40]. Mean within-person variation was determined and two coefficients of variation (CV) were calculated: CVw [(√within-person variation)/mean] × 100, and CVb [(√between-person variation)/mean] × 100. The within-to-between individual variance ratio (CVw^2/CVb^2) was then determined. The number of days (D) required for assessing usual intake of flavonoids or flavonoid subclasses uses a hypothetical correlation coefficient (*r*) between the observed and the true intakes, given by the formula proposed by Black et al. [39, 54]. As *r* increases, the proportion of individuals correctly classified increases [39]. For the current study, $r \geq 0.9$ was selected in order to accurately classify 80% of individuals into thirds of a distribution with 90% confidence and ensure <1% of individuals are misclassified [40]. D is influenced by the variance ratio, whereby if the within-individual variance observed is smaller than the between-individual variation, a smaller number of repeated measures will be needed. D also depends on the selected *r*. Therefore, depending on hypothetical *r* selected, the resulting number of days of dietary assessment needed will increase or decrease, with *r* closer to 1 increasing the number of days required. To solve for D the following formula was applied: $D = [(r^2/1 - r^2) \times (CVw^2/CVb^2)$ [39].

Assessment of seasonality

Each day of WFR data was categorized according to the season in which the data was collected, based on Australian conditions; summer: December – February; autumn: March – May; winter: June – August; spring: September – November. Both parametric (analysis of variance; ANOVA) and non-parametric (Kruskal-Wallis H) analyses were initially conducted to determine seasonality differences in estimated flavonoid intake (mg/day) and intake of flavonoid subclasses (mg/day), with $\alpha = 0.05$. Since the results of these analyses were comparable, only results from the ANOVA are presented [55]. The results from the Kruskal Wallis test are available as supplementary material (Additional file 1).

Results

Days required for assessing usual flavonoid intakes

Table 1 presents the median and mean intakes, as well as presenting the standard deviation (SD) and interquartile range (IQR) to highlight the range of intakes for total flavonoids and each subclass. Coefficients of within- and between- individual variations for flavonoids and flavonoid subclasses are also presented. Overall, between-individual variation was greater than within-individual variation for total flavonoids and all subclasses, resulting in a variance ratio of more than 1. The number of days of dietary assessment required are presented in Table 1 and show that for total flavonoid intake 6 days of WFR data are required, 6 days are required for anthocyanins and flavan-3-ols, 8 days for flavones and flavanones and 10 days for flavonols (Table 1). Total flavonoid intake, anthocyanins and flavan-3-ols required less days of dietary assessment as they showed a smaller variance ratio, resulting from higher between-person variation than the other subclasses.

Table 1 Median, mean, SD and IQR for intake of flavonoid and flavonoid subclasses, coefficients of variation, within-to-between individual variance ratios and number of days to reach $r \geq 0.9$ for 79 older adults

	Median mg/day	Mean	SD	IQR	CVw	CVb	Variance Ratio	D
Flavonoid Total	581.84	678.69	498.53	619.58	136.18	116.74	1.36	6
Anthocyanins	1.05	6.73	12.70	7.88	80.40	72.78	1.22	6
Flavonols	24.06	28.04	33.29	21.21	139.70	91.79	2.32	10
Flavones	0.55	1.87	4.78	2.11	80.41	62.49	1.66	8
Flavan-3-ols	499.72	596.17	494.95	622.95	120.79	109.75	1.21	6
Flavanones	2.15	21.43	61.46	12.14	79.99	59.05	1.83	8

SD Standard Deviation, *IQR* Interquartile range, *CVw* [(√within-person variation)/mean] × 100, *CVb* [(√between-person variation)/mean] × 100, *Variance Ratio* (CVw^2/CVb^2), *D* days of dietary assessment needed, calculated by $D = [(r^2/1 - r^2) \times (CVw^2/CVb^2)$, *Mg* milligram

Seasonal intake

Table 2 shows the seasonal differences in flavonoid intake and intake of flavonoid subclasses. When comparing total flavonoids intakes across seasons, there is > 60 mg difference between seasons, where intakes are highest in spring and lowest in autumn. However, there was no statistically significant difference detected between the seasons for total flavonoid intake using the ANOVA. Additionally, there was no statistically significant difference across seasons for flavonol or anthocyanin (highest in winter), or flavone (highest in autumn) subclasses. However, there were statistically significant differences across seasons for two flavonoid subclasses. For flavan-3-ol intake, a statistically significant difference between seasons was observed ($F(3,944) = 2.79$, $p = 0.039$). Post-hoc analysis using Tukey's test indicated that flavan-3-ol intake was statistically significantly lower in summer than in spring ($p = 0.029$), with interpretation of the raw data showing a mean difference in intake of over 100 mg per day/person. A statistically significant difference between seasons was also detected for flavanone intake ($F(3,944) = 3.85$, $p = 0.009$). Post hoc analysis indicated that flavanone intake was higher in autumn than in summer ($p = 0.017$) and winter ($p = 0.016$), where flavanone intakes doubled in autumn, when compared to winter.

Discussion

This study shows, for the first time, that precise assessment of total flavonoid intake in older adults requires at least 6 days of weighed food records, and between 6 and 10 days to determine intake of specific flavonoid subclasses with an acceptable degree of accuracy. Season appears to influence intake of subclasses flavanones and flavan-3-ols, but not overall total flavonoid intake.

Substantial within-individual variation and between-individual variation was documented for both total flavonoid intake and intake of flavonoid subclasses in the current study. The within-individual variations ranged from around 80–140% and the between individual variation ranged from around 60–117%, which are both considerably greater than the range suggested for energy and macronutrients. Generally, the expected within- and between-individual variation for energy and other macronutrient intakes is around 25% in free-living subjects [56]. A number of studies have examined the between and within-individual variability of both macro and micro-nutrient and food intakes [57–60]. An early review by Bingham [61] identified the mean within-individual CV was lower for energy (23%), and macronutrients (carbohydrate (23%) and protein (27%)). The CV was reported to be greater for vitamins and minerals, such as calcium and iron (34%), ascorbic acid (63%) and retinol (131%). The review concluded that the wider the variation, the greater the number of days required for the reporting period [61]. It was suggested that 13 days of recording are necessary for 90% of the population to calculate mean energy intake with a standard error of ±10% [61]. Day-to-day variation in nutrient intake may be the result of an individual's behaviour [62], such as differing meal patterns and food availability. For flavonoids, this variability may be attributed to the sporadic nature of consumption patterns of flavonoid-rich foods within the different flavonoid subclasses. For example, red wine or berries are major contributors to anthocyanin intake [63] but may not be consumed daily. The variation in flavonoid intakes between individuals is also high, with literature showing that sociocultural, economic and ecological factors may be responsible for the variation [64]. Additionally, small between-person variation may reflect a homogenous population, which does not appear to be the case in the this population, who varied in age and gender [47]. The within- and between-person variation for some dietary nutrients differs between genders, where women have shown higher CVs than males [40].

The major sources of variability when determining the flavonoid content of foods are well-known and include the cultivar, growing, processing, and preparation methods, and the variability associated with the analytical methods of flavonoid quantification [11]. Additionally, differences in a country's food supply may limit the ability of an international flavonoid FCDB to accurately reflect the flavonoid composition of country-specific foods [65]. Studies frequently cite these factors as

Table 2 Mean ± SD intake of flavonoids and subclasses (mg/day) according to season

	n records	Flavonoid Total [a] Mean ± SD	Anthocyanin	Flavonols	Flavones	Flavan-3-ols*	Flavanones*
Summer	177	652.35 ± 487.01	5.90 ± 13.17	26.01 ± 17.34	1.25 ± 2.85	501.93 ± 425.42*	15.26 ± 31.06*
Autumn	195	648.58 ± 400.21	5.95 ± 10.48	26.67 ± 18.32	2.29 ± 8.00	616.02 ± 488.97	34.06 ± 113.14
Winter	280	683.16 ± 548.65	7.78 ± 14.48	30.88 ± 40.94	1.92 ± 3.53	604.08 ± 526.50	17.06 ± 33.23*
Spring	296	710.06 ± 514.09	6.72 ± 11.90	27.48 ± 39.50	1.90 ± 3.77	631.97 ± 502.09	20.94 ± 44.08

All data are reported in milligrams (mg) of intake

SD standard deviation

*One way ANOVA $p \leq 0.05$

[a]for flavonoid and subclass intakes in this population per person, per day, and according to gender please see [17]

limitations in the interpretation of study findings. However, the potential impact of high within-individual variability on estimates of flavonoid intake has not been addressed. Whilst some studies have averaged repeated measures of flavonoid intake [66–68], so as to minimise the potential impact of within-individual variation, there is no description of the extent of the variability across different time points. The current findings suggest that studies collect as many days of dietary data as possible in order to minimize the effect of within-individual variability on estimates of flavonoid intake. However, increasing the number of days of dietary assessment to minimize this bias is associated with an increase in participant burden and may thereby detract from participant compliance with dietary recording. Therefore, statistically correcting for variability may be more appropriate for large epidemiological studies.

Several statistical methods exist to correct for within-individual variability in dietary intake data [69]. One method is to collect multiple days of 24-h recall data on each survey participant and average these data [69]. Another method is to apply a correction factor to the distribution. This method requires estimating the correction factor to be applied, by collecting multiple samples from a representative subset of the survey population for example [69]. This narrows the population distribution at the extreme ends due to accounting for within-individual variation. More sophisticated statistical modelling methods to account for variability include the Multiple Source Method (MSM) [70] and National Cancer Institute (NCI) [71] methods. However, these methods are usually applied to dietary information obtained by repeated short-term instruments, such as a repeated 24-h dietary recalls [70, 71] in large sample sizes.

Given that flavonoid intake is difficult to quantify, and in the absence of a gold standard approach, methods have been developed for application in various settings, including various techniques within the fields of dietary assessment and biomarker analyses [65]. A recent review [65] assessed the available tools to estimate dietary intake of polyphenols, including flavonoids, and identified little consistency across studies when applying FCDBs to estimate intake. Additionally, there is no consensus regarding which dietary assessment tool (e.g. FFQ, 24 h recall, food records etc.) should be utilized to provide the most valid measure of habitual flavonoid intake. However, the use of general FFQs not designed for the purpose of capturing flavonoid intake has been discouraged [12]. Recently, a flavonoid-specific FFQ for older adults was developed and validated [38]. Dietary flavonoid intake can also be determined by quantifying relevant biomarkers (e.g. intact phytochemicals or a related metabolite) found in various biological samples. However, there is currently no standardized protocol of how to perform these analyses or which biomarker to target [12]. Despite the significant problems associated with estimating flavonoid intake using a biomarker (such as within-individual variability in flavonoid metabolism [12]), future research should focus on the identification of appropriate and easily measurable biomarkers of flavonoid intake. This will be imperative in overcoming limitations associated with the estimation of flavonoid intake using dietary assessment.

There was no statistically significant effect of season on total flavonoid intake in the current study, despite flavonoid intake being relatively high in spring and relatively low in autumn. This finding is not aligned with findings from similar research, which showed that total antioxidant intakes in a Japanese population were highest in winter and lowest in summer [44]. The authors of this study were able to document differences in participants' selection of food and beverages across the seasons, and therefore this analysis could be a consideration as a future extension of the current study. The analysis may be crucial to highlight if certain foods are responsible for contributing to the major differences flavanone and flavan-3-ol intakes across seasons. It is possible our lack of seasonal differences for total flavonoid intake reflects, in part, the way in which flavonoid values included in FCDBs are averaged across measurements when determining the flavonoid contents of foods, including different seasons [11, 24]. As flavonoid-specific FCDBs evolve, information on the influence of seasonality on the flavonoid content of foods may become more widely available. A limitation of this analysis is that the WFR data was collected across three seasons for each participant only. Ideally, dietary information would be collected mid-season, and in all seasons for each individual in future research.

The sample used for the current analysis was originally collected for a validation study of a FFQ developed for a prospective cohort study. The burden to participants entailed in the collection of twelve days of weighed food records is substantial and the sample size, while typical of validation studies of this nature, was relatively small. The reason for utilizing this dataset to estimate flavonoid intake in older adults relates to the richness of the dietary data. WFRs are likely to provide a more accurate estimation of flavonoid intake in comparison to other dietary assessment methods, such as repeated 24 h recalls. The dietary data collected in the total BMES sample was a FFQ, which grouped nutritionally similar foods (e.g., apples and pears). Given that such foods have significantly different flavonoid profiles, however, the FFQ may be unsuitable for accurately estimating flavonoid intake. Additionally, several major flavonoid contributing foods were not included in the BMES FFQ. Thus, despite the relatively small sample size, the depth of the dietary data from the WFRs in this group is a major strength when estimating flavonoid intake. We have previously compared flavonoid intake in this population to other national and international estimates for older adults, showing that older adults tend to consume higher amounts of dietary flavonoids when compared with younger age groups [17]. This may be related to higher intakes of tea and wine as people age [17]. It is difficult to compare flavonoid intakes in older adults across populations and studies because of differences in dietary assessment methods and the use of different FCDBs. Nevertheless, flavonoid intakes are reported to range from around 21.2 mg/day to 191.2 mg/day in this population [72].

An additional limitation of the current study is that the data used for this analysis was collected in the 1990s. However, in the BMES population, fruit and vegetable consumption did not significantly change from baseline to the 10-year follow up [73]. Some changes in dietary patterns related to fat (MUFA, PUFA, SFA) and total sugar (not CHO) intake [73] may have occurred during this period, but these macronutrients are not generally associated with flavonoid-rich foods. Nevertheless, the generalizability of the study findings may be limited by the changing food supply. Despite the age of the comprehensive dietary data used by this study. The USDA database chosen as our reference flavonoid FCDB was comprehensive enough to assign the WFR food items flavonoid content values. However, the validity of using a current (present-day) flavonoid FCDB to retrospectively assign flavonoid contents to foods collected approximately two decades earlier is uncertain, and these methodological limitations should be considered when interpreting the findings of this research. This study utilised an international FCDB, and therefore the potential inaccuracy of the flavonoid content of foods for Australian produce is a limitation of this study. The USDA [1] recognises that flavonoid contents in foods are influenced by cultivar types, and the growth and processing conditions of foods, but this is an issue across all flavonoid FCDBs. Therefore the USDA database was an appropriate choice for this study as it is a comprehensive resource and is commonly applied across studies. However, improvements in country-specific flavonoid FCDBs, ideally integrated into existing dietary analysis software, are vital to improve the accuracy and ease of flavonoid intake estimates in future studies.

Lastly, the sample size of the current study did not permit stratification of findings by gender, which is another limitation of the analysis. We have previously reported a significant difference in energy intake between men and women in the current study population [17] but a gender difference was not evident for flavonoid intake [17]. The vast majority of flavonoids are provided by tea, a low energy food, such that accounting for differences in energy intake is unlikely to uncover sex differences in flavonoid intake. Further research is needed to investigate the influence of energy intake, gender, or other confounders for diet, such as age and levels of physical activity on variations in flavonoid intake.

In conclusion, further research is needed to identify the determinants of the day-to-day variation in flavonoid and subclass intake within and between individuals, and whether a high variability in flavonoid intake has any biological implications in terms of metabolism, uptake and excretion [62]. Additionally, given the limitations of our study, further research is required to confirm our findings and to determine the appropriate number of days to accurately determine flavonoid intake. Comprehensive, Australian-specific flavonoid FCDBs are also needed, ensuring flavonoid content values are representative across all seasons. Our study has shown that the within- and between-individual variation in flavonoid intake is considerable and needs to be accounted for in dietary assessment methodology. Additionally, the collection of dietary data in different seasons may not significantly influence estimates of total flavonoid intake but may influence the reported intakes for flavanones and flavan-3-ols. The findings of this study suggest that at least 6 days of weighed food records for total flavonoid intake, and up to 10 days for individual flavonoid subclasses, should be collected to reduce the bias associated with within-individual variations in intake.

Abbreviations

BMES: Blue mountains eye study; CV: Coefficient of variation; CVb: Between-individual variation; CVw: Within-individual variation; FCDB: food composition database; FFQ: Food frequency questionnaire; USDA: United States Department of Agriculture; WFR: Weighed food records

Acknowledgements

None.

Funding

None.

Authors' contributions

KK was responsible for the design of the study, conducting the statistical analysis, and prepared the first draft of the manuscript. KC, SL, and JM provided advice on statistical methods for this study. KC, JR, VF and PM contributed to the flavonoid intake assessment of the Blue Mountains Eye Study. All authors critically revised the manuscript, read and approved the final version of the manuscript. All authors are in agreement with the manuscript and declare the content has not been published elsewhere.

Authors' information

Dr. Katherine Kent (PhD, B.Sc,) is a Postdoctoral Research Fellow in the Centre for Rural Health, School of Health Sciences, University of Tasmania. Associate Professor Karen E Charlton (PhD, Adv APD, RPHNutr) is a nutritional epidemiologist who is Public Health Nutrition domain leader in the Nutrition & Dietetics programme, University of Wollongong. Dr. Simone Lee (PhD, MND, BSc) is a lecturer at the Centre for Rural Health and has a background in public health, nutrition/dietetics, chronic disease risk factors and prevention, and health literacy. Dr. Jonathan M. Mond (BA(Hons), MA(Hons), PhD, MPH) is a Senior Research Fellow in the Centre for Rural Health, University of Tasmania. Dr. Joanna Russell (BSc(Hons) Nutrition, MPH (Nutrition), PhD) is a lecturer in public health subjects at the University of Wollongong. Professor Paul Mitchell (MBBS, MD, PhD, FRANZCO, FRACS, FRCOphth, FAFPHM) is a Professor of Clinical Ophthalmology & Eye Health at Westmead Clinical School. Professor Victoria M Flood (BAppSc, Grad Dip Nutr&Diet, MPH, PhD; APD) holds a conjoint appointment as Professor of Allied Health with Western Sydney Local Health District and Faculty of Health Sciences, University of Sydney.

Competing interests

The authors declare that they have no competing interests.

Author details

[1]Centre for Rural Health, Faculty of Health, University of Tasmania, Locked Bag 1322, Launceston, TAS 7250, Australia. [2]Faculty of Science, Medicine and Health, University of Wollongong, Wollongong, Australia. [3]Illawarra Health and Medical Research Institute, Wollongong, Australia. [4]Faculty of Social Sciences, University of Wollongong, Wollongong, Australia. [5]Centre for Vision Research, University of Sydney, Sydney, Australia. [6]Faculty of Health Sciences, University of Sydney, Sydney, Australia. [7]Western Sydney Local Health District, Sydney, Australia.

References

1. Bhagwat S, Haytowitz DB, Wasswa-Kintu SI, Holden JM. USDA develops a database for Flavonoids to assess dietary intakes. Procedia Food Science. 2013;2:81–6.
2. Romagnolo DF, Selmin OI. Flavonoids and cancer prevention: a review of the evidence. J Nutr Gerontol Geriatr. 2012;31:206–38.
3. Peterson JJ, Dwyer JT, Jacques PF, McCullough ML. Associations between flavonoids and cardiovascular disease incidence or mortality in European and US populations. Nutr Rev. 2012;70:491–508.
4. Dai Q, Borenstein AR, Wu Y, Jackson JC, Larson EB. Fruit and vegetable juices and Alzheimer's disease: the Kame project. Am J Med. 2006;119:751–9.
5. Laurin D, Masaki KH, Foley DJ, White LR, Launer LJ. Midlife dietary intake of antioxidants and risk of late-life incident dementia: the Honolulu-Asia aging study. Am J Epidemiol. 2004;159:959–67.
6. Letenneur L, Proust-Lima C, Le Gouge A, Dartigues JF, Barberger-Gateau P. Flavonoid intake and cognitive decline over a 10-year period. Am J Epidemiol. 2007;165:1364–71.
7. Nurk E, Refsum H, Drevon CA, Tell GS, Nygaard HA, Engedal K, Smith AD. Intake of flavonoid-rich wine, tea, and chocolate by elderly men and women is associated with better cognitive test performance1-3. J Nutr. 2009;139:120–7.
8. Root M, Ravine E, Harper A. Flavonol intake and cognitive decline in middle-aged adults. J Med Food. 2015;18:1327–32.
9. Wengreen HJ, Munger RG, Corcoran CD, Zandi P, Hayden KM, Fotuhi M, Skoog I, Norton MC, Tschanz J, Breitner JCS, Welsh-Bohmer KA. Antioxidant intake and cognitive function of elderly men and women: the Cache County study. J Nutr Health Aging. 2007;11:230–7.
10. Beecher GR. Overview of dietary flavonoids: nomenclature, occurrence and intake. J Nutr. 2003;133:3248s–54s.
11. Haytowitz DB, Bhagwat S, Holden JM. Sources of variability in the Flavonoid content of foods. Procedia Food Science. 2013;2:46–51.
12. Peterson JJ, Dwyer JT, Jacques PF, McCullough ML. Improving the estimation of flavonoid intake for study of health outcomes. Nutr Rev. 2015;73:553–76.
13. Bai W, Wang C, Ren C. Intakes of total and individual flavonoids by US adults. Int J Food Sci Nutr. 2014;65:9–20.
14. Jun S, Shin S, Joung H. Estimation of dietary flavonoid intake and major food sources of Korean adults. Br J Nutr. 2016;115:480.
15. Samieri C, Sun Q, Townsend MK, Rimm EB, Grodstein F. Dietary flavonoid intake at midlife and healthy aging in women. Am J Clin Nutr. 2014;100:1489–97.
16. Kim K, Vance TM, Chun OK. Estimated intake and major food sources of flavonoids among US adults: changes between 1999–2002 and 2007–2010 in NHANES. Eur J Nutr. 2016;55:833–43.
17. Kent K, Charlton KE, Russell J, Mitchell P, Flood VM. Estimation of Flavonoid intake in older Australians: secondary data analysis of the Blue Mountains eye study. J Nutr Gerontol Geriatr. 2015;34:388.
18. Zamora-Ros R, Knaze V, Lujan-Barroso L, Romieu I, Scalbert A, Slimani N, Hjartaker A, Engeset D, Skeie G, Overvad K, et al. Differences in dietary intakes, food sources and determinants of total flavonoids between Mediterranean and non-Mediterranean countries participating in the European prospective investigation into cancer and nutrition (EPIC) study. Sweden: Cambridge University Press; 2013.
19. Vogiatzoglou A, Mulligan AA, Lentjes MAH, Luben RN, Spencer JPE, Schroeter H, Khaw K-T, Kuhnle GGC. Flavonoid intake in European adults (18 to 64 years). PLoS One. 2015;10:e0128132.
20. Mink PJ, Scrafford CG, Barraj LM, Harnack L, Hong C-P, Nettleton JA, Jacobs JDR. Flavonoid intake and cardiovascular disease mortality: a prospective study in postmenopausal women. Am J Clin Nutr. 2007;85: 895–909.
21. Cassidy A, O'Reilly ÉJ, Kay C, Sampson L, Franz M, Forman JP, Curhan G, Rimm EB. Habitual intake of flavonoid subclasses and incident hypertension in adults. Am J Clin Nutr. 2011;93:338–47.
22. Willett W. Nutritional epidemiology. 2nd ed. New York: Oxford University Press; 1998.
23. Igwe E, Neale E, Charlton KE, Morton K, Probst YC. First stage development of an Australian anthocyanin food composition database for dietary studies – A systematic process and itschallenges. J Food Compos Anal. 2017;64(Part 1):33-8.
24. Bhagwat S, Haytowitz DB, Holden JM. USDA database for the Flavonoid content of selected foods release 3.1 edition. Nutrient Data Laboratory, U.S. Department of Agriculture: Maryland; 2013.
25. Witkowska AM, Zujko ME, Waskiewicz A, Terlikowska KM, Piotrowski W. Comparison of various databases for estimation of dietary Polyphenol intake in the population of polish adults. Nutrients. 2015;7:9299–308.
26. Cassidy A, Mukamal KJ, Liu L, Franz M, Eliassen AH, Rimm EB. High anthocyanin intake is associated with a reduced risk of myocardial infarction in young and middle-aged women. Circulation. 2013;127:188–96.
27. Ivey KL, Lewis JR, Prince RL, Hodgson JM. Tea and non-tea flavonol intakes in relation to atherosclerotic vascular disease mortality in older women. Br J Nutr. 2013;110:1648–55.
28. Wang Y, Stevens VL, Shah R, Peterson JJ, Dwyer JT, Gapstur SM, McCullough ML. Dietary flavonoid and proanthocyanidin intakes and prostate cancer risk in a prospective cohort of US men. Am J Epidemiol. 2014;179:974–86.
29. Beking K, Vieira A. An assessment of dietary flavonoid intake in the UK and Ireland. Int J Food Sci Nutr. 2011;62(1):17-9.
30. Chun OK, Chung SJ, Song WO. Estimated dietary flavonoid intake and major food sources of U.S. adults. J Nutr. 2007;137:1244–52.
31. Dwyer J, Peterson J, Winters B, Liu W, Mitchell DC, Atkinson K. Do flavonoid intakes of postmenopausal women with breast cancer vary on very low fat diets? Nutr Cancer. 2008;60:450–60.
32. Hirvonen T, Virtamo J, Korhonen P, Albanes D, Pietinen P. Flavonol and flavone intake and the risk of cancer in male smokers (Finland). Cancer causes & control : CCC. 2001;12(9):789-96.
33. Mursu J, Nurmi T, Tuomainen TP, Ruusunen A, Salonen JT, Voutilainen S. The intake of flavonoids and carotid atherosclerosis: the Kuopio Ischaemic heart disease risk factor study. Br J Nutr. 2007;98:814–8.
34. Ponzo V, Goitre I, Fadda M, Gambino R, De Francesco A, Soldati L, et al. Dietary flavonoid intake and cardiovascular risk: a population-based cohort study. J Translational Med. 2015;13(1):218.
35. Kent K, Charlton K. Relative validity and reproducibility of an interviewer administered 14-item FFQ to estimate Flavonoid intake among older adults with mild-moderate dementia. J Nutr Gerontol Geriatr. 2017;36(2-3):134-47.
36. Burkholder-Cooley NM, Rajaram SS, Haddad EH, Oda K, Fraser GE, Jaceldo-Siegl K. Validating polyphenol intake estimates from a food-frequency questionnaire by using repeated 24-h dietary recalls and a unique method-of-triads approach with 2 biomarkers. Am J Clin Nutr. 2017;105:685–94.
37. Somerset S, Papier K. A food frequency questionnaire validated for estimating dietary Flavonoid intake in an Australian population. Nutr Cancer. 2014;66:1200–10.

38. Kent K, Charlton KE. Development, validation and reproducibility of a food frequency questionnaire to measure flavonoid intake in older Australian adults. Nutr Diet. 2017. doi:10.1111/1747-0080.12371. [Epub ahead of print].
39. Nelson M, AB J, Morris TJ. Cole: between- and within-subject variation in nutrient intake from infancy to old age: estimating the number of days required to rank dietary intakes with desired precision. Am J Clin Nutr. 1989; 50:155–67.
40. Ouellette CD, Yang M, Wang Y, Vance T, Fernandez ML, Rodriguez N, Chun OK. Number of days required for assessing usual nutrient and antioxidant intakes in a sample from a U.S. healthy college population. Nutrition. 2014; 30:1355–9.
41. Johannot L, Somerset SM. Age-related variations in flavonoid intake and sources in the Australian population. Public Health Nutr. 2006;9:1045–54.
42. Stelmach-Mardas M, Kleiser C, Uzhova I, Peñalvo JL, La Torre G, Palys W, Lojko D, Nimptsch K, Suwalska A, Linseisen J, et al. Seasonality of food groups and total energy intake: a systematic review and meta-analysis. Eur J Clin Nutr. 2016;70:700–8.
43. Hitomi S, Keiko A, Satoshi S, Masanori N, Hitomi O, Naoko H, Akiko N, Mitsuru F, Chigusa D. Effect of seasonality on the estimated mean value of nutrients and ranking ability of a self-administered diet history questionnaire. Nutr J. 2014;13:126.
44. Tatsumi Y, Ishihara J, Morimoto A, Ohno Y, Watanabe S. Seasonal differences in total antioxidant capacity intake from foods consumed by a Japanese population. Eur J Clin Nutr. 2014;68:799.
45. Valpiani N, Wilde P, Rogers B, Stewart H. Patterns of fruit and vegetable availability and price competitiveness across four seasons are different in local food outlets and supermarkets. Public Health Nutr. 2015;18:2846.
46. Mitchell P, Smith W, Attebo K, Jie Jin W. Prevalence of age-related maculopathy in Australia: the blue mountains eye study. Ophthalmology. 1995;102:1450–60.
47. Smith W, Mitchell P, Reay EM, Webb K, Harvey PW. Validity and reproducibility of a self-administered food frequency questionnaire in older people. Aust N Z J Public Health. 1998;22:456–63.
48. Barclay AW, Flood VM, Brand-Miller JC, Mitchell P. Validity of carbohydrate, glycaemic index and glycaemic load data obtained using a semi-quantitative food-frequency questionnaire. Public Health Nutr. 2008;11:573–80.
49. Flood VM, Smith WT, Webb KL, Mitchell P. Issues in assessing the validity of nutrient data obtained from a food-frequency questionnaire: folate and vitamin B-12 examples. Public Health Nutr. 2004;7:751–6.
50. Fukumoto A, Asakura K, Murakami K, Sasaki S, Okubo H, Hirota N, Notsu A, Todoriki H, Miura A, Fukui M, Date C. Within- and between-individual variation in energy and nutrient intake in Japanese adults: effect of age and sex differences on group size and number of records required for adequate dietary assessment. J Epidemiol. 2013;23:178–86.
51. Beaton GH MJ, Corey P, McGuire V, Cousins M, Stewart E: Sources of variance in 24-hour dietary recall data: Implications for nutrition study design and interpretation. Am J Clin Nutr. 1979:2546.
52. Manning WG. The logged dependent variable, heteroscedasticity, and the retransformation problem. J Health Econ. 1998;17:283–95.
53. SY O, Hong MH. Within- and between-person variation of nutrient intakes of older people in Korea. Eur J Clin Nutr. 1999;53:625–9.
54. Black AE, Cole TJ, Wiles SJ, White F. Daily variation in food intake of infants from 2 to 18 months. Hum Nutr Appl Nutr. 1983;37:448–58.
55. Sedgwick P. The importance of statistical power. BMJ. 2013;347:f6282.
56. Beaton GH. Approaches to analysis of dietary data: relationship between planned analyses and choice of methodology. Am J Clin Nutr. 1994;59:253s–61s.
57. Palaniappan U, Cue RI, Payette H, Gray-Donald K. Implications of day-to-day variability on measurements of usual food and nutrient intakes. J Nutr. 2003; 133:232–5.
58. Beaton GH, Milner J, McGuire V, Feather TE, Little JA. Source of variance in 24-hour dietary recall data: implications for nutrition study design and interpretation. Carbohydrate sources, vitamins, and minerals. Am J Clin Nutr. 1983;37:986–95.
59. Sempos CT, Johnson NE, Smith EL, Gilligan C. Effects of intraindividual and interindividual variation in repeated dietary records. Am J Epidemiol. 1985; 121:120–30.
60. Marr JW, Heady JA. Within- and between-person variation in dietary surveys: number of days needed to classify individuals. Hum Nutr Appl Nutr. 1986; 40:347–64.
61. Bingham S. The dietary assessment of individuals; methods, accuracy, new techniques and recommendations. Nutr Abstr Rev. 1987;57:705–42.
62. Tarasuk V, Beaton GH. Day-to-day variation in energy and nutrient intake: evidence of individuality in eating behaviour? Appetite. 1992;18:43–54.
63. Manach C, Scalbert A, Morand C, Rémésy C, Jiménez L. Polyphenols: food sources and bioavailability. Am J Clin Nutr. 2004;79:727–47.
64. MdMF C, Takeyama L, Voci SM, Slater B, Silva MV. Within- and between-person variations as determinant factors to calculate the number of observations to estimate usual dietary intake of adolescents. Revista Brasileira de Epidemiologia. 2008;11:541–8.
65. Probst Y, Guan V, Kent K. A systematic review of food composition tools used for determining dietary polyphenol intake in estimated intake studies. Food Chem. 2018;235:146-152
66. Chang S-C, Cassidy A, Willett WC, Rimm EB, O'Reilly EJ, Okereke OI. Dietary flavonoid intake and risk of incident depression in midlife and older women. Am J Clin Nutr. 2016;104:704–14.
67. Bertoia ML, Rimm EB, Mukamal KJ, FB H, Willett WC, Cassidy A. Dietary flavonoid intake and weight maintenance: three prospective cohorts of 124086 US men and women followed for up to 24 years. BMJ. 2016;352:i17.
68. Gao X, Cassidy A, Schwarzschild MA, Rimm EB, Ascherio A. Habitual intake of dietary flavonoids and risk of Parkinson disease. Neurology. 2012;78:1138–45.
69. Dodd KW, Guenther PM, Freedman LS, Subar AF, Kipnis V, Midthune D, Tooze JA, Krebs-Smith SM. Statistical methods for estimating usual intake of nutrients and foods: a review of the theory. J Am Diet Assoc. 2006;106:1640–50.
70. Harttig U, Haubrock J, Knüppel S, Boeing H. The MSM program: web-based statistics package for estimating usual dietary intake using the multiple source method. Eur J Clin Nutr. 2011;65(Suppl 1):S87–91.
71. Tooze JA, Kipnis V, Buckman DW, Carroll RJ, Freedman LS, Guenther PM, et al. A mixed-effects model approach for estimating the distribution of usual intake of nutrients: the NCI method. Stat Med. 2010;29(27):2857-68.
72. Chun OK, Lee SG, Wang Y, Vance T, Song WO. Estimated Flavonoid intake of the elderly in the United States and around the world. J Nutr Gerontol Geriatr. 2012;31:190–205.
73. Flood VM, Burlutsky G, Webb KL, Wang JJ, Smith WT, Mitchell P. Food and nutrient consumption trends in older Australians: a 10-year cohort study. Eur J Clin Nutr. 2010;64:603–13.

2

High phosphorus intake and gut-related parameters – results of a randomized placebo-controlled human intervention study

Ulrike Trautvetter[1*], Amélia Camarinha-Silva[2], Gerhard Jahreis[3,5], Stefan Lorkowski[4,5] and Michael Glei[1,5]

Abstract

Background: In recent years, high phosphate intakes were discussed critically. In the small intestine, a part of the ingested phosphate and calcium precipitates to amorphous calcium phosphate (ACP), which in turn can precipitate other intestinal substances, thus leading to a beneficial modulation of the intestinal environment. Therefore, we analysed faecal samples obtained from a human intervention study regarding gut-related parameters.

Methods: Sixty-two healthy subjects (men, $n = 30$; women, $n = 32$) completed the double-blind, placebo-controlled and parallel designed study (mean age: 29 ± 7 years; mean BMI: 24 ± 3 kg/m^2). Supplements were monosodium phosphate and calcium carbonate. During the first 2 weeks, all groups consumed a placebo sherbet powder, and afterwards a sherbet powder for 8 weeks according to the intervention group: P1000/Ca0 (1000 mg/d phosphorus), P1000/Ca500 (1000 mg/d phosphorus and 500 mg/d calcium) and P1000/Ca1000 (1000 mg/d phosphorus and 1000 mg/d calcium). After the placebo period and after 8 weeks of intervention faecal collections took place. We determined in faeces: short-chain fatty acids (SCFA) and fat as well as the composition of the microbiome (subgroup) and cyto- and genotoxicity of faecal water (FW). By questionnaire evaluation we examined tolerability of the used phosphorus supplement.

Results: Faecal fat concentrations did not change significantly due to the interventions. Concentrations of faecal total SCFA and acetate were significantly higher after 8 weeks of P1000/Ca500 supplementation compared to the P1000/Ca0 supplementation. In men, faecal total SCFA and acetate concentrations were significantly higher after 8 weeks in the P1000/Ca1000 group compared to the P1000/Ca0 one. None of the interventions markedly affected cyto- and genotoxic activity of FW. Men of the P1000/Ca1000 intervention had a significantly different gut microbial community compared to the men of the P1000/Ca0 and P1000/Ca500 ones. The genus *Clostridium* XVIII was significantly more abundant in men of the P1000/Ca1000 intervention group compared to the other groups. Supplementations did not cause increased intestinal distress.

Conclusions: The used high phosphorus diet did not influence cyto- and genotoxicity of FW and the concentrations of faecal fat independent of calcium intake. Our study provides first hints for a potential phosphorus-induced modulation of the gut community and the faecal total SCFA content.

Keywords: Phosphorus intake, Phosphate intake, Calcium intake, Human study, Faecal water, Cytotoxicity, Genotoxicity, Short-chain fatty acids

* Correspondence: Ulrike.Trautvetter@uni-jena.de
[1]Department of Nutritional Toxicology, Institute of Nutrition, Friedrich Schiller University Jena, Dornburger Straße 24, 07743 Jena, Germany

Background

Dietary phosphate and serum phosphate concentrations of healthy people and patients with chronic kidney disease have been discussed critically in the last years, regarding bone, cardiovascular health and mortality [1–4]. Whereas associations of phosphate concentrations in serum with cardiovascular diseases and mortality have been well established [2], it is still unclear whether dietary phosphorus influences serum phosphate concentrations [5, 6].

According to the National Health and Nutrition Examination Survey of the USA, dietary phosphorus intake of Americans exceeds the daily recommended intake of 700 mg phosphorus for adults and the elderly [4, 7]. This is mainly a result of the increased consumption of food prepared or treated with phosphate additives, which ranged from baked goods to cola beverages [8, 9]. In 2014, our department determined the influence of a high phosphorus intake in combination with different calcium supplies on phosphorus, calcium, magnesium and iron metabolism as well as fibroblast growth factor 23 in a human intervention study [10]. In this and in other intervention studies, increased concentrations of phosphorus and calcium in the faeces after high calcium and phosphorus supplementation compared to placebo were found [10–13]. However, up to now, only a few studies dealt with the question, which effects are provoked by higher intestinal concentrations of calcium and phosphorus in the human gut. It is known that calcium and phosphate form amorphous calcium phosphate complexes (ACP) in the small intestine. Intestinal substances and food ingredients, such as bile and fatty acids, can bind to ACP [13, 14]. This leads to several physiological changes in the human gut, e.g. a modulation of the composition of faecal bile acids, faecal short-chain fatty acids (SCFA) and gut microbiota [11, 13]. Furthermore, high phosphorus intakes can lead to disturbances in the gut, like diarrhoea [15].

In the study presented here, we analysed faecal samples from the subjects of the above-mentioned study [10] regarding cytotoxicity and genotoxicity of faecal water (FW), faecal concentrations of SCFA and fat as well as the composition of the gut microbiome (in a subgroup of study subjects). In addition, we examined the tolerability of the used phosphorus supplement with respect to gut distress, such as diarrhoea or stomach ache, by questionnaire evaluation.

Methods

Supplements

In the current study, two supplements were used: monosodium phosphate (NaH_2PO_4; cfb, Budenheim, Germany) and calcium carbonate ($CaCO_3$; cfb, Budenheim, Germany). In order to achieve a supplementation of additional 1000 mg phosphorus/d as well as additional 500 or 1000 mg calcium/d, monosodium phosphate and calcium carbonate were mixed with sherbet powder. Sherbet powder without additional supplements served as placebo. Participants were encouraged to drink the sherbet powder twice a day diluted in 250 ml water and to document when the sherbet powder was not consumed. Detailed information has been published elsewhere [10].

Subjects and study design

The study was conducted by the Institute of Nutrition of the Friedrich Schiller University Jena between March and July 2014.

Sixty six omnivorous healthy subjects (men, $n = 33$; women $n = 33$) participated in this double-blinded, placebo-controlled and parallel designed study. Eligibility criteria for participants were an age between 18 and 60 years as well as mental and physical well-being. Exclusion criteria were regular intake of dietary supplements, renal diseases, pregnancy, nursing as well as post-menopausal age. Renal diseases were determined with the Chronic Kidney Disease Epidemiology Collaboration equation for estimating the glomerular filtration rate [16]. Subjects with baseline glomerular filtration rates of < 80 ml/min/1.73 m^2 were excluded.

The volunteers were provided with detailed information regarding purpose, course, and possible risks of the study. This study was conducted according to the guidelines laid down in the Declaration of Helsinki and all procedures involving human subjects were approved by the Ethical Committee of the Friedrich Schiller University Jena (no. 3987-01/14). Written informed consent was obtained from all subjects. The trial is registered at ClinicalTrials.gov as NCT02095392. Four participants dropped out because of illness and personal reasons. The remaining 62 volunteers (men, $n = 30$; women, $n = 32$) aged 29 ± 7 years and had a mean BMI of 24 ± 3 kg/m^2.

The details of the study design have been published previously [10]. In short, 62 healthy subjects completed a double-blinded, placebo-controlled and parallel designed study. During the first two weeks, all groups consumed a placebo sherbet powder and afterwards, for eight weeks, a supplemented sherbet powder according to the intervention group: P1000/Ca0 (1000 mg/d phosphorus), P1000/Ca500 (1000 mg/d phosphorus and 500 mg/d calcium) and P1000/Ca1000 (1000 mg/d phosphorus and 1000 mg/d calcium). Dietary records, fasting blood samplings and urine collections took place (after placebo, four and eight weeks of supplementation). After two weeks of placebo and eight weeks of intervention subjects collected one faeces sample. Figure 1 shows the flow chart with the number of subjects included and excluded on each analysis.

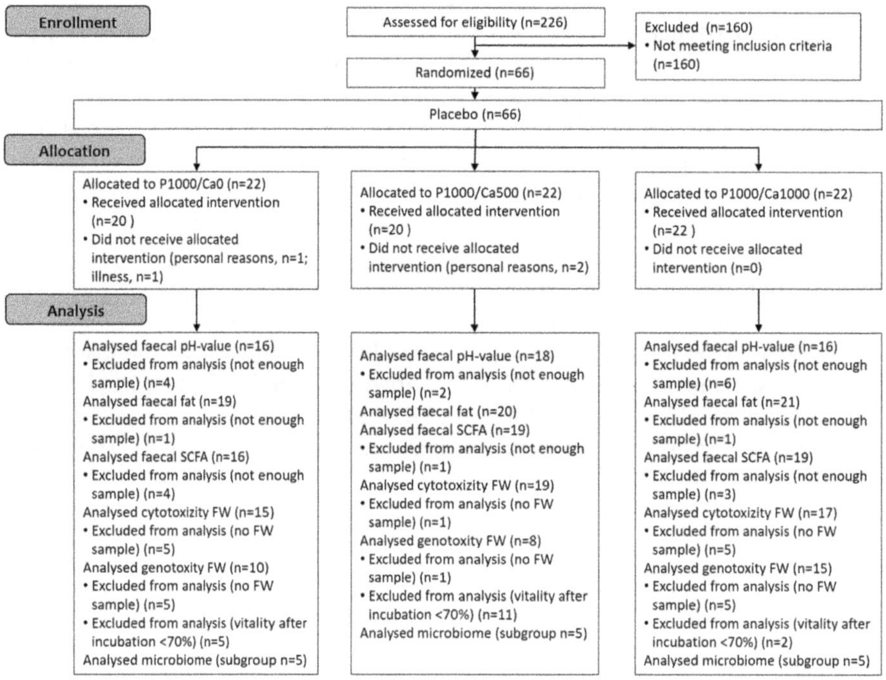

Fig. 1 Flow chart of the study concept. P1000/Ca0: 1000 mg phosphorus; P1000/Ca500: 1000 mg phosphorus/500 mg calcium; P1000/Ca1000: 1000 mg phosphorus/1000 mg calcium; SCFA: short-chain fatty acids; FW: faecal water

Supplement tolerance questionnaire

After placebo as well as after four and eight weeks of supplementation, subjects were encouraged to fill out a questionnaire about diverse health aspects for the last weeks. One question aimed to assess complaints regarding gut health. The subjects should report, whether they had problems with diarrhoea, obstipation, flatulence or undefined stomach ache. In the case of such problems, the subjects were asked to state, whether these problems could be due to the consumption of the test products (supplemented or non-supplemented powder).

Faecal analysis

At the evening before or at the morning of the blood sampling, the subjects were encouraged to collect one whole defecation in provided boxes and to store the sample in a cool dark place. The faecal samples were transported to the study centre at the day of the blood sampling after placebo and eight weeks of intervention. Each specimen was weighed and homogenised. Faecal pH value was measured using a glass pH electrode (InLab 420 electrode MP 225, Mettler Toledo GmbH, Giessen, Germany). Faeces samples were aliquoted for the respective analysis (faecal fat and FW preparation) and stored at − 20 °C until use. For SCFA analysis, 1 g fresh faeces were diluted with 2 ml distilled water, mixed and stored at − 20 °C until use.

Faecal fat

Faecal fat was measured as ether extract after acid hydrolysis by conventional Soxhlet Extraction on a SOXTHERM 2000 automatic (C. Gerhardt, Königswinter, Germany) [13].

Short-chain fatty acids in faeces

SCFA analysis was performed as published by [17]. Briefly, faeces-water mixtures were thawed and thoroughly mixed. After centrifugation (6000 x g, 15 min), 500 μl of the supernatant were added with 50 μl *i*-caproic acid (internal standard), mixed and centrifuged (6000 x g, 15 min). For gas chromatographic measurements, 1 μl of the solution was used (Shimadzu model GC 17A, Shimadzu, Kyoto, Japan).

Faecal water preparation

Fresh faeces samples were homogenised and diluted 1:1 with phosphate buffered saline (PBS) according to Klinder et al. [18]. Afterwards the faeces-PBS mixture was centrifuged for 4 h at 51500 x g at 4 °C. The supernatant (FW) was aliquoted and stored at − 80 °C.

Cell culture and cytotoxicity of faecal water

In the present analysis, the human colorectal adenocarcinoma cell line HT29 (American Type Culture Collection no. HTB-38, Rockville, MD, USA) was used for in vitro experiments. The specific properties and cell culture conditions have been described previously [19].

Briefly, cells were grown in Dulbecco's modified eagle medium (DMEM, Biochrom, Berlin, Germany), which was supplemented with 10% (*v*/v) fetal bovine serum (FBS Superior, Biochrom, Berlin, Germany) and 1% (v/v) antibiotics (penicillin/streptomycin, Biochrom, Berlin, Germany). Within about 24 h the cells doubled their number under given laboratory conditions. In the experiments, passages 10-15 were used. To exclude contamination with mycoplasma, a mycoplasma test (MycoAlert Detection Kit, Lonza, Cologne, Germany) was performed [20].

To determine the cellular vitality after FW incubation, the trypan blue exclusion test, which is based on changes in membrane integrity of the treated cells, was used [21]. For this, the harvested HT29 cell suspension was incubated with trypan blue (Trypan Blue Solution, Sigma Aldrich, Steinheim, Germany) in a 1:1 dilution, followed by automatically counting of viable and dead cells using the ViCell XR (Beckman Coulter, Brea, CA, USA).

Genotoxicity of faecal water

Genotoxicity of FW was tested in HT29 cells as proposed by Oberreuther-Moschner et al. [22]. Briefly, cells were harvested and incubated with FW for 30 min at 37 °C. Single cell microgel electrophoresis (comet assay) was used to analyse genotoxic activity of FW. For this, cells were embedded into agarose on microscopical slides, lysed and subjected to electrophoresis [17, 23]. Each FW sample was analysed in triplicates. PBS as negative control and 75 μM H_2O_2 as positive control were included for each assay, in order to ensure the performance of the comet assay. Microscopic evaluation was performed using the Comet Assay IV image analysis system (Perceptive Instruments, Suffolk, UK). The extent of DNA migration was determined for 60 spots per slide. The tail intensity (TI) was used as the marker for evaluation. The TI is defined as the proportion of tail fluorescence intensity of total comet fluorescence intensity.

DNA extraction and sequencing

A total of 30 faecal samples (five of each intervention group, thereof three men and two women) were extracted with PowerSoil® DNA Isolation Kit (MO BIO, Carlsbad, CA, USA) following the manufacturer's protocol. DNA was quantified using a NanoDrop 2000 spectrophotometer (Thermo Scientific, Waltham, MA, USA) and stored at − 20 °C until further analysis. Illumina library preparation was performed according to Camarinha-Silva et al. [24] with a slightly modified sequence of the primer 27F (AGRGTTHGATYMTGGCTCAG). Amplicons were verified by agarose gel electrophoresis, purified and normalized using SequalPrep Normalization Kit (Invitrogen, Carlsbad, CA, USA). Samples were sequenced using 250 bp paired-end sequencing chemistry on an Illumina MiSeq platform. Raw reads were quality filtered, assembled and aligned using the Mothur pipeline [25]. A total of 36,915 ± 1233 sequencing reads were obtained per sample. The UCHIME algorithm was used to find possible chimeras, and reads were clustered at 97% identity into 832 operative taxonomic units (OTU). Only OTUs present on average abundance higher than 0.002% and a sequence length > 250 bp were considered for further analysis. The closest representative was manually identified with seqmatch from the Ribosomal Database Project classifier [26]. Sequences were submitted to the European Nucleotide Archive under the accession number PRJEB2203.

Statistics

Data analysis was performed using the SPSS Statistics 21 statistical software package (IBM, Chicago, IL, USA). Power calculation for the primary outcome (plasma phosphate concentration) of the human intervention study was published elsewhere [10]. Variance homogeneity and normal distribution were tested using the Levene and the Kolmogorov-Smirnov test, respectively. The effect of supplementation between groups was tested using univariate analysis of variance followed by Bonferroni *post-hoc* test. Effects of time and gender were tested with paired and unpaired Students t-test, respectively. Differences were considered significant at $p \leq 0.05$. Values in the text and tables are means with standard deviations.

The amplicon sequencing data set was standardised by total, and the community similarity structure was depicted through non-metric multidimensional scaling plots and Principal Coordinate Analysis by calculating the Bray-Curtis similarity matrix using PRIMER version 7.0.9 (PRIMER-E, Plymouth Marine Laboratory, Plymouth, UK) [27]. PERMANOVA routine, based on the pair-wise tests using a permutation method under a reduced model, was used to study the significant differences and interactions between factors (diet, time point and gender). Similarity percentages analysis (SIMPER) identified the species contribution to the Bray-Curtis similarity among samples within each diet [27]. Differences in the abundance of OTUs of interest between diets were evaluated using the unpaired Welch's t-test that can handle unequal variances, unequal sample sizes and non-parametric data [28]. OTU abundances were considered significantly different for $p < 0.05$.

Results

Baseline characteristics of subjects who completed the study and nutrient intake (three-day dietary record) have been published elsewhere [10]. Briefly, age, BMI, serum 25-hydroxyvitamin D, kidney function as well as intake of fat, protein and carbohydrates were not significantly different between the three study groups. Phosphorus and calcium intake increased significantly after the respective supplementations.

Supplement tolerance questionnaire

After consumption of placebo and the test products, 20-40% of subjects in each intervention group and at each time point reported complaints with gut health in the last four weeks (Fig. 2a). The majority of these subjects established a subjectively connection to the sherbet powder. This was independent of the respective phosphorus/calcium supplementation or placebo (Fig. 2b). The main complaints according to the questionnaire were diarrhoea and flatulence; a few subjects also reported obstipation and undefined stomach ache (Fig. 2c).

Faecal pH value and fat concentration

After P1000/Ca0 and P1000/Ca500 intervention, the faecal pH value did not change (Table 1). In the whole study collective and in male subjects, the pH value decreased significantly due to P1000/Ca1000 intervention after eight weeks compared to placebo (Table 1). Noteworthy, this effect was likely caused by one male subject with a faecal pH value of 9.1 after placebo.

Faecal fat concentrations did not change significantly due to the interventions (Table 1).

Concentration of faecal SCFA

Considering men and women together, the interventions did not affect the concentrations of total SCFA or the concentrations of the main SCFA acetate, propionate and butyrate compared to placebo (Fig. 3). Certainly, concentrations of total SCFA and acetate were significantly higher after eight weeks of P1000/Ca500 supplementation compared to the P1000/Ca0 (Fig. 3). A gender-specific analysis revealed that acetate and total SCFA concentrations were significantly higher in the P1000/Ca1000 group compared to the P1000/Ca0 group after eight weeks, but only in male subjects (Additional file 1: Figure S1). The faecal concentrations of SCFA in the female subjects did not change (Additional file 2: Figure S2).

Cytotoxicity and genotoxicity of faecal water

After incubation with FW, vitality of the HT29 cells ranged on average between 73 and 83%. For the P1000/Ca1000 intervention group, incubation of HT29 cells with FW from the eight-week time-point resulted in a significantly higher vitality of the cells compared to placebo (Fig. 4a). The interventions with phosphorus did not significantly affect the TI as a marker for genotoxic activity of the FW (Fig. 4b), considering men and women together and separately. Certainly, FW obtained from P1000/Ca0 subjects

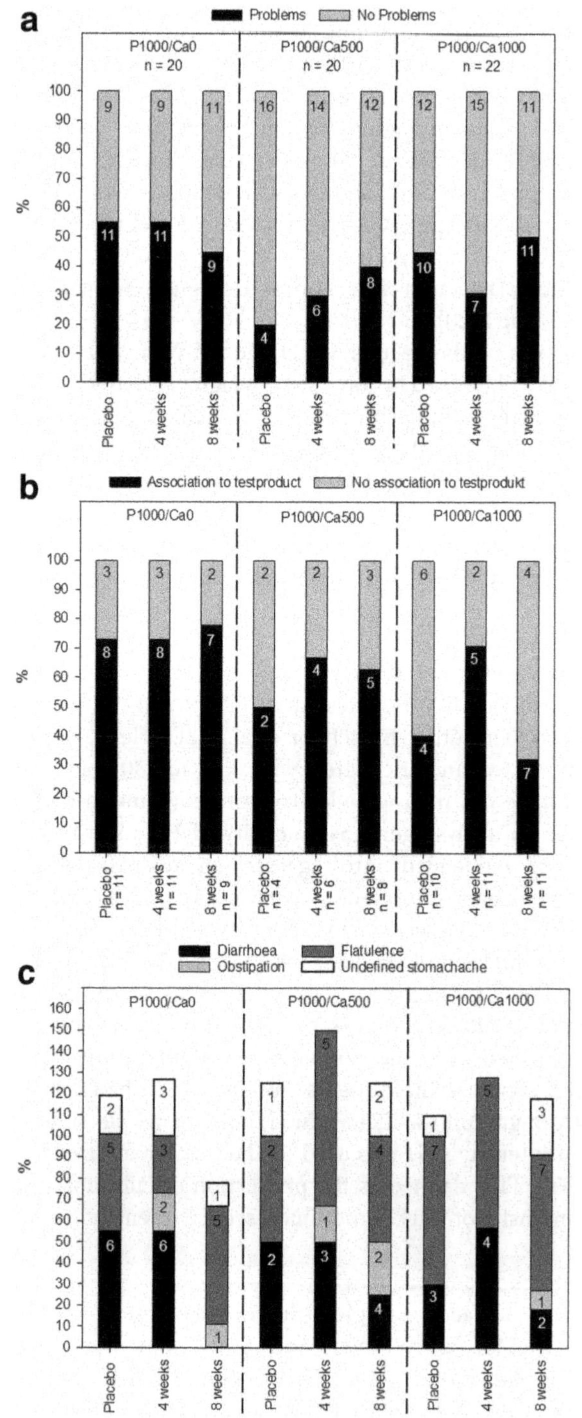

Fig. 2 Overview of intestinal disturbances after supplementation with phosphorus and calcium. **a**: Proportional (y-axis) and absolute (numbers in the bars) distribution of subjects reporting problems with gut health or not; **b**: proportional (y-axis) and absolute (numbers in the bars) distribution of reported associations with the test product, when subjects reported complaints; **c** proportional (y-axis) and absolute (numbers in the bars) distribution of types of reported problems; P1000/Ca0: 1000 mg phosphorus/0 mg calcium; P1000/Ca500: 1000 mg phosphorus/500 mg calcium; P1000/Ca1000: 1000 mg phosphorus/1000 mg calcium

Table 1 Faecal pH values and faecal fat concentrations after intervention with phosphorus and calcium

Parameter	P1000/Ca0	P1000/Ca500	P1000/Ca1000
Faecal pH value			
n	16	18	16
Placebo	6.7 ± 0.7	6.6 ± 0.5	7.0 ± 0.7
8 weeks	6.5 ± 0.5	6.3 ± 0.5	6.5* ± 0.6
Faecal fat [g/100 g fresh faeces]			
n	19	20	21
Placebo	5.9 ± 2.8	5.6 ± 3.2	4.1 ± 1.7
8 weeks	5.5 ± 3.1	5.6 ± 2.5	4.0 ± 2.3

Data are expressed as mean ± standard deviation

P1000/Ca0 1000 mg phosphorus/0 mg calcium, *P1000/Ca500* 1000 mg phosphorus/500 mg calcium, *P1000/Ca1000* 1000 mg phosphorus/1000 mg calcium

*significantly different to placebo ($p \leq 0.05$); effect of time was tested with paired Students t-test

showed significantly higher genotoxic activity before the intervention compared to those from the P1000/Ca1000 group (Fig. 4b). Based on our results that PBS (negative control) caused no genotoxic damages (TI 7 ± 2%) and H_2O_2 caused strong genotoxic effects (TI 59 ± 15%), the FW matrix showed only moderate genotoxicity independent of the phosphorus and calcium interventions (mean TI for all subjects 25 ± 13%).

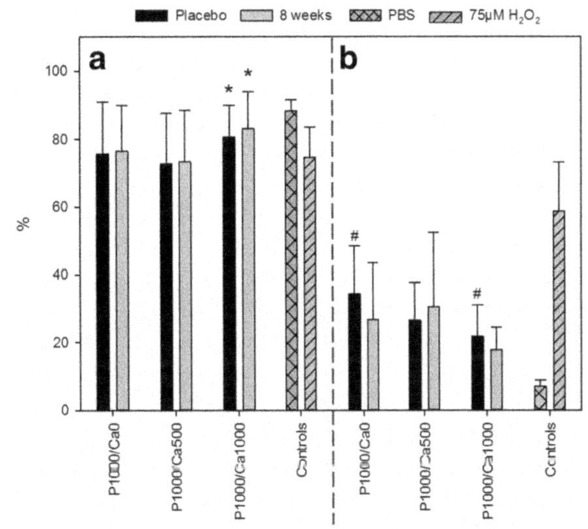

Fig. 4 Cell vitality (**a**) and tail intensity (**b**) of HT29 cells. **a** P1000/Ca0: $n = 15$; P1000/Ca500: $n = 19$; P1000/Ca1000: $n = 17$; **b** P1000/Ca0: $n = 10$; P1000/Ca500: $n = 8$; P1000/Ca1000: $n = 15$; cell vitality and tail intensity after treatment of HT29 cells with faecal water collected following supplementation with phosphorus and calcium; data are expressed as means + standard deviations; #, * mean values with similar symbols are significantly different ($p \leq 0.05$); effect of time was tested with paired Students t-test, effect of supplementation was tested using univariate analysis of variance followed by Bonferroni *post-hoc* test; P1000/Ca0: 1000 mg phosphorus; P1000/Ca500: 1000 mg phosphorus/500 mg calcium; P1000/Ca1000: 1000 mg phosphorus/1000 mg calcium; PBS: phosphate buffered saline

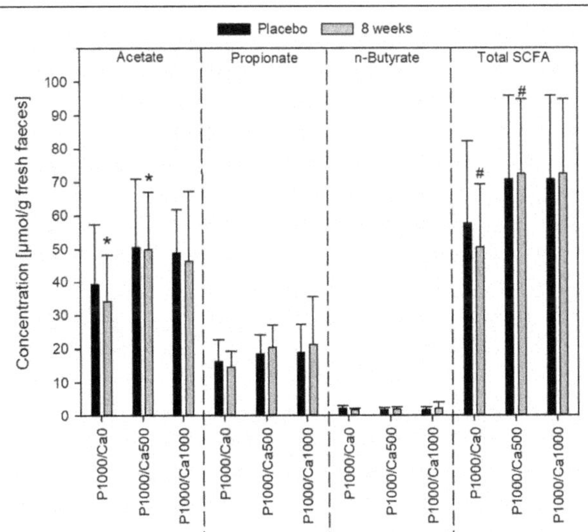

Fig. 3 Faecal concentrations of short-chain fatty acids after supplementation with phosphorus and calcium. P1000/Ca0: $n = 16$; P1000/Ca500: $n = 19$; P1000/Ca1000: $n = 19$; data are expressed as means + standard deviations; #, * mean values with similar symbols are significantly different ($p \leq 0.05$); effect of supplementation was tested using univariate analysis of variance followed by Bonferroni *post-hoc* test; P1000/Ca0: 1000 mg phosphorus; P1000/Ca500: 1000 mg phosphorus/500 mg calcium; P1000/Ca1000: 1000 mg phosphorus/1000 mg calcium; SCFA: short-chain fatty acids

Microbial composition in faeces

Considering all subjects of the study subgroups ($n = 5$ for each intervention), no differences of the microbiome were observed between placebo and eight weeks of intervention as well as between the different intervention groups after eight weeks. Interestingly, men of the P1000/Ca1000 intervention had a significantly different gut microbial community compared to the men of the P1000/Ca0 ($R = 0.778$, $p = 0.01$) and the P1000/Ca500 groups ($R = 0.593$, $p = 0.01$) (Fig. 5). Abundance of the genus *Acetivibio* and of the family *Coriobacteriaceae* were significantly lower in men after eight weeks of P1000/Ca500 intervention when compared to P1000/Ca0 intervention ($p < 0.05$). *Clostridium* XVIII was significantly more abundant in men of the P1000/Ca1000 intervention group compared to men of the P1000/Ca500 ($p = 0.04$) and P1000/Ca0 ($p = 0.04$) groups. The OTUs belonging to *Bifidobacterium* genus were significantly less abundant in faeces of men of the P1000/Ca1000 intervention compared to the faeces of men of the P1000/Ca500 group ($p = 0.04$). Figure 6 shows the relative abundance of the OTUs contributing to the group separation of the men per intervention after eight weeks. OTU4, an uncultured bacterium related to *Clostridium* XVIII, was significantly more abundant in the

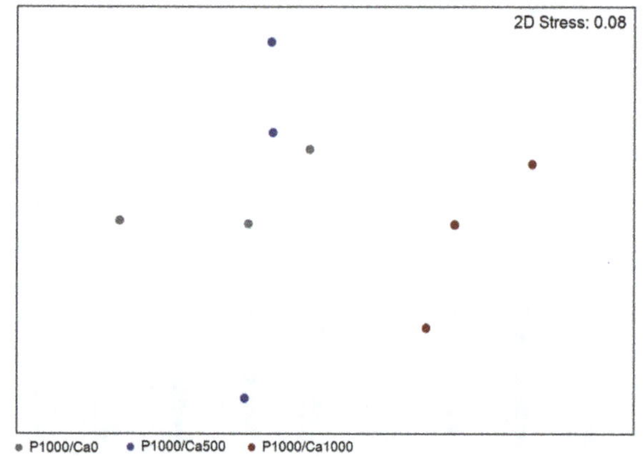

Fig. 5 Global bacterial community structure of men after eight weeks of intervention with phosphorus and calcium. Sequencing data were standardized prior to the use of Bray-Curtis similarity algorithm, the symbols represent a unique sample comprising all OTUs and its abundance information, the data of the red symbols (P1000/Ca1000) are significantly different from the grey (P1000/Ca0, $R = 0.778$, $p = 0.01$) and blue (P1000/Ca500, $R = 0.593$, $p = 0.01$) ones, P1000/Ca0: 1000 mg phosphorus; P1000/Ca500: 1000 mg phosphorus/500 mg calcium; P1000/Ca1000: 1000 mg phosphorus/1000 mg calcium, $n = 9$; ns: not significant, OTU: operational taxonomic unit

men of P1000/Ca1000 intervention group compared to P1000/Ca500 ($p = 0.03$) and P1000/Ca0 ($p = 0.04$). OTU2, a butyrate-producing bacterium, was significantly more abundant in men of the P1000/Ca0 intervention group compared to the men with P1000/Ca1000 supplementation ($p = 0.01$). A trend was observed when the microbial community of men was compared with the one of women (P1000/Ca1000) ($p = 0.1$). OTU 4 was more abundant in men while OTU 19 and OTU 28 were more abundant in women ($p < 0.03$) (Additional file 3: Figure S3). Dietary interventions in women did not cause any significant differences of the microbial community.

Discussion

Already in the 1980s, Newmark et al. hypothesized that calcium ions, bile and fatty acids form insoluble soaps in the human gut, which are detectable in the faeces [29]. Initially, phosphate was considered as a competitor of bile and fatty acids, but Van der Meer et al. showed that phosphate did not compete with bile and fatty acids, but was rather necessary for the

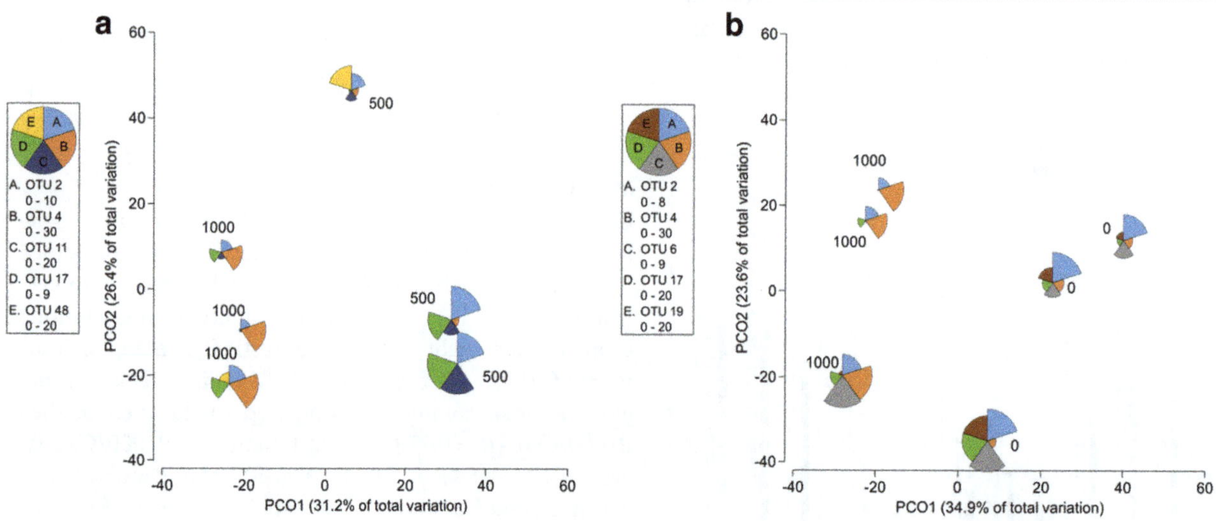

	Species	P1000/Ca0 vs P1000/Ca1000	P1000/Ca500 vs P1000//Ca1000
OTU 2	butyrate-producing bacterium (AJ270475)	p = 0.01	ns
OTU 4	uncultured bacterium (DQ793270)	p = 0.04	p = 0.03
OTU 6	*Bifidobacterium longum* (AY151399)	ns	ns
OTU 11	uncultured bacterium (AY981842)	ns	ns
OTU 17	*Collinsella aerofaciens* (AB011816)	ns	ns
OTU 19	*Bifidobacterium pseudocatenulatum* (D86187)	Ns	ns
OTU 48	*Prevotella copri* (AB064923)	ns	ns

Fig. 6 Principal coordinate analysis ordination of the global microbial community structure of men. **a** Data of men after eight weeks of P1000/Ca1000 vs. P1000/Ca500 intervention; **b** data of men after eight weeks of P1000/Ca1000 vs. P1000/Ca0 intervention, $n = 6$; bubbles were superimposed to visualise the relative abundance of the most relevant OTUs; P1000/Ca0: 1000 mg phosphorus; P1000/Ca500: 1000 mg phosphorus/500 mg calcium; P1000/Ca1000: 1000 mg phosphorus/1000 mg calcium, ns: not significant, OTU: operational taxonomic unit; PCO: principal coordinate

precipitation with calcium [30]. At a molar calcium-to-phosphate ratio of 3:2 and a pH value of 5.6, one part of the ingested dietary calcium and phosphate precipitates as ACP in the small intestine [31]. ACP are able to precipitate both glycine-conjugated and free bile acids by ionic absorption of their negatively charged carboxyl group to the positively charged calcium ions on the surface of the ACP [31]. The hydrophobic tail of the bile acid is exposed to the aqueous phase, which in turn leads to the formation of hydrophobic aggregates. These aggregates are able to bind other hydrophobic ligands [31]. This and the facts that calcium from milk and fermented milk products increases the resistance of rats to salmonella infections [32] and stimulates intestinal lactobacilli colonisation [33], leads to the assumption that dietary calcium and phosphorus can beneficially modify the intestinal environment.

Our human intervention study showed that the faecal concentrations of phosphorus and calcium increased significantly after eight weeks of phosphorus and calcium supplementation [10]. This increase could be due to the formation of ACP. However, even in the group supplemented only with phosphorus indications for ACP formation were observed. We found increasing concentrations of faecal phosphorus without increasing calcium concentrations, but decreasing renal calcium excretion [10]. These results led to the assumption that dietary calcium partly precipitates with phosphate to ACP and cannot be absorbed in the gut. In order to maintain calcium homeostasis of the body, fewer calcium was excreted via urine.

Formation of ACP is a well-known process in the human gut [12, 13, 28], and could be a prerequisite for a beneficial modulation of gut health. A decrease of the available intestinal bile acids by precipitation with ACP can lead to a modified microbiota composition and accordingly to a change in SCFA production and composition [34, 35]. The faecal SCFA concentrations of our subjects showed no effect over time (placebo vs. eight weeks of each intervention). But, after eight weeks, the P1000/Ca0 group showed the lowest concentrations of total SCFA (55 ± 18 µmol/g faeces) compared to P1000/Ca500 (76 ± 22 µmol/g faeces, $p \leq 0.05$) and P1000/Ca1000 (73 ± 31 µmol/g faeces, $p = 0.081$). This higher concentration of total SCFA in the calcium supplemented groups is likely due to a higher acetate concentration. Furthermore, men showed significantly higher total SCFA and acetate concentrations after eight weeks of P1000/Ca1000 intervention compared to the P1000/Ca0 one. These effects are independent of the water content of the faeces, since faecal dry matter did not change due to the interventions (data not shown). In a study of Ditscheid, total SCFA ($p = 0.065$) and acetate concentrations ($p = 0.019$) increased after supplementation with calcium phosphate (β-tricalciumphosphate) compared to placebo [36]. The author assumed that either an increased production or a decreased absorption of acetate could be the reason for the higher faecal concentrations after calcium phosphate supplementation. Trinidad et al. showed that bioavailable calcium supports intestinal acetate absorption [37]. Therefore, Ditscheid hypothesized that bioavailability of calcium decreased due to ACP formation and thus acetate absorption is diminished [36]. But, calcium phosphate supplementation has been shown to modulate the intestinal gut community by changing the intestinal environment [11, 33]. This shift of the gut microbiota could lead to an increased production of SCFA, such as acetate [34].

In the present study, we determined in a subgroup of five subjects per intervention the microbial community in faeces by DNA extraction and amplicon sequencing. Interestingly, men of the P1000/Ca1000 group showed a shift of the microbial community compared to men of the two other intervention groups. *Clostridium* XVIII was significantly more abundant in men of the highest calcium group. Furthermore, men of the P1000/Ca1000 intervention group had significantly higher acetate concentrations compared to men of the P1000/Ca0 one. In general, *Clostridium spp.* are known to produce acetate by microbial fermentation of carbohydrates in the human gut [34]. Although, the detected *Clostridium* XVIII is an uncultured bacterium and not characterised so far, it could exhibit similar acetate producing properties. Moreover, OTU2, a butyrate-producing bacterium, was significantly more abundant in men of the P1000/Ca0 intervention group and tended to be more abundant in the P1000/Ca500 group compared to the men of the P1000/Ca1000 ($p = 0.01$) one. But whether these associations depend on the calcium and phosphorus supplementation remains unclear, since we were only able to study the microbial community of a subgroup of five subjects per intervention. The partly gender-specific effects might be a result of sex-specific diet effects on the human microbiome as proposed by Bolnick et al. [38]. Animal and human studies showed, that gender influences microbial composition in the gut [38–41] and, thus, the formation of SCFA [42], too.

A modulation of the cyto- and genotoxicity of the FW after calcium and phosphorus supplementation is discussed since ACP are known to precipitate secondary bile acids in the gut [29, 43]. Secondary bile acids showed cyto- and genotoxic effects on human normal and tumour colon cells [44–46]. Our results indicate that the phosphorus supplementation with and without calcium did not affect the genotoxicity of FW and did not markedly effect the vitality of HT29 cells. Similar results were provided by Ditscheid et al., which could not show changes in the genotoxicity of FW after calcium phosphate supplementation [47]. Glinghammer et al. reported that cytotoxicity of FW increased after subjects switched from a dairy product-rich (high calcium) to a dairy product-free diet (lower calcium), but genotoxicity did not alter [48]. The authors suggested that the mechanism by which dairy products may act colon cancer protective are at the level of tumour promotion and indicated that dairy products, especially calcium and phosphate, exert protective effects by precipitating bile and fatty acids [48]. Gomes et al. summarised in a review that high calcium diets reduce FW cytotoxicity by precipitating cytotoxic surfactants, which results in a lower colonic epithelium damage and higher resistance against infections [49]. All studies cited in this context used a calcium phosphate supplement, but almost all are based on animal models. Furthermore, the cell model systems and methods used were different to the ones used here, e.g. cytotoxicity was tested with erythrocytes [43] instead of intestinal cells. Besides, maybe a more realistic picture of the FW genotoxicity would be displayed by a quantitative stool sampling over one or more days. Unfortunately, parameters in faeces were not the main outcome of our human intervention study and so only one stool sample was collected.

Like the precipitation of bile acids, ACP are in principle able to precipitate fatty acids as well [49]. The resulting increased faecal excretion of fat could favour weight control [50]. Our study did not show changes in faecal fat concentrations in response to the phosphorus and calcium supplementation. Ditscheid et al. also reported no significant changes in faecal fat excretion after supplementation with β-tricalciumphosphate compared to a normal calcium intake (approx. 2200 vs. 1200 mg calcium/d and 2000 vs. 1600 mg phosphorus/d) [13]. In contrast, Boon et al. showed a non-significant 57% increase in faecal fat after high compared to low calcium intakes (2500 vs 400 mg calcium/d, low-fat dairy) [51]. Furthermore, in a study by Bendsen et al. faecal fat increased from 5.4 to 11.5 g/d after intake of 1600 mg calcium/d (by dairy supplementation) [52]. Another study comparing low (approx. 500 mg calcium/d) with high calcium diets (approx. 1800 mg calcium/d, low-fat dairy products) showed a 2.5-fold increase in faecal fat after the high calcium intake [53]. One reason for the discrepancies could be the standardising of the diet and stool collection time. In the study presented here a dietary record for three days was done and one faecal sample was collected. However, the study of Ditscheid et al. included a standardised diet and a five-day faecal collection. But, nevertheless they also found no effect on faecal fat concentration. Possibly, this could be caused by the normal calcium intake that was used as placebo here (approx. 900 mg calcium/d) [10] and by Ditscheid et al. (approx. 1200 mg calcium/d) [13], whereas in the studies by Boon et al. (400 mg calcium/d) [51] and Jacobsen et al. (500 mg calcium/d) [53] low calcium diets were used as controls. It is therefore possible that the observed changes in faecal fat concentrations were caused by decreasing the intake of calcium in the controls to levels below the norm.

In a phosphate supplementation study of Grimm et al., a phosphate-rich diet (additional 1436 mg phosphorus/d) was associated with intestinal distress, soft stool or mild diarrhoea. The authors concluded that the symptoms are a consequence of an osmotic effect of the added polyphosphates in the intestinal lumen [15]. In our study 20-40% of the subjects in each intervention group and at each time point reported intestinal disturbances. The majority of the subjects mentioned a connection to the test product. Analysis of the questionnaires showed that the reported disturbances were independent of the phosphorus and calcium supplementation and time-point of intervention. Therefore, we consider the gut problems as a result of the sherbet powder consumption in general and not as a result of the phosphorus and calcium supplementation. Another reason could be the focus of the subjects on the new diet component (sherbet powder) and a resulting overestimation of intestinal distress in case of gut problems. Furthermore, the interpretation of the questionnaires is limited, since the subjects reported only whether they had problems but not the frequency and intensity of disturbances.

The most important limitations of our study are (i) the restricted one portion faecal collection and (ii) the determination of gut community in a limited subgroup with only a few subjects.

To the best of our knowledge, this is the first human intervention study in the field of high phosphorus and calcium intakes, which also paid attention on gut health. As the main part of the additional phosphorus and calcium passes the whole gut via ACP and seems to modulate gut physiology, further human intervention studies in this context are needed.

Conclusions

In conclusion, the high phosphorus supplementation did not influence cyto- and genotoxicity of FW as well as the concentrations of faecal fat independent of calcium intake. Our study provides first hints for a potential phosphorus-induced modulation of the gut community and the faecal total SCFA content. Since additional dietary phosphorus and calcium passes the gut as ACP, further studies are needed to evaluate the effect of high phosphorus and calcium diets on gut-related parameters.

Additional files

Additional file 1: Figure S1. Faecal concentrations of short-chain fatty acids after supplementation with phosphorus and calcium of men. P1000/Ca0: $n = 7$; P1000/Ca500: $n = 9$; P1000/Ca1000: $n = 8$; data are expressed as means + standard deviations; #,* mean values with similar symbols are significant different ($p \leq 0.05$); effect of supplementation was tested using univariate analysis of variance followed by Bonferroni *post-hoc* test; a, b significantly different (Wilcoxon sign-rank test); P1000/Ca0: 1000 mg phosphorus; P1000/Ca500: 1000 mg phosphorus/500 mg calcium; P1000/Ca1000: 1000 mg phosphorus/1000 mg calcium; SCFA: short-chain fatty acids.

Additional file 2: Figure S2. Faecal concentrations of short-chain fatty acids after supplementation with phosphorus and calcium of women. P1000/Ca0: $n = 9$; P1000/Ca500: $n = 10$; P1000/Ca1000: $n = 11$; data are expressed as means + standard deviations; #,* mean values with similar symbols are significant different ($p \leq 0.05$); effect of time was tested with paired Students t-test; effect of supplementation was tested using univariate analysis of variance followed by Bonferroni *post-hoc* test; P1000/Ca0: 1000 mg phosphorus; P1000/Ca500: 1000 mg phosphorus/500 mg calcium; P1000/Ca1000: 1000 mg phosphorus/1000 mg calcium; SCFA: short-chain fatty acids.

Additional file 3: Figure S3. Principal coordinate analysis ordination of the global community structure of men and women after eight weeks of P1000/Ca1000 intervention. $n = 5$, bubbles were superimposed to visualise the relative abundance of the most relevant OTUs; P1000/Ca1000: 1000 mg phosphorus/1000 mg calcium, ns: not significant, OTU: operational taxonomic unit; PCO: principal coordinate.

Abbreviations
ACP: Amorphous calcium phosphate; FW: Faecal water; OTU: Operational taxonomic unit; P1000/Ca0: 1000 mg phosphorus; P1000/Ca1000: 1000 mg phosphorus/1000 mg calcium; P1000/Ca500: 1000 mg phosphorus/500 mg calcium; PBS: Phosphate buffered saline; PCO: Principal coordinate; SCFA: Short-chain fatty acids; TI: Tail intensity

Acknowledgements
Technical assistance is greatly appreciated from Ute Helms, Esther Woschee, Kerstin Kalmring-Raspe und Carsten Rohrer.

Funding
Phosphoric Acid & Phosphate Producers Associations (PAPA) funded the project. PAPA was not involved in the study design and did not influence the interpretation of the results.

Authors' contributions
All authors made substantial contributions to one or more of the following: study conception and design, acquisition of data, analysis and interpretation of data, drafting and/or critically revising the manuscript for important intellectual content. Each author has seen and approved the contents of the submitted manuscript. None of the authors had any personal or financial conflicts of interests. UT conducted research, analysed data, performed statistical analysis and wrote the manuscript; ACS extracted samples and performed statistical and bioinformatics analysis of sequencing data; SL analysed SCFA data; UT, GJ and MG designed research and had primary responsibility for final content. All authors were responsible for the critical revision of the manuscript. All authors read and approved the final manuscript.

Competing interests
The authors declare that they have no competing interests.

Author details
[1]Department of Nutritional Toxicology, Institute of Nutrition, Friedrich Schiller University Jena, Dornburger Straße 24, 07743 Jena, Germany. [2]Institute of Animal Science, University of Hohenheim, Emil-Wolff-Straße. 10, 70599 Stuttgart, Germany. [3]Department of Nutritional Physiology, Institute of Nutrition, Friedrich Schiller University Jena, Dornburger Straße 23, 07743 Jena, Germany. [4]Department of Nutritional Biochemistry and Physiology, Institute of Nutrition, Friedrich Schiller University Jena, Dornburger Straße 25, 07743 Jena, Germany. [5]Competence Cluster for Nutrition and Cardiovascular Health (nutriCARD) Halle-Jena-Leipzig, Jena, Germany.

References
1. Calvo MS, Uribarri J. Public health impact of dietary phosphorus excess on bone and cardiovascular health in the general population. Am J Clin Nutr. 2013;98:6–15.
2. Dhingra R, Sullivan LM, Fox CS, Wang TJ, D'Agostino RB, Gaziano JM, Vasan RS. Relations of serum phosphorus and calcium levels to the incidence of cardiovascular disease in the community. Arch Intern Med. 2007;167:879–85.
3. Eddington H, Hoefield R, Sinha S, Chrysochou C, Lane B, Foley RN, Hegarty J, New J, O'Donoghue DJ, Middleton RJ, Kalra PA. Serum phosphate and mortality in patients with chronic kidney disease. Clin J Am Soc Nephrol. 2010;5:2251–7.
4. Chang AR, Lazo M, Appel LJ, Gutierrez OM, Grams ME. High dietary phosphorus intake is associated with all-cause mortality: results from NHANES III. Am J Clin Nutr. 2014;99:320–7.
5. de Boer IH, Rue TC, Kestenbaum B. Serum phosphorus concentrations in the third National Health and Nutrition Examination Survey (NHANES III). Am J Kidney Dis. 2009;53:399–407.
6. Selamet U, Tighiouart H, Sarnak MJ, Beck G, Levey AS, Block G, Ix JH. Relationship of dietary phosphate intake with risk of end-stage renal disease and mortality in chronic kidney disease stages 3-5: the modification of diet in renal disease study. Kidney Int. 2016;89:176–84.
7. Adatorwovor R, Roggenkamp K, Anderson JJ. Intakes of calcium and phosphorus and calculated calcium-to-phosphorus ratios of older adults: NHANES 2005-2006 data. Nutrients. 2015;7:9633–9.
8. Calvo MS, Uribarri J. Contributions to total phosphorus intake: all sources considered. Semin Dial. 2013;26:54–61.
9. Ritz E, Hahn K, Ketteler M, Kuhlmann MK, Mann J. Phosphate additives in food–a health risk. Dtsch Arztebl Int. 2012;109:49–55.
10. Trautvetter U, Jahreis G, Kiehntopf M, Glei M. Consequences of a high phosphorus intake on mineral metabolism and bone remodeling in dependence of calcium intake in healthy subjects - a randomized placebo-controlled human intervention study. Nutr J. 2016;15:7.
11. Trautvetter U, Ditscheid B, Kiehntopf M, Jahreis G. A combination of calcium phosphate and probiotics beneficially influences intestinal lactobacilli and cholesterol metabolism in humans. Clin Nutr. 2012;31:230–7.
12. Trautvetter U, Neef N, Leiterer M, Kiehntopf M, Kratzsch J, Jahreis G. Effect of calcium phosphate and vitamin D3 supplementation on bone remodelling and metabolism of calcium, phosphorus, magnesium and iron. Nutr J. 2014;13:6.
13. Ditscheid B, Keller S, Jahreis G. Cholesterol metabolism is affected by calcium phosphate supplementation in humans. J Nutr. 2005;135:1678–82.
14. Van der Meer R, Lapre JA, Govers M, Kleibeuker JH. Mechanisms of the intestinal effects of dietary fats and milk products on colon carcinogenesis. Cancer Lett. 1997;114:75–83.
15. Grimm M, Müller A, Hein G, Fünfstück R, Jahreis G. High phosphorus intake only slightly affects serum minerals, urinary pyridinium crosslinks and renal function in young women. Eur J Clin Nutr. 2001;55:153–61.
16. Matsushita K, Tonelli M, Lloyd A, Levey AS, Coresh J, Hemmelgarn BR. Clinical risk implications of the CKD Epidemiology Collaboration (CKD-EPI) equation compared with the Modification of Diet in Renal Disease (MDRD) study equation for estimated GFR. Am J Kidney Dis. 2012;60:241–9.
17. Roessler A, Forssten SD, Glei M, Ouwehand AC, Jahreis G. The effect of probiotics on faecal microbiota and genotoxic activity of faecal water in patients with atopic dermatitis: a randomized, placebo-controlled study. Clin Nutr. 2012;31:22–9.

18. Klinder A, Karlsson PC, Clune Y, Hughes R, Glei M, Rafter JJ, Rowland I, Collins JK, Pool-Zobel BL. Fecal water as a non-invasive biomarker in nutritional intervention: comparison of preparation methods and refinement of different endpoints. Nutr Cancer. 2007;57:158–67.
19. Glei M, Kirmse A, Habermann N, Persin C, Pool-Zobel BL. Bread enriched with green coffee extract has chemoprotective and antigenotoxic activities in human cells. Nutr Cancer. 2006;56:182–92.
20. Munjal U, Scharlau D, Glei M. Gut fermentation products of inulin-type fructans modulate the expression of xenobiotic-metabolising enzymes in human colonic tumour cells. Anticancer Res. 2012;32:5379–86.
21. Knoll N, Weise A, Claussen U, Sendt W, Marian B, Glei M, Pool-Zobel BL. 2-Dodecylcyclobutanone, a radiolytic product of palmitic acid, is genotoxic in primary human colon cells and in cells from preneoplastic lesions. Mutat Res. 2006;594:10–9.
22. Oberreuther-Moschner DL, Jahreis G, Rechkemmer G, Pool-Zobel BL. Dietary intervention with the probiotics lactobacillus acidophilus 145 and Bifidobacterium longum 913 modulates the potential of human faecal water to induce damage in HT29clone19A cells. Br J Nutr. 2004;91:925–32.
23. Glei M, Matuschek M, Steiner C, Böhm V, Persin C, Pool-Zobel BL. Initial in vitro toxicity testing of functional foods rich in catechins and anthocyanins in human cells. Toxicol in Vitro. 2003;17:723–9.
24. Camarinha-Silva A, Jauregui R, Chaves-Moreno D, Oxley AP, Schaumburg F, Becker K, Wos-Oxley ML, Pieper DH. Comparing the anterior nare bacterial community of two discrete human populations using Illumina amplicon sequencing. Environ Microbiol. 2014;16:2939–52.
25. Kozich JJ, Westcott SL, Baxter NT, Highlander SK, Schloss PD. Development of a dual-index sequencing strategy and curation pipeline for analyzing amplicon sequence data on the MiSeq Illumina sequencing platform. Appl Environ Microbiol. 2013;79:5112–20.
26. Wang Q, Garrity GM, Tiedje JM, Cole JR. Naive Bayesian classifier for rapid assignment of rRNA sequences into the new bacterial taxonomy. Appl Environ Microbiol. 2007;73:5261–7.
27. Clarke KR, Warwick RM: Change in Marine Communities: an approach to statistical analysis and Interpretation. Plymouth marine laboratory, Natural environment research council; 1994.
28. Welch BL. The generalization of 'Student's' problem when several different population variances are involved. Biometrika. 1947;34:28–35.
29. Newmark HL, Wargovich MJ, Bruce WR. Colon cancer and dietary fat, phosphate, and calcium: a hypothesis. J Natl Cancer Inst. 1984;72:1323–5.
30. Van der Meer R, Termont DS, De Vries HT. Differential effects of calcium ions and calcium phosphate on cytotoxicity of bile acids. Am J Phys. 1991;260:G142–7.
31. Govers MJAP, Termont DSML, Van der Meer R. Mechanism of the antiproliferative effect of milk mineral and other calcium supplements on colonic epithelium. Cancer Res. 1994;54:95–100.
32. Bovee-Oudenhoven I, Termont D, Dekker R, Van der Meer R. Calcium in milk and fermentation by yoghurt bacteria increase the resistance of rats to salmonella infection. Gut. 1996;38:59–65.
33. Bovee-Oudenhoven IM, Wissink ML, Wouters JT, Van der Meer R. Dietary calcium phosphate stimulates intestinal lactobacilli and decreases the severity of a salmonella infection in rats. J Nutr. 1999;129:607–12.
34. Koh A, De Vadder F, Kovatcheva-Datchary P, Bäckhed F. From dietary fiber to host physiology: short-chain fatty acids as key bacterial metabolites. Cell. 2016;165:1332–45.
35. Bovee-Oudenhoven IM, Termont DS, Weerkamp AH, Faassen-Peters MA, Van der Meer R. Dietary calcium inhibits the intestinal colonization and translocation of salmonella in rats. Gastroenterology. 1997;113:550–7.
36. Ditscheid B: In vivo investigation into the physiologic effects of pentacalcium hydroxy-triphosphate supplementation in humans and in vitro model for the adsorption of bile acids and neutral sterols to different calcium phosphates. Dissertation; 2006.
37. Trinidad TP, Wolever TM, Thompson LU. Effects of calcium concentration, acetate, and propionate on calcium absorption in the human distal colon. Nutrition. 1999;15:529–33.
38. Bolnick DI, Snowberg LK, Hirsch PE, Lauber CL, Org E, Parks B, Lusis AJ, Knight R, Caporaso JG, Svanbäck R. Individual diet has sex-dependent effects on vertebrate gut microbiota. Nat Commun. 2014;5:4500.
39. Org E, Mehrabian M, Parks BW, Shipkova P, Liu X, Drake TA, Lusis AJ. Sex differences and hormonal effects on gut microbiota composition in mice. Gut Microbes. 2016;7:313–22.
40. Neuman H, Debelius JW, Knight R, Koren O. Microbial endocrinology: the interplay between the microbiota and the endocrine system. FEMS Microbiol Rev. 2015;39:509–21.
41. Most J, Goossens GH, Reijnders D, Canfora EE, Penders J, Blaak EE. Gut microbiota composition strongly correlates to peripheral insulin sensitivity in obese men but not in women. Benefic Microbes. 2017;8:557–62.
42. Wong JMWRD, de Souza RRD, Kendall CWCP, Emam AM, Jenkins DJAMD. Colonic health: fermentation and short chain fatty acids. J Clin Gastroenterol. 2006;40:235–43.
43. Govers MJ, Termont DS, Lapre JA, Kleibeuker JH, Vonk RJ, Van der Meer R. Calcium in milk products precipitates intestinal fatty acids and secondary bile acids and thus inhibits colonic cytotoxicity in humans. Cancer Res. 1996;56:3270–5.
44. Rosignoli P, Fabiani R, De Bartolomeo A, Fuccelli R, Pelli MA, Morozzi G. Genotoxic effect of bile acids on human normal and tumour colon cells and protection by dietary antioxidants and butyrate. Eur J Nutr. 2008;47: 301–9.
45. Tong JL, Ran ZH, Shen J, Fan GQ, Xiao SD. Association between fecal bile acids and colorectal cancer: a meta-analysis of observational studies. Yonsei Med J. 2008;49:792–803.
46. Powolny A, Xu J, Loo G. Deoxycholate induces DNA damage and apoptosis in human colon epithelial cells expressing either mutant or wild-type p53. Int J Biochem Cell Biol. 2001;33:193–203.
47. Ditscheid B, Keller S, Jahreis G. Faecal steroid excretion in humans is affected by calcium supplementation and shows gender-specific differences. Eur J Nutr. 2009;48:22–30.
48. Glinghammar B, Venturi M, Rowland IR, Rafter JJ. Shift from a dairy product-rich to a dairy product-free diet: influence on cytotoxicity and genotoxicity of fecal water–potential risk factors for colon cancer. Am J Clin Nutr. 1997; 66:1277–82.
49. Gomes JM, Costa JA, Alfenas RC. Could the beneficial effects of dietary calcium on obesity and diabetes control be mediated by changes in intestinal microbiota and integrity? Br J Nutr. 2015;114:1756–65.
50. Christensen R, Lorenzen JK, Svith CR, Bartels EM, Melanson EL, Saris WH, Tremblay A, Astrup A. Effect of calcium from dairy and dietary supplements on faecal fat excretion: a meta-analysis of randomized controlled trials. Obes Rev. 2009;10:475–86.
51. Boon N, Hul GBJ, Stegen JHCH, Sluijsmans WEM, Valle C, Langin D, Viguerie N, Saris WHM. An intervention study of the effects of calcium intake on faecal fat excretion, energy metabolism and adipose tissue mRNA expression of lipid-metabolism related proteins. Int J Obes. 2007;31:1704–12.
52. Bendsen NT, Hother AL, Jensen SK, Lorenzen JK, Astrup A. Effect of dairy calcium on fecal fat excretion: a randomized crossover trial. Int J Obes. 2008; 32:1816–24.
53. Jacobsen R, Lorenzen JK, Toubro S, Krog-Mikkelsen I, Astrup A. Effect of short-term high dietary calcium intake on 24-h energy expenditure, fat oxidation, and fecal fat excretion. Int J Obes. 2005;29:292–301.

3

Western and Modern Mexican dietary patterns are directly associated with incident hypertension in Mexican women

Adriana Monge[1,2], Martín Lajous[1,4], Eduardo Ortiz-Panozo[1], Beatriz L. Rodríguez[2,3], José Juan Góngora[2] and Ruy López-Ridaura[1*]

Abstract

Background: Research has found that diet and dietary patterns are associated with blood pressure and hypertension. Limited research in this area has been conducted in a Mexican population.

Methods: We investigated the relation between dietary patterns (principal component analysis) and the incidence of self-reported treated hypertension in 62,913 women from the Mexican Teachers' Cohort, a large population-based cohort of female Mexican teachers, who were free of hypertension at baseline in 2006–2008 when diet was assessed using a food frequency questionnaire. Dietary patterns were categorized into quartiles and logistic regression models were fit.

Results: Participants were 42.1 ± 7.3 years old, had a BMI 27.0 ± 4.4 and a cumulative incidence of hypertension of 4.6%. Between baseline and first follow-up (2011–2014) we identified 2916 incident cases of hypertension. We identified three major components. The first was loaded heavily with vegetables, fruits and legumes; the second component was loaded heavily with processed meats, fast foods, and red meat; and finally the third component was loaded heavily with corn tortillas, hot peppers, and sodas. We named the components as Fruits & Vegetables (FV), Western (W), and Modern Mexican (MM).

The multivariable-adjusted odds of hypertension in the highest quartile of the W pattern were 24% higher than the odds for individuals in the lowest quartile (95%CI = 1.10, 1.40; *P*-trend = 0.0004); women in the highest quartile of the MM pattern had 15% higher odds than women in the lowest quartile (95%CI = 1.02, 1.29; *P*-trend = 0.01). The FV pattern was not significantly associated with hypertension (OR for extreme quartiles = 0.94; 95%CI = 0.84, 1.05; *P*-trend = 0.19).

Conclusion: The Western pattern and the Modern Mexican pattern, which showcases an undergoing nutrition transition, may affect the incidence of hypertension, whereas the FV pattern was not associated with hypertension. These findings are important in the prevention of hypertension and cardiovascular diseases in Mexico and possibly among Mexican people living in the US.

Keywords: Diet, Dietary patterns, Hypertension, Women, Mexican

* Correspondence: rlridaura@insp.mx
[1]Center for Research on Population Health, National Institute of Public Health, Cuernavaca, Mexico

Background

Hypertension is an important public health concern in Mexico where the prevalence in adult women is 30% [1]. High blood pressure is a marker of cardiovascular risk and has important health impacts, such as on cardiovascular and cerebrovascular disease, renal failure, retinopathy and optic neuropathy. Diet is a modifiable risk factor for hypertension, however results from studies on individual foods and nutrients (i.e. coffee and caffeine, dairy, cruciferous vegetables, etc.) have been controversial [2–8]. Evaluating dietary patterns has been proposed as a strategy that captures the overall manner in which individuals consume foods [9–11]. Dietary patterns overcome the challenge of collinearity of studying single foods or nutrients and potentially considering their joint effects [10].

Dietary patterns based on a priori indices have been associated to decreased risk of chronic disease. While there is robust scientific evidence on the benefits of the DASH diet (Dietary Approaches to Stop Hypertension) and the Mediterranean diet on lowering blood pressure [12–14], these a priori indices have been generated from studies done mostly in Caucasian populations, with little representation of Mexicans, one of the largest minorities in the US. It is questionable whether these indices are appropriate for the Hispanic population, specifically Mexicans, since evidence shows low adherence to these indices [15]. In contrast, empirically derived dietary patterns are data driven and allow for the examination of eating behaviors without prior knowledge or assumption of the existence of dietary patterns in the population.

There is a need to understand dietary patterns within the Mexican population and comprehend which of these patterns are associated with hypertension risk and subsequently target culturally appropriate public health messages of healthy diets. In this study we derived dietary patterns using principal component analysis to explore the association between the Mexican dietary patterns and incident hypertension in a population-based study.

Methods

Study population

The Mexican Teachers' Cohort (MTC) was established in 2006–08, when 115,315 female teachers aged 25 years and older responded to a scannable paper questionnaire on demographic and reproductive characteristics, diet, lifestyle, and medical conditions. Women participate in a well-established voluntary economic incentives program and the study questionnaire was delivered and collected in collaboration with public education authorities from 12 states in Mexico [16]. All women signed an informed consent form to take part in the study. This study was approved by the Institutional Review Board at National Institute of Public Health of Mexico (INSP). Between December 2011 and February 2014, a follow-up questionnaire was released. Sixty-nine percent of participants responded to a paper-based questionnaire, 2% to an online questionnaire and 11% to a short telephone interview for an overall response of 82% for the 2011–2014 questionnaire.

After a feasibility phase in 2006, 106,466 participants responded a questionnaire in 2008 that included a previously validated dietary questionnaire [17]. We excluded women with unrealistic energy intake (500 > calories> 3500) or an invalid questionnaire (70 or more items missing, or cereals and grains section missing) (n = 18,396). Prevalent cases of hypertension (n = 11,292), myocardial infarction, stroke or cancer (n = 1772) were also excluded. Finally, we excluded 12,093 participants for whom information after baseline was unavailable. The final study sample included 62,913 participants.

Dietary assessment

We collected dietary information with a 140-item semi-quantitative food frequency questionnaire (FFQ). Participants were asked to specify the average frequency of consumption over the previous year of each food item in a commonly used unit or portion size. The consumption frequencies were never, once a month or less, two to three times a month, once a week, two to four times a week, five to six times a week, once a day, two to three times a day, four to five times a day and six or more times a day. With the USDA food-composition database [18] and the database used in the National Health and Nutrition Survey in Mexico we calculated nutrient and energy intakes by multiplying the nutrient content of the pre-defined portion sizes by the frequency of consumption. A similar version of our FFQ was previously validated amongst 134 Mexico City female residents in a 12-month study [17]. Pearson correlation coefficients for total energy, carbohydrate, protein, and total fat intakes between the FFQ and four 4-day 24-h recalls were 0.52, 0.57, 0.32, and 0.63, respectively.

Hypertension assessment

At follow-up, we asked participants to report whether a clinician had made a diagnosis of elevated blood pressure in the previous two years, if treatment was received, and the year of diagnosis. We defined hypertension as self-reported physician diagnosed elevated blood pressure under drug treatment. We assessed the validity of self-reported hypertension diagnosis in a random subsample of 101 participants who reported elevated blood pressure, using a structured phone interview to confirm the diagnosis, year of diagnosis and treatment. We confirmed the presence of hypertension in 89% of participants who reported a clinical diagnosis of elevated blood pressure under treatment, whereas only 50% of cases were confirmed in those who reported a diagnosis without treatment.

Dietary patterns

Dietary patterns were derived using all valid FFQs at baseline (n = 88,082). Food items in the FFQ were collapsed into 37 food groups (Table 1) based on similarity of nutrient content by a trained dietitian. Some individual foods were retained because they represented distinct dietary patterns or constituted a distinct item on their own (e.g. corn tortillas, atole, and eggs). Gram amounts of food groups were converted to calories and divided by total energy intake of each individual, resulting in food groups standardized as percent of total energy intake plus one and log transformed to normalize the distribution.

We defined dietary patterns on the 37 food groups with principal component analysis (PCA) using the factor procedure in SAS. PCA reduces the number of observed variables to a smaller number of principal components that account for most of the variance of the observed variables. Components were rotated by an orthogonal transformation (*Varimax* rotation function) to achieve simpler structures with greater interpretation. The number of components retained were determined using a combination of the eigenvalues (> 1.5), the scree plot, and the interpretability of the components. The cut-off value for eigenvalues is arbitrary, some have used eigenvalues > 1.25 [11, 19] however, the usual value is > 1.0 but this cut-off generated too many factors. We decided not use the percentage of variance explained to determine the number of components to retain because this depends on the number of variables entered into the analysis [20, 21]. There are two approaches to calculate the factor scores per participant, one is to compute the score by summing the observed intakes of the component food items weighted by its factor loading. The second approach is a simpler approach to sum only the factors that load higher than a certain value [19]. We chose to use the more elaborate approach to calculate factor scores for this analysis (results were similar). Factor loadings >|0.30| were considered to contribute to the component and were used to name the dietary patterns.

Covariates

Covariate information was based on self-reports from the baseline questionnaire. Responses to ownership of seven household assets (phone, car, computer, vacuum cleaner, microwave oven, cell phone and internet) were summed and classified into low, medium and high socioeconomic status tertile. Participant's education was classified as having a high-school degree or less, an undergraduate degree, or a graduate degree or higher. To account for income and health disparities between different regions in Mexico we categorized individuals based on their State of residence (Baja California, Chiapas, Durango, Guanajuato, Hidalgo, Jalisco, Mexico City, Mexico State, Nuevo Leon, Sonora, Yucatan and Veracruz). Physical activity was defined as self-reported minutes per week spent on moderate and vigorous recreational physical activity calculated from responses to eight categories that ranged from none to more than 10 h per week. Menopausal status was based on self-reported information related to last menstruation, hot flushes, hysterectomy, oophorectomy, and hormonal treatments; if these data were unknown then an algorithm using current age was used to determine status where possible. Smoking status was classified into never, past or current smokers. Diabetes and hypercholesterolemia were defined by self-reported treated disease. Body mass index (BMI) was calculated as self-reported weight in kg over height in meters squared.

Statistical analyses

Continuous variables were summarized as means ±SD and categorical variables as percentages. Our main exposures were the three major dietary patterns derived from PCA. We categorized individuals into quartiles of each dietary pattern using the lowest category as the referent. We estimated age-adjusted and multivariable-adjusted odds ratios (OR) and 95% confidence intervals (CI) using logistic regression models (SAS 9.4, SAS Institute Inc., Cary, NC). The median value for each quartile was used as a continuous variable to test for linear trend. A complete-case analysis was conducted.

In multivariable models we adjusted for age (continuous), socioeconomic status (tertiles), education (high-school or less, undergraduate, graduate or more), state of residence (12 States), menopausal status (premenopausal, postmenopausal, unknown), smoking (never, past, current, and unknown), recreational physical activity (minutes/week), diabetes, hypercholesterolemia, and energy intake (quartiles). In an exploratory model we also adjusted for BMI (kg/m^2) as a potential mediator to conduct an exploratory mediation analysis.

In sensitivity analyses we conducted the analyses among non-diabetics because diabetics could have altered their diet after diagnosis but they are still at a higher risk of hypertension. We also repeated analyses among never-smokers because smoking is a strong risk factor for hypertension and could mask the association between diet and hypertension. To take into account that deriving dietary patterns through PCA has arbitrary decisions which may affect the reproducibility of the findings, we repeated the analyses 1) rotating the patterns using an oblique factor rotation (*promax* rotation), 2) retaining different number of factors (n = 2), 3) using all individual food items (n = 140) instead of collapsing

Table 1 Thirty-seven food groups derived from the 140-item food frequency questionnaire of the Mexican Teachers' Cohort[a]

Food group	Description
Carrots	Carrots
Tomato	Red tomato cooked and raw
Green vegetables	Lettuce, dark leafy greens, broccoli or cauliflower, cabbage
Starchy vegetables	Potatoes and corn
Other vegetables	Onions, tomatillo, cucumber, squash/chayote, avocado, nopal, jicama, green beans, beets, pumpkin flowers
Hot peppers	Hot peppers sauce, hot peppers canned, dried hot peppers
Fruits	Lime, orange/mandarin, apple, papaya, banana, mango, guava, pear, pineapple, melon, watermelon, apricot, grapes, prickly pear, strawberries, grapefruit, raisins, plum, mamey, sapodilla
Legumes	Beans, Green peas, lentils, broad beans
Nuts	Peanuts, walnuts, almonds - unprocessed
Milk and yogurt	Whole, skim and semi milk, soy milk, yogurt or bulgurs
Cheese	Fresh cheese, Oaxaca, Cream cheese, Other types of cheese, Manchego/Chihuahua cheese
Egg	Egg
Seafood	Canned tuna, white fish, shrimp, fatty fish, other seafood, canned sardines, and dry fish
Poultry	Chicken
Red meat	Beef, pork, barbacoa, carnitas, dry beef, birria
Organs	Liver, pancita or menudo
Pozole	Pozole
Corn tortilla	Corn tortilla
Pasta and rice	Rice and pasta
Refined grains	French style baguette, ready to eat cereals, white loaf of bread, wheat flour tortilla, saltine crackers
Whole grain	Whole loaf of bread, high fiber ready to eat cereals
Atole	Atole with and without milk
Breakfast and cereal bars	Oats, granola bars
Candies and jams	Candy, jams, chocolate
Pastries	Sweet bread, cookies, donuts, cakes
Milk desserts	Jello or flan, fermented milk drink, Ice cream, petit suisse,
Fast foods	Pizza, hotdog, hamburguers
Meat by products	Turkey ham, pork ham, sausage, chorizo/longaniza, pork skins, bacon, other cold meats
Antojitos	Sopes/quesadillas, tacos, tamales, tortas
Butter, margarine and cream	Cream, butter, margarine
Snacks	Fried snacks, processed snack nuts
Coffee and tea	Regular or decaf coffee and tea
Soda	Regular soda
SSBs	Fruit waters, hibiscus water
Juice	Orange juice
Alcohol	Beer, tequila, brandy, whisky, rum, pulque, mezcal, aguardiente
Wine	Wine

[a]Foods within food groups appear in increasing frequency of consumption

into food groups, 4) running the analysis using the maximum likelihood method as an alternate method to PCA, and 5) dividing the whole cohort randomly into two groups to show whether the major dietary patterns were similar for the two groups and closely resembled those for the overall sample. The two component solution was used as an alternative exposure in sensitivity analyses. To assess whether our findings were sensible to the hypertension definition, we also used an alternative definition of hypertension as those participants who responded having had a diagnosis of hypertension regardless of medication use (n = 3650 incident cases).

Results

The mean age of participants was 42.1 ± 7.3 years. We identified 2916 incident cases of hypertension and three dietary patterns. The cumulative incidence of hypertension was 4.6% over 1.7 ± 1.1 years. Factor-loading matrixes for these patterns are shown in Fig. 1, positive loadings indicate a positive association with the component, while negative loadings indicate an inverse association with it. The first component was loaded positively with other vegetables, green vegetables, tomatoes, carrots and fruits, while pastries loaded negatively; the second component was loaded positively with processed meats, fast foods, and red meat, and negatively with fruit and corn tortilla; and finally the third component was loaded positively with corn tortillas, hot peppers and sodas, and negatively on whole grains, dairy and fruits. The first component explained 8.6% of the total variance, while the second and third component explained 5.9% and 5.1% of the total variance, respectively. We named the component as Fruits & Vegetables, Western,

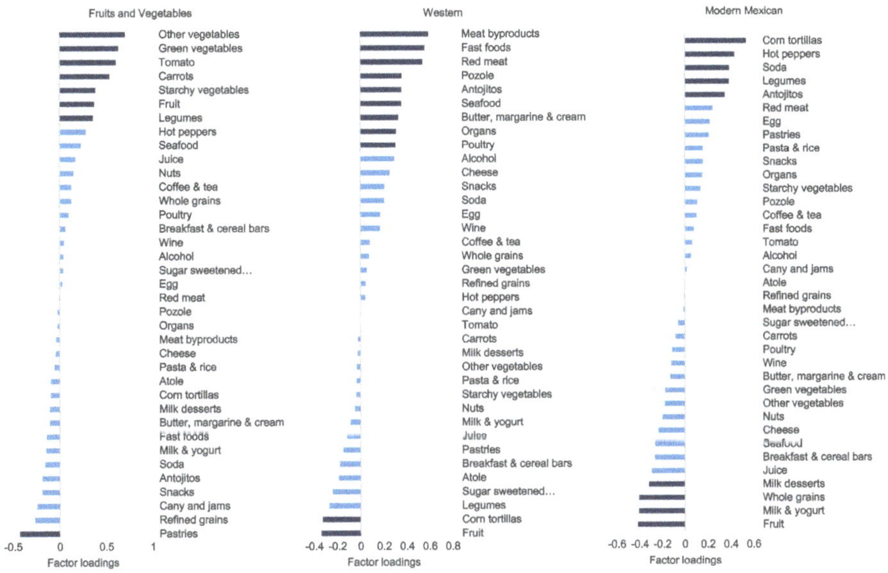

Fig. 1 Factor loadings of dietary patterns derived from the Mexican Teachers' Cohort. Rotated factor loadings of the three dietary patterns derived in 88,082 Mexican women who responded the 2008 food frequency questionnaire from the Mexican Teachers' Cohort. The first dietary pattern was named Fruits and Vegetables, the second Western, and the third Modern Mexican. The variability explained by each factor was 8.6%, 5.9% and 5.1%

and Modern Mexican. PCA performed on the FFQs responded during the feasibility phase in 2006 resulted in similar dietary patterns.

Age-adjusted baseline characteristics of participants according to quartiles of each dietary pattern are shown in Table 2. Women in the highest quartile of the Fruits & Vegetables pattern were more likely to come from Northern Mexico and less from Mexico City, were more likely to have a graduate education, diabetes and hypercholesterolemia, and reported a higher physical activity than women in the lowest quartile. In the Western pattern, women with the highest category were less likely to be indigenous, more likely to be from Northern Mexico and less from the south and have a higher socioeconomic status and graduate education, they were also more likely to be current smokers and have a lower energy intake. In contrast, women in the highest quartile of the Modern Mexican pattern were more likely to be indigenous, live in Northern and Southern Mexico, and be current smokers, however they were less likely to live in Mexico City, they had a lower socioeconomic status, and reported lower physical activity and energy intake.

Age-adjusted results showed a statistically significant direct association between the Western dietary pattern and the odds of hypertension (Table 3). After adjustment for confounders the association between the Western pattern and the odds of hypertension remained significant. Women in the highest quartile of Western dietary pattern had 24% higher odds of hypertension (95% CI: 1.10, 1.40; *P*-trend 0.0004) relative to those in the lowest quartile. We also adjusted for BMI, a potential mediator of the association between the Western pattern and hypertension. As expected, the association was attenuated but remained significant (OR: 1.17, 95% CI: 1.03, 1.32; *P*-trend 0.03). Adherence to the Modern Mexican pattern was directly associated with the odds of hypertension. Women in the highest quartile of the Modern Mexican pattern had 15% higher odds (95% CI: 1.02, 1.29; *P*-trend 0.01) of hypertension compared to the lowest quartile. After adjusting for BMI the association became null. The Fruits & Vegetables pattern was not significantly associated with hypertension. However, there was an indication of a protective effect when the pattern score was modeled as a continuous variable (OR: 0.96; 95% CI: 0.92, 1.00).

To explore the consistency of the empirical dietary patterns we randomly divided the cohort into two groups and the dietary patterns derived in both groups resembled the three dietary patterns from the whole cohort. When we used an oblique rotation method and ran a maximum likelihood method it resulted in similar dietary patterns and similar associations with hypertension (data not shown). When we retained two components we obtained a similar Fruits & Vegetables pattern and Western pattern, also with similar associations with hypertension. However, using all individual food items on the food frequency questionnaire resulted in slightly different dietary patterns. The first component was similar (heavily loaded with fruits but also with nuts), the second component was different (loading heavily on

Table 2 Age-adjusted characteristics of 62,913 Mexican women from the MTC at baseline by dietary pattern quartiles[a-d]

	Fruits & Vegetables Dietary Pattern		Western Dietary Pattern		Modern Mexican Dietary Pattern	
	Q1	Q4	Q1	Q4	Q1	Q4
Age at questionnaire[b], years	41.1 ± 7.3	43.2 ± 7.1	42.7 ± 7.3	41.3 ± 7.4	42.9 ± 7.5	41.5 ± 7.1
Indigenous[c], %	7	7	15	5	5	11
Regions in Mexico						
- Northern Mexico, %	17	23	12	31	15	26
- Central Mexico, %	16	18	17	13	18	14
- Mexico City and State of Mexico, %	30	22	21	25	33	17
- Southern Mexico, %	37	37	50	31	34	42
Graduate education, %	13	17	11	17	15	13
Highest socioeconomic status tertile, %	41	47	28	56	47	40
Menopausal status						
- Premenopausal, %	77	76	75	78	76	77
- Postmenopausal, %	14	14	15	13	14	14
- Missing, %	9	10	10	9	10	9
Body mass index, kg/m^2	27.3 ± 4.6	26.9 ± 4.2	26.7 ± 4.2	27.2 ± 4.6	26.3 ± 4.0	27.7 ± 4.7
Current smokers, %	10	9	4	15	7	12
Diabetes mellitus, %	2	4	3	3	2	4
Hypercholesterolemia, %	9	12	11	10	11	10
Recreational physical activity, min/week	30(0,180)	90(0,270)	60(0,210)	60(0,210)	120(30,330)	30(0,150)
Total energy, kcal/day	1796(1405,2276)	1712(1335,2180)	1825(1409,2322)	1556(1210,1978)	1928(1510,2430)	1550(1216,1961)

[a]Values are mean ± SD for continuous variables and percent for categorical variables. Physical activity and total energy intake are expressed as median (IQR). Values are age standardized to the age distribution of the study population. Values of polytomous variables may not sum to 100% due to rounding. N = 15,728 per quartile in all patterns (except Q3: 15,729)
[b]Variable is not age adjusted
[c]Participants who reported speaking an indigenous language or having a parent who did were defined as indigenous
[d]Abbreviations: MTC: Mexican Teachers' Cohort; Q1-Q4: quartile1-quartile4

vegetables), and the third component was similar to the Western pattern (loading heavily on processed meats and fast foods). The variance explained by these three components was 6.8%, 3.9%, and 3.3%, respectively. The third component was directly associated with hypertension while the first two were not (data not shown).

In sensitivity analyses we ran the multivariable adjusted model only in non-diabetics and non-smokers to reduce confounding (Additional file 1: Table S1). We also ran the multivariable adjusted model using the dietary patterns derived from the two component solution as the exposure. Among non-diabetics and using the two factor solution as the exposure results remained the same as in the main analyses. Among non-smokers results were slightly strengthened in the Fruits & Vegetables pattern as a protector factor and the Western pattern as high risk factor but were attenuated in the Modern Mexican pattern and results were no longer significant. When we used the less strict definition of hypertension, the associations with dietary patterns were stronger, in the same direction, and significant with all dietary patterns without changes in our main conclusions. Fruits & Vegetables pattern OR comparing extreme quartiles: 0.87 (95%CI: 0.79,0.96), P-trend: 0.002; Western pattern OR comparing extreme quartiles: 1.20 (95%CI: 1.08,1.34), P-trend: 0.0009; Modern Mexican pattern OR comparing extreme quartiles: 1.19 (95%CI: 1.07,1.32), P-trend: 0.001. Moreover, after further adjustment by BMI, as in the main analysis, the association with the Modern Mexican dietary pattern lost significance.

Discussion

In this prospective study, the Western and Modern Mexican dietary patterns were directly associated with the incidence of hypertension in Mexican women. However, we did not observe an inverse association with the Fruits & Vegetables pattern (Prudent pattern) after adjusting for risk factors for hypertension.

The dietary patterns (Fruits & Vegetables and Western) we derived from PCA are consistent with Prudent and Western dietary patterns found in other studies [22–24] and in a previous MTC study [25]. However, besides these two globally similar patterns we also derived

Table 3 Multivariate adjusted OR of incident hypertension by dietary pattern quartiles in women from the MTC[a-e]

Model	Q1	Q2	Q3	Q4	*P*-trend	Continuous[a]
Fruits & Vegetables						
Cases	713	737	736	730		
Non-cases	15,015	14,991	14,993	14,998		
Age-adjusted [b]	1	1.00(0.90,1.11)	0.96(0.87,1.07)	0.91(0.82,1.01)	0.06	0.96(0.92,0.99)
Multivariable [c]	1	1.03(0.92,1.14)	0.97(0.87,1.09)	0.94(0.84,1.05)	0.19	0.96(0.92,1.00)
Multivariable+BMI[d]	1	1.07(0.96,1.20)	0.99(0.88,1.11)	1.00(0.89,1.13)	0.71	0.98(0.94,1.02)
Western						
Cases	679	729	736	772		
Non-cases	15,049	14,999	14,993	14,956		
Age-adjusted [b]	1	1.10(0.99,1.22)	1.14(1.02,1.26)	1.23(1.11,1.37)	<0.0001	1.08(1.04,1.12)
Multivariable [c]	1	1.10(0.98,1.23)	1.12(1.00,1.26)	1.24(1.10,1.40)	0.0004	1.09(1.04,1.13)
Multivariable+BMI[d]	1	1.10(0.98,1.23)	1.06(0.94,1.20)	1.17(1.03,1.32)	0.03	1.06(1.01,1.11)
Modern Mexican						
Cases	705	752	750	709		
Non-cases	15,023	14,976	14,979	15,019		
Age-adjusted [b]	1	1.12(1.01,1.24)	1.15(1.03,1.27)	1.10(0.99,1.22)	0.08	1.03(0.99,1.07)
Multivariable [c]	1	1.11(1.00,1.24)	1.18(1.06,1.32)	1.15(1.02,1.29)	0.01	1.05(1.00,1.09)
Multivariable+BMI[d]	1	1.03(0.92,1.15)	1.08(0.97,1.22)	0.99(0.88,1.12)	0.95	0.99(0.95,1.03)

[a]Multivariate adjusted odds (95% CI) of incident hypertension by dietary patterns (continuous)
[b]Model 1: adjusted for age (continuous)
[c]Model 2: adjusted as in model 1 plus socioeconomic status (tertiles), education (high school, college, graduate), State (12 states of Mexico), menopausal status (premenopausal, postmenopausal, unknown), diabetes, hypercholesterolemia (yes/no), smoking (never, past, current, and missing), recreational physical activity (minutes/week), and energy intake (quartiles)
[d]Model 3: adjusted as in model 2 plus body mass index (kg/m^2)
[e]Abbreviations. MTC: Mexican Teachers' Cohort; Q1-Q4: quartile1-quartile4

a third pattern which exemplifies the nutritional transition in Mexicans, who have low adherence to dietary recommendations [26]. Adherence to this pattern is characterized by eating traditional foods (i.e. corn tortillas and hot peppers) together with unhealthy foods (i.e. sodas) and low intake of fruits. The variance explained by the three dietary patterns (8.6%, 5.9% and 5.1%) is slightly lower than other dietary patterns derived by PCA in other studies [21, 22, 24]. However, when summing the variance explained by the three of them (19.6%), the total variance explained is within the range from other studies (17.4%–24%) [21, 22, 24].

It is difficult to compare empirically derived and a priori dietary patterns. Some of the advantages of using empirically derived dietary patterns are that they are data driven and allow for the examination of eating behaviors. Previous studies have shown inverse and direct associations between Prudent and Western patterns and cardiovascular risk, respectively [15, 21, 23]. Other studies have focused on the association between diet and blood pressure [12–14]. However, few have studied the relation between diet and incident hypertension and findings have been controversial [27–29]. While Schulze et al. did not find an association between exploratory dietary patterns and incident hypertension they did find an inverse association with the DASH diet (quartile 3 vs. 1) [27]. Li et al. found strong inverse associations between three commonly used index scores (Dietary Approaches to Stop Hypertension, alternative Mediterranean diet, alternative Healthy Eating Index) and hypertension but Toledo et al. found no association with fifteen hypothesis-oriented dietary patterns [28, 29]. However, all of them adjusted for BMI which we hypothesize is a mediator in the association between diet and hypertension. Adjusting for a mediator, in this case BMI, would cause collider bias [30] so the direct association between the dietary patterns and hypertension would not be valid.

Nutrients in fruits and vegetables hypothesized to lower blood pressure include fiber, potassium, magnesium, folate, vitamin C and flavonoids; however, other nutrient(s) or interactions among nutrients may be responsible for decreasing hypertension risk [31–35]. In our study we found no association between the Fruits & Vegetables pattern and hypertension; although we did find a suggestion of a protective effect only when the pattern score was modeled as a continuous variable. This was perhaps due to the fact that the beneficial effect of fruits and vegetables could have been obscured by grouping different types of fruits and vegetables, some of which may not have a beneficial effect on blood pressure [7, 8, 35]. Moreover, methods of cooking or added fats and seasonings could be counterbalancing the beneficial effects of vegetables. Additionally, the overall effect of fruits and vegetables on hypertension could be relatively small after considering other risk factors. The possibility of misclassification of the outcome and a short follow-up time may have also underestimated the association. Meat, processed meats, sweets and pastries have been associated with increased blood pressure [5, 35] perhaps due to their higher content of saturated fat, sodium, and sugar than fruits and vegetables [36–38]. Consistent with this literature, we found a direct association between both the Western pattern and the Modern Mexican pattern and incident hypertension. These findings are relevant because these patterns show frequently consumed foods (e.g. meat, processed meats, sweets and pastries) that can be targeted by public policy and decrease their intake.

Strengths and limitations

Our study has several strengths, it is a prospective population-based study, with a large sample size, and multiple risk factors for hypertension were available to adjust for confounding, including smoking and other lifestyle factors. However, confounding by unmeasured or poorly measured factors cannot be ruled out. Self-reported diagnosis of hypertension has been used in other cohort studies and has been shown to be a valid indicator in Hispanics [39, 40]. The positive predictive value of self-report of treated hypertension was moderately high, thus measurement error is likely. This measurement error is probably non-differential since the exposure was ascertained before the outcome occurred. This error may have resulted in an underestimation of the association between dietary patterns and hypertension. A short follow-up time may have decreased the power to detect an association between the dietary patterns and hypertension, especially in the association with the Fruits & Vegetables pattern whose effect size may be smaller. However, this study has 80% power to detect an OR of 1.17 between Q4 and Q1 of each food pattern. The large sample size and population-based population were crucial in finding distinct dietary patterns which would be otherwise missed. However, dietary patterns derived by PCA depend on some arbitrary decisions that may affect the reproducibility of our findings such as the consolidation of food items into food groups, the number of components to retain, the rotation method, and the labeling of the components. We conducted sensitivity analyses to examine whether these decisions affected the consistency of our results by choosing alternatives and found similar dietary patterns and associations. We also split the sample into two groups and conducted the PCA in these random samples and found similar results. Using all food items changed the patterns derived. We hypothesize that when we used all food items in the PCA, results were different because we have many single vegetables ($n = 20$) and fruits ($n = 20$).

Since we did not have the certainty of the time of hypertension diagnosis we could not conduct a survival analysis, thus we had to exclude all participants which were lost to follow-up on the 2011 questionnaire and had to model the association with logistic regression as an alternative. Seventeen percent of the study population did not answer the 2011 follow-up questionnaire, which could cause selection bias. However, comparing response vs no response in the 2011 questionnaire (Additional file 1: Table S2) there were no major differences between these two groups, including the distribution of the dietary patterns scores. Since this study is restricted to Hispanic women, generalizability to other populations could be affected.

Conclusions

In conclusion, we found evidence of a relation between the Western and Modern Mexican dietary patterns and hypertension in a population of Mexican women. These results are consistent with prior reports showing an association between a Western diet and coronary heart disease. However, our study also shows that a higher adherence to a nutritional transition diet, the Modern Mexican pattern, is also associated with hypertension. In contrast to previous findings, the Fruits & Vegetables pattern was not significantly associated with hypertension, probably due to misclassification of the outcome. Also, underestimation of the associations may have resulted from a short follow-up time. Our results should be confirmed in other Mexican based studies and evaluate longer term adherence to these dietary patterns. These finding have important public health implications, as improved dietary habits are crucial in the prevention of hypertension and other cardiovascular diseases among Mexicans living in Mexico, and possibly also Mexicans living in the USA.

Acknowledgements

We would like to thank Victor Sastré, Director of Promoción de la Función por Incentivos de la SEP, and the State Coordinators for their support in contacting the MTC's participants and assisting with logistics operations during the questionnaire distribution. We are also grateful to the Mexican Teachers' Cohort participants, the American Institute for Cancer Research, and Consejo Nacional de Ciencia y Tecnología (CONACyT).

Funding

This work is supported by the American Institute for Cancer Research Grant 05B047 and Consejo Nacional de Ciencia y Tecnología (CONACyT) grant S0008–2009-1: 000000000115312.

Authors' contributions

Authors' contributions to manuscript: ML, RLR designed research; JJG provided statistical guidance; AM analyzed data; AM, ML wrote first draft; RLR, BLR and EOP revised manuscript; AM had primary responsibility for final content. All authors read and approved the final manuscript.

Consent for publication

Not applicable

Competing interests

The authors declare that they have no competing interests.

Author details

[1]Center for Research on Population Health, National Institute of Public Health, Cuernavaca, Mexico. [2]Escuela de Medicina, Tecnológico de Monterrey, Monterrey, Mexico. [3]University of Hawaii at Manoa, Honolulu, HI, USA. [4]Department of Global Health and Population, Harvard T.H. Chan School of Public Health, Boston, USA.

References

1. Campos-Nonato I, Hernández-Barrera L, Rojas-Martínez R, Pedroza A, Medina-García C, Barquera-Cervera S. Hipertensión arterial: prevalencia, diagnóstico oportuno, control y tendencias en adultos mexicanos. Salud Publica Mex. 2013;55:S144–50.
2. Winkelmayer WC, Stampfer MJ, Willett WC, Curhan GC. Habitual caffeine intake and the risk of hypertension in women. JAMA. 2005;294:2330–5.
3. Rhee JJ, Qin F, Hedlin HK, Chang TI, Bird CE, Zaslavsky O, Manson JE, Stefanick ML, Winkelmayer WC. Coffee and caffeine consumption and the risk of hypertension in postmenopausal women. Am J Clin Nutr. 2016;103: 210–7.
4. Hartley TR, Sung BH, Pincomb GA, Whitsett TL, Wilson MF, Lovallo WR. Hypertension risk status and effect of caffeine on blood pressure. Hypertension. 2000;36:137–41.
5. Steffen LM, Kroenke CH, Yu X, Pereira MA, Slattery ML, Van Horn L, Gross MD, Jacobs DR. Associations of plant food, dairy product, and meat intakes with 15-y incidence of elevated blood pressure in young black and white adults: the coronary artery risk development in young adults (CARDIA) study. Am J Clin Nutr. 2005;82:1169–77.
6. Wang H, Fox CS, Troy LM, McKeown NM, Jacques PF. Longitudinal association of dairy consumption with the changes in blood pressure and the risk of incident hypertension: the Framingham heart study. Br J Nutr. 2015;114:1887–99.
7. Borgi L, Muraki I, Satija A, Willett WC, Rimm EB, Forman JP. Fruit and vegetable consumption and the incidence of hypertension in three prospective cohort studies. Hypertension. 2016;67:288–93.
8. Wang L, Manson JE, Gaziano JM, Buring JE, Sesso HD. Fruit and vegetable intake and the risk of hypertension in middle-aged and older women. Am J Hypertens. 2012;25:180–9.
9. Jacques PF, Tucker KL. Are dietary patterns useful for understanding the role of diet in chronic disease? Am J Clin Nutr. 2001;73:1–2.
10. Hu FB. Dietary pattern analysis: a new direction in nutritional epidemiology. Curr Opin Lipidol. 2002;13:3–9.
11. Slattery ML, Boucher KM, Caan BJ, Potter JD, Ma K-N. Eating patterns and risk of colon cancer. Am J Epidemiol. 1998;148:4–16.
12. Appel LJ, Brands MW, Daniels SR, Karanja N, Elmer PJ, Sacks FM. Dietary approaches to prevent and treat hypertension: a scientific statement from the American Heart Association. Hypertension. 2006;47:296–308.
13. Nissensohn M, Roman-Vinas B, Sanchez-Villegas A, Piscopo S, Serra-Majem L. The effect of the Mediterranean diet on hypertension: a systematic review and meta-analysis. J Nutr Educ Behav. 2016;48:42–53 e41.
14. Gay HC, Rao SG, Vaccarino V, Ali MK. Effects of different dietary interventions on blood pressure: systematic review and meta-analysis of randomized controlled trials. Hypertension. 2016;67:733–9.
15. Harmon BE, Boushey CJ, Shvetsov YB, Ettienne R, Reedy J, Wilkens LR, Le Marchand L, Henderson BE, Kolonel LN. Associations of key diet-quality indexes with mortality in the multiethnic cohort: the dietary patterns methods project. Am J Clin Nutr. 2015;101:587–97.
16. Lajous M, Ortiz-Panozo E, Monge A, Santoyo-Vistrain R, Garcia-Anaya A, Yunes-Diaz E, Rice MS, Blanco M, Hernandez-Avila M, Willett WC, et al. Cohort profile: the Mexican teachers' cohort (MTC). Int J Epidemiol. 2017;46:e10.
17. Hernandez-Avila M, Romieu I, Parra S, Hernandez-Avila J, Madrigal H, Willett W. Validity and reproducibility of a food frequency questionnaire to assess dietary intake of women living in Mexico City. Salud Publica Mex. 1998;40: 133–40.
18. Gebhardt S, Lemar L, Pehrsson P, Exler J, Haytowitz D, Patterson K: USDA National Nutrient Database for standard reference, release 22. USDA National Nutrient Database for standard reference 2009.
19. Schulze MB, Hoffmann K, Kroke A, Boeing H. An approach to construct simplified measures of dietary patterns from exploratory factor analysis. Br J Nutr. 2003;89:409–19.
20. Kim J-O, Mueller CW. Introduction to factor analysis: what it is and how to do it. Newbury Park: Sage; 1978.
21. Hu FB, Rimm EB, Stampfer MJ, Ascherio A, Spiegelman D, Willett WC. Prospective study of major dietary patterns and risk of coronary heart disease in men. Am J Clin Nutr. 2000;72:912–21.
22. Hu FB, Rimm E, Smith-Warner SA, Feskanich D, Stampfer MJ, Ascherio A, Sampson L, Willett WC. Reproducibility and validity of dietary patterns assessed with a food-frequency questionnaire. Am J Clin Nutr. 1999;69:243–9.
23. Fung TT, Rimm EB, Spiegelman D, Rifai N, Tofler GH, Willett WC, Hu FB. Association between dietary patterns and plasma biomarkers of obesity and cardiovascular disease risk. Am J Clin Nutr. 2001;73:61–7.
24. Khani BR, Ye W, Terry P, Wolk A. Reproducibility and validity of major dietary patterns among Swedish women assessed with a food-frequency questionnaire. J Nutr. 2004;134:1541–5.
25. Romieu I, Escamilla-Nunez MC, Sanchez-Zamorano LM, Lopez-Ridaura R, Torres-Mejia G, Yunes EM, Lajous M, Rivera-Dommarco JA, Lazcano-Ponce E. The association between body shape silhouette and dietary pattern among Mexican women. Public Health Nutr. 2012;15:116–25.
26. Batis C, Aburto TC, Sánchez-Pimienta TG, Pedraza LS, Rivera JA. Adherence to dietary recommendations for food group intakes is low in the Mexican population. J Nutr. 2016;146:1897S–906S.
27. Schulze MB, Hoffmann K, Kroke A, Boeing H. Risk of hypertension among women in the EPIC-Potsdam study: comparison of relative risk estimates for exploratory and hypothesis-oriented dietary patterns. Am J Epidemiol. 2003; 158:365–73.
28. Li S, Zhu Y, Chavarro JE, Bao W, Tobias DK, Ley SH, Forman JP, Liu A, Mills J, Bowers K, et al. Healthful dietary patterns and the risk of hypertension among women with a history of gestational diabetes mellitus: a prospective cohort study. Hypertension. 2016;67:1157–65.
29. Toledo E, FdA C-T, Alonso A, Puchau B, Zulet MA, Martinez JA, Martinez-Gonzalez MA. Hypothesis-oriented food patterns and incidence of hypertension: 6-year follow-up of the SUN (Seguimiento Universidad de Navarra) prospective cohort. Public Health Nutr. 2010;13:338–49.
30. Cole SR, Platt RW, Schisterman EF, Chu H, Westreich D, Richardson D, Poole C. Illustrating bias due to conditioning on a collider. Int J Epidemiol. 2010; 39:417–20.
31. Eliasson K, Ryttig KR, Hylander B, Rössner S. A dietary fibre supplement in the treatment of mild hypertension. A randomized, double-blind, placebo-controlled trial. J Hypertens. 1992;10:195–9.
32. Whelton PK, Klag MJ. Magnesium and blood pressure: review of the epidemiologic and clinical trial experience. Am J Cardiol. 1989;63:26G–30G.
33. Cassidy A, O'Reilly EJ, Kay C, Sampson L, Franz M, Forman JP, Curhan G, Rimm EB. Habitual intake of flavonoid subclasses and incident hypertension in adults. Am J Clin Nutr. 2011;93:338–47.
34. Macready AL, George TW, Chong MF, Alimbetov DS, Jin Y, Vidal A, Spencer JP, Kennedy OB, Tuohy KM, Minihane A-M, et al. Flavonoid-rich fruit and vegetables improve microvascular reactivity and inflammatory status in men at risk of cardiovascular disease—FLAVURS: a randomized controlled trial. Am J Clin Nutr. 2014;99:479–89.

35. Ascherio A, Hennekens C, Willett WC, Sacks F, Rosner B, Manson J, Witteman J, Stampfer MJ. Prospective study of nutritional factors, blood pressure, and hypertension among US women. Hypertension. 1996;27:1065–72.
36. Wang L, Manson JE, Forman JP, Gaziano JM, Buring JE, Sesso HD. Dietary fatty acids and the risk of hypertension in middle-aged and older women. Hypertension. 2010;56:598–604.
37. Medicine Io. Sodium intake in populations: assessment of evidence. Washington, DC: The National Academies Press; 2013.
38. Brown IJ, Stamler J, Van Horn L, Robertson CE, Chan Q, Dyer AR, Huang C-C, Rodriguez BL, Zhao L, Daviglus ML, et al. Sugar-sweetened beverage, sugar intake of individuals, and their blood pressure: international study of macro/micronutrients and blood pressure. Hypertension. 2011;57:695–701.
39. Vargas CM, Burt VL, Gillum RF, Pamuk ER. Validity of self-reported hypertension in the National Health and nutrition examination survey III, 1988–1991. Prev Med. 1997;26:678–85.
40. de Menezes TN, Oliveira ECT, de Sousa Fischer MAT. Validity and concordance between self-reported and clinical diagnosis of hypertension among elderly residents in northeastern Brazil. Am J Hypertens. 2014;27: 215–21.

4

Utility of eButton images for identifying food preparation behaviors and meal-related tasks in adolescents

Margaret Raber[1]*, Monika Patterson[2], Wenyan Jia[3], Mingui Sun[3] and Tom Baranowski[2]

Abstract

Background: Food preparation skills may encourage healthy eating. Traditional assessment of child food preparation employs self- or parent proxy-reporting methods, which are prone to error. The eButton is a wearable all-day camera that has promise as an objective, passive method for measuring child food preparation practices.

Purpose: This paper explores the feasibility of the eButton to reliably capture home food preparation behaviors and practices in a sample of pre- and early adolescents (ages 9 to 13).

Methods: This is a secondary analysis of two eButton pilot projects evaluating the dietary intake of pre- and early adolescents in or around Houston, Texas. Food preparation behaviors were coded into seven major categories including: browsing, altering food/adding seasoning, food media, meal related tasks, prep work, cooking and observing. Inter-coder reliability was measured using Cohen's kappa and percent agreement.

Results: Analysis was completed on data for 31 participants. The most common activity was browsing in the pantry or fridge. Few participants demonstrated any food preparation work beyond unwrapping of food packages and combining two or more ingredients; actual cutting or measuring of foods were rare.

Conclusions: Although previous research suggests children who "help" prepare meals may obtain some dietary benefit, accurate assessment tools of food preparation behavior are lacking. The eButton offers a feasible approach to food preparation behavior measurement among pre- and early adolescents. Follow up research exploring the validity of this method in a larger sample, and comparisons between cooking behavior and dietary intake are needed.

Keywords: Food preparation, Nutritional assessment, All-day imaging, Cooking, Adolescents

Background

Diet is a modifiable risk factor for several chronic diseases including heart disease, obesity and cancer [1–3]. Child and adolescent-targeted prevention efforts are vital to establishing healthy dietary habits early in life [4, 5]. Understanding child eating habits is critical for the design and evaluation of nutrition education programs, however, measurement of dietary intake and related factors has proven challenging [6]. Traditionally, self- or parent proxy-reported methods have been used to measure child and adolescent dietary intakes [7], food preparation skills and practices [8], knowledge [9] and preferences [8, 9]. These assessment tools, while widely used, have demonstrated modest validity when compared to observation and biomarker verification [10–12]. Novel technologies such as all day cameras and other wearable devices have been utilized to develop more sensitive lifestyle assessment tools for children [13–15]. All day cameras show promise as a passive mechanism for measuring child diet [15] and may also provide valuable information regarding food preparation practices.

Home cooked meals are generally lower in saturated fat, sugar and calories and higher in fruit and vegetables compared to foods eaten out of the home [16–18]. Increased frequency of home cooked meals has been associated with better healthy eating index (HEI-2010)

* Correspondence: mpraber@mdanderson.org
[1]Department of Pediatrics Research, University of Texas MD Anderson Cancer Center, Houston, USA

scores [19] and lower meal costs [19], making food preparation skill development an attractive target for healthy diet promotion.

Frequent family meals may promote healthier diets, emotional well-being and lower weight status of children [20–22]. The benefits of family meals and home cooking may be amplified by the inclusion of children in food preparation. For example, adolescent involvement in meal preparation has been associated with increased fruit, vegetable, iron, calcium, vitamins D and C, and folate intake, however these trends were not detected when parents prepared meals without their child's assistance [23]. Similarly promising effects have been observed in younger children [24–26].

Programs to promote food preparation skills among youth have gained popularity worldwide [27–30]. Youth cooking programs, however, are extremely variable in curriculum content and evaluation approach [8]. Attempts to measure cooking skills tend to assess simple cooking frequency [31] or cooking of specific items (e.g. ability to bake a cake) [32]. Youth participation in food preparation is typically gauged through self- or parent-reported items that focus on frequency of assistance [23, 33]. More objective measures may illuminate the details of how youth engage in food preparation, which is currently absent in extant self-report tools. This deeper understanding of youth cooking behavior may in turn support practical nutrition intervention development and evaluation.

The eButton is a wearable electronic device for passive assessment (i.e. requires no volitional effort to initiate assessment once the device has been successfully turned on) of diet, physical activity and lifestyle behaviors for both adults and children. It uses a small camera located on the chest to take images at four-second intervals throughout the day [34]. Analysis of these images has been used to objectively assess children's dietary intake [15]. The collection of passive, observational images of child food preparation activities offers promise as a more precise measure of child cooking behaviors. This paper explores the ability of eButton image analysis to capture home food preparation behaviors/practices in a sample of pre- and early adolescents. A secondary aim was to describe the meal and food preparation habits observed in the sample.

Methods

This study employed observational methods and is presented as per STROBE (a checklist to Strengthen the Reporting of Observational Studies in Epidemiology) research guidelines [35].

Participants

Data from two eButton pilot projects evaluating dietary intake of pre- and early adolescents who lived in or around Houston, Texas were re-analyzed for food preparation and meal-related tasks. The recruitment strategies were comparable between the two studies. Child-parent dyads were recruited by phone from an institutional volunteer participant database, flyers posted across the Texas Medical Center campus, and online announcements promoting the study. Inclusion criteria for the first study included: children aged 8–13, who spoke and read English and were willing to complete all measures. Further, parents needed to give permission for children to wear the eButton, be willing to answer questions about the eButton and have sufficient Internet access at home to download resulting data [15]. Inclusion criteria were similar for the second study, except that only children aged 9–13 were recruited. Ten participants were recruited for the first pilot study, and 31 participants recruited for the second. Although 8 year olds were eligible for the first study, none were included in this analysis.

eButton description and procedures

The eButton is a multi-sensor device that attaches around the collar, to the shirt of a participant and includes a camera, a 9-axis motion sensor (including an accelerometer, a gyroscope and a magnetometer, each providing three-dimensional measurements), a barometer, a temperature sensor, and a light sensor. It also includes data storage on a MiniSD flash card and a lithium-ion battery. The camera recorded pictures of everything in front of the wearer at four-second intervals throughout the wearing period. The images were automatically encrypted upon taking and therefore safely sent via email from participants. Upon retrieval, the images were de-encrypted and de-identified (visible faces blurred using specialized software) by study staff in preparation for analysis [14, 15, 34].

Children and parents were given a full explanation of the eButton device and detailed instructions for its use. Participants in the first study were instructed to wear the eButton for one day only as this was an early pilot study of the eButton in children. Participants in the second study were instructed to wear the device for two days. Participants were encouraged to wear the device from waking until bed-time, including at school if during a weekday. Participants were given a letter for their school principals that explained the study and eButton device. Only one day per participant was used in this analysis for consistency. Parents emailed encrypted image files to research staff at the end of each day. Participants also kept a log of any software issues they encountered while using the device [15].

Measurement tools

The eButton hardware was complemented by software for data processing, including one for dietary intake assessment and another focused on activity categorization. The activity categorization software used accelerometer data to divide the images into homogenous events, allowing researchers to view the photos in clusters of common activity [14]. This project utilized the activity categorization software to identify food preparation events. One day of images for each participant was viewed in its entirety to ensure all food preparation events were analyzed.

Food preparation behaviors identified in the images were encompassed by seven major categories (Table 1) including browsing, altering food on plate/adding seasoning, food media, tasks, prep work, observing and cooking. "Browsing" specifies moments when a participant is facing food storage, either in the fridge, freezer, pantry, on the kitchen counter, at the grocery store, at school in the lunch line or at a convenience store or café. The browsing subcategories focus on where participants were most likely to be exposed to food options. This information is pertinent to initiatives to improve healthy food choices, improve food labeling, or restrict high sugar/high calorie food in the home and at school [36–38].

"Altering food or adding seasoning" specifies the actions adolescents took to subtly alter foods once they were plated, mainly through seasoning or condiment use. This behavior could occur at home or outside the home (at restaurants or school). The addition of certain seasonings and condiments can impact the final nutrient content of foods and the use of herbs and spices has become a target for healthy cooking interventions [39].

The category "food media" specifies how children were exposed to images of foods during the day. Food media activities ranged from the child taking a photo of foods they were eating to watching a food show, visiting a food-related website or reading a cookbook. Food advertisements were not included as they were not identified in images during preliminary review. Increased knowledge of how this sample employed food media may reveal targets for interventions utilizing new technology to promote food preparation in youth [40–42].

The category "meal related tasks" specifies non-food preparation behaviors that are relevant to meal times, such as clearing dishes or getting drinks. While slightly outside of "food preparation" as a concept, these activities may be relevant to understanding the range of behaviors that can be captured through questionnaires examining how children help with meals.

"Prep work" and "Cooking" categories include actual food preparation behaviors demonstrated by the sample and range from washing vegetables to using the stove. These categories classify instances where basic culinary ability is demonstrated with regard to both cold and hot preparations. Adolescents who were classified as demonstrating any of these behaviors were deemed to have demonstrated cooking skills and food preparation habits. Reliable assessment of these behaviors enables the determination of successful transmission of skills from youth-focused cooking classes to the home food environment.

"Observing" specifies the child witnessing the food preparation behaviors of others including adults or peers. This category is important since most food skills are likely transmitted within the home [43]. Modeling positive food behaviors and involving children while cooking are considered powerful parenting tools for encouraging healthy eating [44].

Data analysis

The first author generated a basic codebook of behaviors, including definitions and examples, to capture the non-consumption food related behaviors of the participants in this project based on prior research on food preparation [45] and a preliminary review of the images. Codes were kept broad to accommodate the range of activities and limited culinary literacy demonstrated by the sample. During the preliminary review, codes were added if participants demonstrated previously uncategorized behaviors to ensure all food preparation activities demonstrated were captured. Once the codebook was developed, 20 % of the final total sample was coded by a second coder and inter coder reliability assessed using Cohen's Kappa. After the initial double coding, inconsistencies were resolved through discussion between the two coders. Final categories were clarified (broadened or made more specific) and recoding was completed and analyzed to reflect the refined behavior classifications. Parent-reported participant demographics were assessed using descriptive statistics. Contingency tables were generated for age groups (9–11) and (12–13) to explore age-related trends in food/meal behavior.

Results

Participants

Forty-one participants provided image data for at least one day across the two studies. Data from 10 participants was excluded. Exclusions were made if the resulting images could not be analyzed using the activity software developed for the eButton, i.e. missing files ($n = 2$), software malfunction ($n = 6$) or file storage issues ($n = 2$). Analysis was completed on data for 31 participants. Each day of images took approximately one to two hours to code. Demographics of participants are shown in Table 2.

One set of participants ($n = 25$) included all day camera images for two different days. The other set of participants ($n = 6$) provided only one day of images. Given the exploratory nature of this study, one day per participant was used for analysis. To address possible differences in the days selected for inclusion, day one

Table 1 Description of activity categories used during analysis

Activity category	Subcategory	Description
Browsing: Any apparent moments when the child is actively looking at or for food in various locations. Does not include just walking through kitchen without pausing.	Pantry	Standing in front of open unit containing dry stored foodstuffs. May be a shelf, walk in pantry, or extra pantry (in garage for example)
	Fridge	Standing in front of open fridge or freezer
	Grocery Store	Walking through grocery store and/or looking at items. Includes most types of food markets and specialty food shops, does not include convenience store or gas station
	Convenience Store or Café Counter	Walking through and/or looking at items in convenience store or café including: gas station, corner store, ice cream shop display, coffee shop display, other sorts of retailers with display cases of food to select. Does not include sit-down restaurants.
	Kitchen Counter	Standing in front of counter space containing food (i.e.: bowl of fruit on counter)
	At School	Walking through and/or looking at items in school lunch line
Altering Food on Plate/sAdding Seasoning: Making any alterations to food already plated in front of child such as adding salt or other seasonings, hot sauce, ketchup or other condiments. Also includes removing elements of already plated food such as taking crusts off of bread or removing candies from cereal. Does not include seasoning food while cooking.		
Food Media, Recipes, Cookbooks, Photo: Child takes photo of food using any camera device, reads or looks at cookbooks/recipes, visits food/cooking related websites/apps or appears to be watching a cooking-related tv show		
Meal Related Tasks: Activities related to meal behaviors that do not include working with food directly	Plating	Moving food from cooking or serving vessels to one's own or another's plate. Includes getting second servings. Does not include a parent or peer putting food onto plate in front of the child.
	Getting Drinks	Pouring beverage into a cup for oneself or for another. Includes getting up to get the beverage from the kitchen or pouring from a container on the table/in the eating space. Includes retrieving a squeeze pack or bottled drink. Does not include a parent or peer pouring a drink for the child.
	Clearing and/or washing dishes	Moving used dishes from table or eating space to the kitchen, either directly to the sink or dishwasher or to the counter. Also includes rinsing dishes, washing dishes, and/or moving dishes into the dishwasher as well as wiping down the sink space. Includes putting clean dishes away.
	Setting the Table	Placing napkins, plates, cutlery, serving vessels or other necessary dining accessories on a table or in eating space.
Prep Work: Includes all preparation of food for eating or cooking. Does not include heating of any food items.	Washing and/or Peeling Produce	Includes rinsing of all types of fruits and vegetables with water. Also includes peeling produce by hand (i.e. orange) or by peeler (i.e. potatoes).
	Cutting	Includes all cutting of food products with knives regardless of size or apparent sharpness. Also includes use of graters/mandolins or other sharp cutting equipment.
	Cracking Eggs	Cracking eggs by hand. Does not include any other activity.
	Combining 2+ ingredients by hand	Combining of two or more ingredients by hand in a range of settings including preparing cereal (combination of cereal and milk), making sandwiches (combination of bread and other products), mixing together a salad, and all general mixing of ingredients by hand. Includes mixing beverages such as chocolate sauce/powder with milk or hot tea with honey. Does not include placing ingredients in small appliance.

Table 1 Description of activity categories used during analysis *(Continued)*

Activity category	Subcategory	Description
	Measuring	Demonstrated use of measuring tools including measuring cups, spoons and liquid measures. Does not include rough estimates or "eyeballing".
	Unwrapping	Removing packaging from foods. Includes all snacks such as chips, granola bars, ice cream bars etc. Also includes unwrapping raw packaged meat, fruit/ vegetables, cheese and other staples before preparation.
	Using Blender/Small appliance	Placing items in kitchen stand mixer, in bowl fitted with electric mixer, blender, or food processor. Does not include using a small cooking appliance such as a counter grill or electric kettle.
Cooking: Any direct use of heat-based cooking methods.	Stove	Includes any cooking done on stove top burners including boiling water or helping adult cooking, also includes cooking on stove independently. Does not include using small cooking appliances.
	Oven (Baking)	Includes any cooking done in oven including baking of cookies/cakes etc., reheating of left-overs or frozen snacks, and any other baking/roasting/broiling.
	Microwave	Includes any use of microwave for food such as heating water/milk, making microwave popcorn, reheating pre-prepared foods, defrosting foods or cooking foods fully in microwave.
Observing: Any apparent witnessing of food / meal behaviors by adults and/or peers. Does not include adults and/or peers simply being present in kitchen/near food. Does not include observing consumption.	Food Selection by Adults	Witnessing any adults in household select foods to consume or prepare from home. Includes selection from pantry, fridge, counter and stores.
	Food Selection by Peers	Witnessing any child (not apparent adult) select foods to consume or prepare from home. Includes selection from pantry, fridge, counter, stores and school.
	Any Food Preparation by Adults	Any food preparation or cooking undertaken by adults including combining ingredients, using appliances, using heat-application methods. Also includes unwrapping of food products as well as heating of pre-prepared meals and plating of foods. Does not include consumption.
	Any Food Preparation by Peers	Any food preparation or cooking undertaken by children (not adults) including combining ingredients, using appliances, using heat-application methods. Also includes unwrapping of food as well as heating of pre-prepared meals and plating of foods. Does not include consumption.

and day two images were coded and compared for eleven participants. Frequency of overall food preparation behaviors and meal related tasks across the two days matched 81.4% of the time, although this mainly indicated that participants were similarly uninvolved in food preparation on both days. The number of demonstrated behaviors were similar, as those who did three or fewer behaviors (any activities) on day one, did three or fewer behaviors on day two 66.7% of the time. Those who demonstrated four or more behaviors (any activities) on day one, did four or more behaviors on day two 87.5% of the time.

Reliability for the recorded observations (yes/no for the day per individual behavior) was measured between two independent coders. Overall percent agreement between the two coders across all subcategories was high (agreement = 89.1%), with moderate/high inter-coder reliability (Cohen's Kappa = .667). The main category disagreement centered around "observing", specifically observing the food preparation of adults and food selection by peers. This category may need to be further refined with more specific definitions given that a wide spectrum of preparation and selection behaviors exist.

Activities by age group (Table 3)

Observed activities are reported by age group in Table 3 (details of these behaviors are available in Table 1), given the potential variability in food preparation behavior between older and younger groups [46]. Each behavior was coded as either exhibited or not exhibited, regardless of the number of times demonstrated. The most common activities among the entire group included browsing in

Table 2 Participant Demographics ($N=31$)

Age	N	%
9	3	9.7
10	9	29.0
11	6	19.4
12	6	19.4
13	7	22.6
Gender		
Male	15	48.4
Female	16	51.6
Household Highest Education		
< High School Grad	2	6.5
High School Grad	1	3.2
Some College	4	12.9
College Graduate	6	19.4
Post Graduate	16	51.6
Annual Reported Income (USD)		
20,000 to 39,999	3	9.7
40,000 to 59,999	5	16.1
60,000 to 79,999	6	19.4
80,000 to 100,000	3	9.7
Over 100,000	12	38.7

the pantry (51.6%) or fridge (71.0%). With regard to meal related tasks, getting drinks (58.1%) and clearing/washing dishes (71.0%) were the most common in the sample. Less than half of participants demonstrated food preparation work, with the most common activities being combining two or more ingredients (45.2%), and unwrapping of food packages (41.9%) while actual cutting or measuring ingredients was less common (12.9% each). Just over half the sample witnessed food preparation by adults according to the eButton image data (51.6%). Using a heat source to cook was uncommon in this sample, with the most common cooking method being microwaving (22.6%).

No statistically significant differences were found between the older and younger age groups with regard to food preparation behaviors, possibly due to the small sample size. Post hoc power analysis shows variable power depending on activity observed, ranging from very low (3.1%) to moderately-low (70.4%) power. However, some slight differences between the groups were identified. In this sample, younger children browsed for foods at school more often than the older group (16.7% vs 0%). The older group demonstrated more use of food media (23.1% vs 0%), more meal plating (46.2% vs 16.7%) and more observation of food selection by adults (30.8% vs 0%) than the younger group. The older participants also showed more food preparation behaviors than the younger group with regard to washing/peeling produce (30.8% vs 0%) and measuring ingredients (23.1% vs 5.6%).

Approximately one to two hours per participant was required to process images, and identify and classify food activity behaviors. Technical difficulties with the software developed for the eButton caused delays and some photo sets were not usable. The software was still in early stages and therefore updated on a regular basis, making later analysis more time-effective as issues were resolved with developers.

Discussion

Food preparation and related activities were consistently identifiable using eButton all-day images in this sample of pre- and early adolescents. Participants were frequently seen browsing for food around their homes, but were less frequently seen actually preparing foods for cooking or cooking foods themselves. The most common food preparation activities were unwrapping, combining two or more ingredients, and microwaving, indicating participants were more likely to work with pre-packaged foods when at home as opposed to meals made from scratch. When food preparation and related activities did occur, they were clearly identifiable from the angle of the eButton camera. Further, the eButton activity software allowed for efficient classification of food preparation activities, as the software automatically segmented photos into homogenous events.

Previous research has explored all day camera and other image-generating technologies to measure food intake and physical activity [47–49]. Most such studies validated their method through concordance with a reference intake measure. A systematic review of the new technologies concluded these tools supported adult self-report data by giving more information about under-reported foods [13]. The authors noted, however, the importance of supporting images with information about food preparation including ingredients and cooking method [13]. Our findings suggest such information can be gleaned from passive all-day camera data, which may support dietary assessments.

Research on food preparation among 4746 adolescents found 49.8% assisted with food shopping [46]. Our sample showed 6.5% of participants had images that appeared to be in grocery stores or markets on the day they wore the eButton. One reason for the discrepancy may be the sample size/selection, or the broader time-frame of the original study, which consisted of a single item: "In the past week, how many times did you help shop for groceries?". Most participants in the original study only helped with grocery shopping a maximum of one time per week (82.2%) [46]. Thus, all day cameras need to be worn for an entire week or longer to obtain

Table 3 Food/meal related activities by age ($N = 31$)

Activity	Age range		
	9 to 11[a]	12 to 13[b]	Ttl (%)[c]
Sample Size	18 (100%)	13 (100%)	31 (100%)
Browsing			
Pantry	7 (38.9)	9 (69.2)	16 (51.6)
Fridge	11 (61.6)	11 (84.6)	22 (71)
Grocery Store	2 (11.1)	0 (0)	2 (6.5)
Convenience Store or Café Counter	4 (22.2)	1 (7.7)	5 (16.1)
Kitchen Counter	3 (16.7)	2 (15.4)	5 (16.1)
At School	3 (16.7)	0 (0)	3 (9.7)
Altering Food on Plate/Adding Seasoning	4 (22.2)	3 (23.1)	7 (22.6)
Food Media, Recipes, Cookbooks, Photo	0 (0)	3 (23.1)	3 (9.7)
Tasks			
Plating	3 (16.7)	6 (46.2)	9 (29)
Getting Drinks	10 (55.6)	8 (61.5)	18 (58.1)
Clearing and/or washing dishes	13 (72.2)	9 (69.2)	22 (71)
Setting the Table	1 (5.6)	0 (0)	1 (3.2)
Prep Work			
Washing and/or Peeling Produce	0 (0)	4 (30.8)	4 (12.9)
Cutting	2 (11.1)	2 (15.4)	4 (12.9)
Cracking Eggs	0 (0)	1 (7.7)	1 (3.2)
Combining 2+ ingredients by hand	8 (44.4)	6 (46.2)	14 (45.2)
Measuring	1 (5.6)	3 (23.1)	4 (12.9)
Unwrapping	7 (38.9)	6 (46.2)	13 (41.9)
Using Blender, Mixer, Small appliance	0 (0)	1 (7.7)	1 (3.2)
Observing			
Food Selection by Adults	0 (0)	4 (30.8)	4 (12.9)
Food Selection by Peers	3 (16.7)	2 (15.4)	5 (16.1)
Any Food Preparation by Adults	9 (50.0)	7 (53.8)	16 (51.6)
Any Food Preparation by Peers	0 (0)	2 (15.4)	2 (6.5)
Cooking			
Stove	3 (16.7)	2 (15.4)	5 (16.1)
Oven (Baking)	0 (0)	1 (7.7)	1 (3.2)
Microwave	3 (16.7)	4 (30.8)	7 (22.6)

Table 3: Food/meal related activities by age. Table showing frequencies of activity by major and sub category. Totals indicate number of children who demonstrated each individual behavior at least one time through the course of a day
[a]= # of participants between the ages of 9–11 demonstrating behavior (# participants/total number of 9–11 year olds ($n = 18$))
[b]= # of participants between the ages of 12–13 demonstrating behavior (# participants/total number of 12–13 year olds ($n = 13$))
[c]= total # of participants demonstrating behavior in all age groups (# participants/total sample ($n = 31$))

accurate data on this behavior consistent with the questionnaire.

In the same survey study, a high percentage of adolescents reported helping with dinner (68.6%), based on a single item: "In the past week, how many times did you help prepare food for dinner?" [46]. This item is open to broad interpretation. Our results show that while most participants did at least one food or meal related activity during the day, they demonstrated little actual food preparation. Camera technology may enhance self-report studies by identifying what adolescents are referring to when they report helping with meals, or help improve the specification of behaviors targeted in study questionnaires.

Another survey study of 2029 Minnesota adolescents used a similar general frequency of food preparation assessment as above, and found 42.2% of girls and 28.4% of boys reported helping prepare meals at least 3 times per week [23]. Future studies with imaging technology using larger sample sizes should consider examining food and meal behaviors by sex over longer periods of time.

A smaller survey of 289 African American adolescents in Maryland used a similar frequency item: "In the past 7 days, how often did you prepare food for yourself or others (including making yourself lunch)?", followed with space to report foods prepared and preparation method (classified as fried, baked, microwaved, not cooked, or other). While most participants reported some food preparation, the most commonly noted food was cereal, with noodles and sandwiches also being widely reported. The most common food preparation method was "not cooked" followed by "microwaved" [50]. These findings are consistent with our data. Sandwiches, cereal and instant variety noodles are essentially prepared by combining two ingredients, an activity which was demonstrated by 45.2% of our sample. Of the heat based cooking methods used, microwaving was the most common in our study (22.6%). Thus, while adolescents are indeed helping prepare meals, they may not be demonstrating cooking skills beyond those needed for convenience foods.

The inactivity of adolescents in regard to more complex food preparations highlights the need for cooking skill interventions in youth. The coding system developed for this study is unique in that it encompasses details of food preparation. This system could be further expanded to assess the duration and quality of food preparation in response to a cooking intervention. Such an evaluation tool could identify the frequency of using intervention resources (e.g. recipe books) in the home and/or reflect an evaluation scale of positive (e.g. reducing added sugars) to more negative (e.g. deep frying) food preparation behaviors [45].

This is the first study to use all day camera images to classify food preparation and meal related behaviors in a sample of pre- and early adolescents. When food preparation behaviors were identified, camera angles offered the ability to clearly see behaviors in action. A wide range of behavior classifications allowed for details to be gathered well beyond standard self-report assessments of food preparation behavior in youth. Our findings support the use of image-based technology in food preparation intervention evaluations targeting adolescents.

Limitations include the small volunteer sample and reliance on secondary analysis. Single day images are also a limitation, as the recorded day may not be representative of normal behavior. The lack of a reference assessment method, such as direct observation, with which to compare both eButton and self reported values, limits our ability to say whether the eButton provides a better method than self report. A subsequent study is in progress to compare eButton images with direct observation and self-report assessments of food preparation events. Reactivity bias is also a potential issue, as participants may have altered behavior due to the knowledge that they were being recorded. However, previous research has shown acceptability and feasibility of using this technology for dietary assessment in adolescents [15]. Although the eButton camera angle is wider than most cameras utilized in smartphones (120° angle of view), it may still miss certain scenes of interest. Food advertisement exposure, for example, was not commonly seen in the sample, potentially due to the downward angle of the camera and four second interval between images. This angle appears to capture extended mobile phone activity, book/magazine reading and most television, but not billboards, posters or restaurant signage. In addition, the camera has a fixed orientation with respect to the vertical line (the line orthogonal to the surface of the earth). The orientation may not be optimal for every child because of variability in body height. These technical issues need to be investigated further to improve device performance in a food preparation study. Further, 24% of our data could not be analyzed due to issues with the software. The activity categorization software is still in a nascent stage, and therefore software updates will be continually needed to ensure all data collected can be processed.

Future research can build on this study by integrating self-report questions regarding food preparation into study design to better understand the relationship between self-reported and actual behaviors. Audio information may also be important, and was not available in the version of the eButton device used in this study. Audio would be useful to understand how a child responds when being taught or helping during active food preparation. Analysis of the camera images was time consuming, requiring one to two hours per participant per day of images. This type of work will benefit from automating all day image processing, and such automation software is currently in development at the University of Pittsburg [14]. Once automated to identify eating events, researchers could target images just before consumption to identify food preparation events more quickly and code food preparation practices. This would allow for more detailed analysis of cooking behaviors, while reducing the overall amount of data for analysis. Thus, all day cameras may be valuable evaluation tools for nutrition education programs, especially those that include food preparation skill development.

Conclusions

Youth cooking programs have gained in popularity but it is unclear if children are cooking at home or otherwise learning positive food or meal related behaviors. Although children who "help" prepare meals may obtain some dietary benefit, most relevant measurement tools are questionnaires that rely on simple single items (i.e.: Did you help make dinner?). Self-report questionnaires, while useful, offer limited detail and unknown validity regarding preparation practices. The eButton shows promise to identify food preparation behaviors in pre- and early adolescents. More work integrating this technology into nutrition intervention evaluations for adolescents and other populations is needed.

Abbreviations

HEI: Healthy Eating Index; STROBE: Strengthen the Reporting of Observational Studies in Epidemiology

Acknowledgements

The authors thank all participants and parents.

Funding

This research was funded by a grant from the National Institutes of Health, National Cancer Institute (5 R21 CA172864) (R01CA165255), National Heart, Lung and Blood Institute (U01HL91736) and institutional support from the U.S. Department of Agriculture, Agricultural Research Service (Cooperative Agreement 58–3092–5-001). MR is supported by the National Cancer Institute of the National Institutes of Health under Award Number R25CA057730 (PI: Shine Chang, PhD). The content is solely the responsibility of the authors and does not necessarily represent the official views of the NIH.

Authors' contributions

MR: Conceptualized this project, developed the codebook, completed coding and analysis and wrote the majority of the manuscript. MP: Served as second coder and assisted with analysis and supported the development of this manuscript. WJ: Developed the eButton software and assisted as technical issues arose during analysis, and supported the development of this manuscript. MS: Developed the eButton hardware and software and supported the development of this manuscript. TB: Oversaw the complete development of this project including conceptualization, analysis and manuscript development.

Competing interests

The authors declare that they have no competing interests.

Author details

[1]Department of Pediatrics Research, University of Texas MD Anderson Cancer Center, Houston, USA. [2]USDA/ARS Children's Nutrition Research Center, Baylor College of Medicine, Houston, USA. [3]Department of Neurological Surgery, University of Pittsburg, Pittsburg, USA.

References

1. Segal LM, Rayburn J, Martin A. State of obesity: better policies for a healthier America: 2015. Trust for America's Health. 2016;
2. Kushi LH, Doyle C, McCullough M, Rock CL, Demark-Wahnefried W, Bandera EV, Gapstur S, Patel AV, Andrews K, Gansler T. American Cancer Society guidelines on nutrition and physical activity for cancer prevention. CA Cancer J Clin. 2012;62(1):30–67.
3. Micha R, Kalantarian S, Wirojratana P, Byers T, Danaei G, Elmadfa I, Ding E, Giovannucci E, Powles J, Smith-Warner S, Ezzati M, Mozaffarian D. Estimating the global and regional burden of suboptimal nutrition on chronic disease: methods and inputs to the analysis. Eur J Clin Nutr. 2012;66(1):119–29.
4. I. Darnton-Hill, C. Nishida, and W. James, "A life course approach to diet, nutrition and the prevention of chronic diseases," Public health nutrition, vol. 7, no. 1A; SPI, pp. 101–122, 2004.
5. Flynn M, McNeil D, Maloff B, Mutasingwa D, Wu M, Ford C, Tough S. Reducing obesity and related chronic disease risk in children and youth: a synthesis of evidence with 'best practice'recommendations. Obes Rev. 2006;7(s1):7–66.
6. Livingstone MBE, Robson P, Wallace J. Issues in dietary intake assessment of children and adolescents. Br J Nutr. 2004;92(S2):S213–22.
7. Magarey A, Watson J, Golley RK, Burrows T, Sutherland R, McNaughton SA, DENNEY-WILSON E, Campbell K, Collins C. Assessing dietary intake in children and adolescents: considerations and recommendations for obesity research. Pediatric Obesity. 2011;6(1):2–11.
8. Hersch D, Perdue L, Ambroz T, Boucher JL. The impact of cooking classes on food-related preferences, attitudes, and behaviors of school-aged children: a systematic review of the evidence, 2003-2014. Prev Chronic Dis. 2014;11:E193.
9. Cairns G, Angus K, Hastings G, Caraher M. Systematic reviews of the evidence on the nature, extent and effects of food marketing to children. A retrospective summary. Appetite. 2013;62:209–15.
10. Diep CS, Hingle M, Chen T, Dadabhoy HR, Beltran A, Baranowski J, Subar AF, Baranowski T. The automated self-administered 24-hour dietary recall for children, 2012 version, for youth aged 9 to 11 years: a validation study. J Acad Nutr Diet. 2015;115(10):1591–8.
11. Schoeller DA. Limitations in the assessment of dietary energy intake by self-report. Metabolism. 1995;44:18–22.
12. Burrows TL, Martin RJ, Collins CE. A systematic review of the validity of dietary assessment methods in children when compared with the method of doubly labeled water. J Am Diet Assoc. 2010;110(10):1501–10.
13. Gemming L, Utter J, Mhurchu CN. Image-assisted dietary assessment: a systematic review of the evidence. J Acad Nutr Diet. 2015;115(1):64–77.
14. Sun M, Burke LE, Baranowski T, Fernstrom JD, Zhang H, Chen HC, Bai Y, Li Y, Li C, Yue Y, Li Z, Nie J, Sclabassi RJ, Mao ZH, Jia W. An exploratory study on a chest-worn computer for evaluation of diet, physical activity and lifestyle. Journal of healthcare engineering. 2015;6(1):1–22.
15. Beltran A, Dadabhoy H, Chen T, Lin C, Jia W, Baranowski J, Yan G, Sun M, Baranowski T. "adapting the eButton to the abilities of children for diet assessment," *Proceedings of Measuring Behavior 2016 - 10th International Conference on Methods and Techniques in Behavioral Research.* May. 2016;25-27(2016):72–81.
16. Laska MN, Larson NI, Neumark-Sztainer D, Story M. Does involvement in food preparation track from adolescence to young adulthood and is it associated with better dietary quality? Findings from a 10-year longitudinal study. Public Health Nutr. 2012;15(7):1150–8.
17. McLaughlin C, Tarasuk V, Kreiger N. An examination of at-home food preparation activity among low-income, food-insecure women. J Am Diet Assoc. 2003;103(11):1506–12.
18. Monsivais P, Aggarwal A, Drewnowski A. Time spent on home food preparation and indicators of healthy eating. Am J Prev Med. 2014;47(6):796–802.
19. Tiwari A, Aggarwal A, Tang W, Drewnowski A. Cooking at home: a strategy to comply with US dietary guidelines at no extra cost. Am J Prev Med. 2017;52(5):616–24.
20. Fulkerson JA, Kubik MY, Story M, Lytle L, Arcan C. Are there nutritional and other benefits associated with family meals among at-risk youth? J Adolesc Health. 2009;45(4):389–95.
21. J. Utter, S. Denny, R. Peiris-John, E. Moselen, B. Dyson, and T. Clark, "Family Meals and Adolescent Emotional Well-Being: Findings From a National Study," J Nutr Educ Behav, vol. 49, no. 1, pp. 67–72. e1, 2017.
22. Hammons AJ, Fiese BH. Is frequency of shared family meals related to the nutritional health of children and adolescents? Pediatrics. 2011;127(6):e1565–74.
23. Berge JM, MacLehose RF, Larson N, Laska M, Neumark-Sztainer D. Family food preparation and its effects on adolescent dietary quality and eating patterns. J Adolesc Health. 2016;59(5):530–6.
24. van der Horst K, Ferrage A, Rytz A. Involving children in meal preparation. Effects on food intake. Appetite. 2014;79:18–24.

25. Allirot X, da Quinta N, Chokupermal K, Urdaneta E. Involving children in cooking activities: a potential strategy for directing food choices toward novel foods containing vegetables. Appetite. 2016;103:275–85.
26. Ritchie B, O'Hara L, Taylor J. Kids in the Kitchen'impact evaluation: engaging primary school students in preparing fruit and vegetables for their own consumption. Health Promot J Austr. 2015;26(2):146–9.
27. Caraher M, Seeley A, Wu M, Lloyd S. When chefs adopt a school? An evaluation of a cooking intervention in English primary schools. Appetite. 2013;62:50–9.
28. Davis JN, Ventura EE, Cook LT, Gyllenhammer LE, Gatto NM. LA sprouts: a gardening, nutrition, and cooking intervention for Latino youth improves diet and reduces obesity. J Am Diet Assoc. 2011;111(8):1224–30.
29. Brown BJ, Hermann JR. Cooking classes increase fruit and vegetable intake and food safety behaviors in youth and adults. J Nutr Educ Behav. 2005;37(2):104–5.
30. Hawkes C, Jewell J, Allen K. A food policy package for healthy diets and the prevention of obesity and diet-related non-communicable diseases: the NOURISHING framework. Obes Rev. 2013;14(S2):159–68.
31. Sweetman C, McGowan L, Croker H, Cooke L. Characteristics of family mealtimes affecting children's vegetable consumption and liking. J Am Diet Assoc. 2011;111(2):269–73.
32. Hartmann C, Dohle S, Siegrist M. Importance of cooking skills for balanced food choices. Appetite. 2013;65:125–31.
33. Larson NI, Perry CL, Story M, Neumark-Sztainer D. Food preparation by young adults is associated with better diet quality. J Am Diet Assoc. 2006;106(12):2001–7.
34. Sun M, Fernstrom JD, Jia W, Hackworth SA, Yao N, Li Y, Li C, Fernstrom MH, Sclabassi RJ. A wearable electronic system for objective dietary assessment. J Am Diet Assoc. 2010;110(1):45–7.
35. Von Elm E, Altman DG, Egger M, Pocock SJ, Gøtzsche PC, Vandenbroucke JP, Initiative S. The strengthening the reporting of observational studies in epidemiology (STROBE) statement: guidelines for reporting observational studies. Int J Surg. 2014;12(12):1495–9.
36. Amini M, Djazayery A, Majdzadeh R, Taghdisi M, Jazayeri S. Effect of school-based interventions to control childhood obesity: a review of reviews. International journal of preventive medicine. 2015;1(6):68.
37. Story M, Kaphingst KM, Robinson-O'Brien R, Glanz K. Creating healthy food and eating environments: policy and environmental approaches. Annu Rev Public Health. 2008;29:253–72.
38. Williamson DA, Han H, Johnson WD, Martin CK, Newton RL. Modification of the school cafeteria environment can impact childhood nutrition. Results from the wise mind and LA health studies. Appetite. 2013;61:77–84.
39. D'Adamo CR, McArdle PF, Balick L, Peisach E, Ferguson T, Diehl A, Bustad K, Bowden B, Pierce BA, Berman BM. Spice MyPlate: nutrition education focusing upon spices and herbs improved diet quality and attitudes among urban high school students. Am J Health Promot. 2016;30(5):346–56.
40. Li R, Raber M, Chandra J. Developing a healthy web-based cookbook for pediatric cancer patients and survivors: rationale and methods. JMIR research protocols. 2015;4(1):e37.
41. Cunningham-Sabo L, Lohse B, Smith S, Browning R, Strutz E, Nigg C, Balgopal M, Kelly K, Ruder E. Fuel for Fun: a cluster-randomized controlled study of cooking skills, eating behaviors, and physical activity of 4th graders and their families. BMC public health. 2016;16(1):444.
42. Nour M, Chen J, Allman-Farinelli M. Efficacy and external validity of electronic and mobile phone-based interventions promoting vegetable intake in young adults: systematic review and meta-analysis. J Med Internet Res. 2016;18(4):e58.
43. Wolfson JA, Frattaroli S, Bleich SN, Smith KC, Teret SP. Perspectives on learning to cook and public support for cooking education policies in the United States: a mixed methods study. Appetite. 2017;108:226–37.
44. Birch LL, Fisher JO. Development of eating behaviors among children and adolescents. Pediatrics. 1998;101(3 Pt 2):539–49.
45. Raber M, Chandra J, Upadhyaya M, Schick V, Strong LL, Durand C, Sharma S. An evidence-based conceptual framework of healthy cooking. Preventive Medicine Reports. 2016;
46. Larson NI, Story M, Eisenberg ME, Neumark-Sztainer D. Food preparation and purchasing roles among adolescents: associations with sociodemographic characteristics and diet quality. J Am Diet Assoc. 2006;106(2):211–8.
47. Stumbo PJ. New technology in dietary assessment: a review of digital methods in improving food record accuracy. Proc Nutr Soc. 2013;72(01):70–6.
48. Boushey CJ, Kerr DA, Wright J, Lutes KD, Ebert DS, Delp EJ. Use of technology in children's dietary assessment. Eur J Clin Nutr. 2009;63:S50–7.
49. Boushey C, Spoden M, Zhu F, Delp E, Kerr D. New mobile methods for dietary assessment: review of image-assisted and image-based dietary assessment methods. Proc Nutr Soc. 2016:1–12.
50. Sattler M, Hopkins L, Anderson Steeves E, Cristello A, Mccloskey M, Gittelsohn J, Hurley K. Characteristics of youth food preparation in low-income, African American homes: associations with healthy eating index scores. Ecology of Food and Nutrition. 2015;54(4):380–96.

5

Development and relative validation of a food frequency questionnaire for French-Canadian adolescent and young adult survivors of acute lymphoblastic leukemia

Sophia Morel[1,3], Olivia Portolese[1], Yasmine Chertouk[1], Jade Leahy[1], Laurence Bertout[2], Caroline Laverdière[2], Maja Krajinovic[2], Daniel Sinnett[2], Emile Levy[1,3] and Valérie Marcil[1,3]*

Abstract

Background: Survivors of childhood acute lymphoblastic leukemia (cALL) experience cardiometabolic and bone complications after treatments. This study aimed at developing and validating an interview-administrated food frequency questionnaire (FFQ) that will serve to estimate the impact of nutrition in the development of long-term sequalea of French-Canadian cALL survivors.

Methods: The FFQ was developed to assess habitual diet, Mediterranean diet score, nutrients promoting bone health and antioxidants. It was validated using a 3-day food record (3-DFR) in 80 cALL survivors (50% male) aged between 11.4 and 40.1 years (median of 18.0 years). Reproducibility was evaluated by comparing FFQs from visit 1 and 2 in 29 cALL survivors.

Results: When compared to 3-DFR, the mean values for macro- and micronutrient intake were overestimated by our FFQ with the exception of lipid-related nutrients. Correlations between nutrient intakes derived from the FFQs and the 3-DFRs showed moderate to very good correlations (0.46–0.74). Intraclass correlation coefficients assessing FFQ reproducibility ranged from 0.62 to 0.92, indicating moderate to good reliability. Furthermore, classification into quartiles showed more than 75% of macro- and micronutrients derived from FFQs 1 and 2 classified into the same or adjacent quartile.

Conclusions: Overall, our results support the reproducibility and accuracy of the developed FFQ to appropriately classify individuals according to their dietary intake. This validated tool will be valuable for future studies analyzing the impact of nutrition on cardiometabolic and bone complications in French-speaking populations.

Keywords: Dietary assessment, Food frequency questionnaire, Dietary intake, Adolescent, Young adults, Quebec

Background

Acute lymphoblastic leukemia (ALL) accounts for approximately one fourth of all childhood malignancies [1]. Fortunately, cure rates now exceed 80%, which allows a growing number of childhood survivors to live into adulthood [1]. However, survivors may face severe long-term sequelae years after the end of treatments [2, 3]. In particular, studies on childhood ALL (cALL) survivors have reported a high prevalence of the typical components of the metabolic syndrome (MetS), namely obesity [4], hypertension [5], glucose intolerance [6] and dyslipidemia [7]. Furthermore, cALL treatments can affect bone growth and development leading to musculoskeletal morbidities that can compromise bone health [8]. Inadequate nutrition has been associated with an increased risk of developing long-term sequelae in cALL survivors [9–11], while the inclusion of specific nutrients or dietary patterns was found protective [10, 11]. Key nutrients for bone health include proteins,

* Correspondence: valerie.marcil@umontreal.ca
[1]Research Centre, Sainte-Justine University Health Center, Department of Nutrition, Université de Montréal, Montreal, QC H3T 1C5, Canada
[3]Institute of Nutrition and Functional Foods, Laval University, Quebec City, QC G1V 0A6, Canada

calcium and vitamin D [12]. In addition to their anti-inflammatory actions [13, 14], antioxidants (polyphenols, vitamins and minerals: e.g. vitamins A, C, E and selenium) mainly found in plant foods and whole grains can improve blood pressure and lipid profile [14–16]. Food scores have been developed to evaluate the adherence to Mediterranean diet and are mainly used in nutritional epidemiologic studies [17]. This diet is characterized by high intake of fruits, vegetables, legumes, fish, whole grains, nuts, and olive oil along with moderate consumption of dairy products and wine, as well as low intake of red and processed meats and foods that contain high amounts of added sugars [18]. The cardio protective properties of a Mediterranean dietary pattern have been widely reviewed [18–20].

Food frequency questionnaires (FFQs) and food records are tools that can be used to estimate individual food intake. Both tools have limitations and are subjected to measurement error and bias. Quantifying precise food intakes with FFQs require challenging respondents with complex and difficult cognitive tasks (e.g., recall and abstraction/estimation of averages over time) [21]. Also, because FFQs are limited by food list content, they need to be adapted to the study objectives and specific populations. On the other hand, self-reported food records might be incomplete or lack details regarding quantities or types of foods consumed. A participant may modify his diet to simplify the task or may report what is, in his perspective, an ideal diet. Poor response rates can also be problematic. Interviewed-administrated FFQs ensure participant's response but are time-consuming for both the participant and the interviewer. The interviewer can also assist the participant with the task of quantifying intakes. FFQs are common tools to estimate usual food intake and are used in epidemiologic studies to investigate associations between diet and diseases [22].

Currently, there is a great need for a reliable tool to assess the impact of dietary habits in cALL survivors. Therefore, the aim of this work is to develop and validate an interview-administrated FFQ in a population of French-Canadian cALL survivors from the Province of Quebec that assesses habitual diet, Mediterranean diet score, bone health-promoting nutrients, and antioxidants.

Methods

Study design

The study design includes 3 phases (Fig. 1): the first consists in the 5-step development of the FFQ; the second reflects the validation of the questionnaire in a cohort of 80 participants; and the third tests the reproducibility of the tool by comparing FFQs collected during 2 different visits.

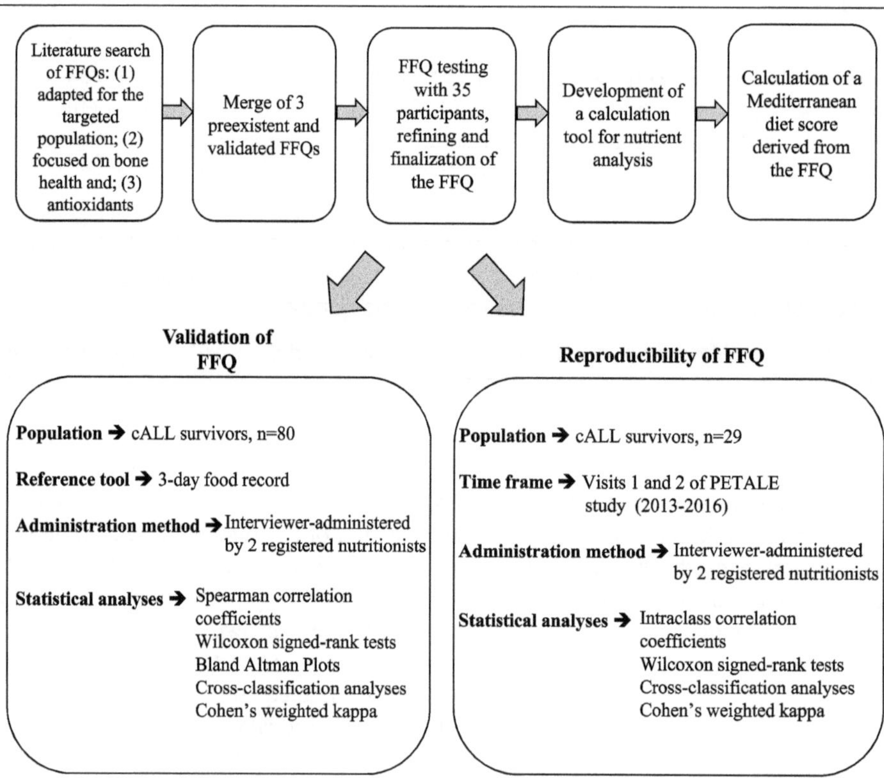

Fig. 1 Study design for the development, validation and reproducibility of the FFQ for adolescent and young adult survivors of acute lymphoblastic leukemia living in the Province of Quebec. FFQ: food-frequency questionnaire; cALL: childhood acute lymphoblastic leukemia

Study population

Participants enrolled in this study were recruited between January 2013 and December 2016 as part of the PETALE program at Sainte-Justine University Health Center in Montreal [8]. The PETALE study allowed the evaluation of long-term sequelae of cALL survivors, namely cardiotoxicity, cardiometabolic complications, neurocognitive problems, bone morbidity and quality of life issues [8]. Participants were recruited from European-descent cALL survivors living in the Province of Quebec. The PETALE study comprised of two phases. All participants were met in Phase 1 ($n = 246$). Participants identified with extreme phenotypes at Phase 1 (those with best and worst outcomes relative to long-term sequelea) were contacted for additional studies (Phase 2, $n = 100$). Visits of Phases 1 and 2 were, on average, 1 year *(± 21 weeks)* apart. In both phases, the FFQ was administrated to participants on the visit day by registered nutritionists (2 interviewers) and a 3-day food record (3-DFR) was handed out to complete at home. For validation of the FFQ, we included participants who fully completed and returned their 3-DFR. If the 3-DFR was incomplete (e.g., missing day or unspecified quantity of food), the participant was excluded from the validation step. A total of 80 FFQs and the associated 3-DFRs from either phase 1 or 2 were randomly selected for the validation, $n = 40$ for each FFQ interviewer (10 men, 10 boys, 10 women and 10 girls). For assessing FFQ reproducibility, 29 participants who took part in the two phases of the study (visits 1 and 2) and who were interviewed by both nutritionists were selected. The Institutional Review Board of Sainte-Justine University Health Center approved the study and investigations were carried out in accordance with the principles of the Declaration of Helsinki. Written informed consent was obtained from study participants and/or parents/guardians.

Development of the food frequency questionnaire

The FFQ was derived from 3 validated and published questionnaires. The first one was developed by Goulet et al., was structured to reflect French-Canadians' dietary habits and was validated among healthy women aged between 30 and 65 years [21]. The second FFQ was developed by Pritchard et al. and targeted nutrients affecting bone health. It was validated in postmenopausal women aged 70.3 ± 4.7 years and mainly Caucasian [23]. The third FFQ was an antioxidant nutrient questionnaire published by Satia et al. in which food items were selected based on the most commonly consumed antioxidant-rich foods. The mean age of participants was 31.9 years, 51% were African American, 52% were female and all were free of chronic disease [24]. The final result consisted of an interviewer-administered FFQ, which comprised 190 items with at least 106 having sub-questions to more accurately describe the nature of the food consumed. The developed FFQ was pre-tested in 35 participants and the tool was then modified accordingly, after addressing issues relating to content and comprehension.

Administration of the Food Frequency Questionnaire

Two registered nutritionists alternately administered the FFQ to participants using measuring cups to facilitate portion size estimation. Importantly, a portion size was specified for each food item. The standard portion size was adjustable by using fractions in the frequency column. An extra column was also available to indicate any other unit of measurement. Quantities were converted when the FFQ was analyzed. Participants were surveyed regarding the frequency each item was consumed during the past 2 months on a daily, weekly or monthly basis. Supplementary open- and closed-ended questions were added to support and complete participants' reported food intake by addressing usual foods that might have been forgotten, recent modifications in eating habits, weekly frequency of the main food groups, as well as use, dosage and frequency of dietary supplements.

3-day food record

At each visit (Phases 1 and 2), instructions were given to participants to complete a 3-DFR at home in the following weeks. Participants were asked to report their food and beverage intake for 1 day over the weekend and 2 days of the week. They were encouraged to choose days that reflected their usual diet and to not restrict their food intake. Emphasis was placed on providing comprehensive information relative to the portion size. While food did not have to be weighed, participants were encouraged to use measuring cups and spoons to estimate portions. A section for dietary supplements gathered information on dosage, frequency and brand.

Nutrient calculation tools

Food frequency questionnaire

To evaluate nutrient intakes derived from the FFQs, a nutrient calculation tool was built in-house using Microsoft® Excel® 2011. Nutrient values were obtained from the 2010 Canadian Nutrient File (CNF) that includes about 5500 food items commonly consumed in Canada [25]. If a food item was not found in the CNF, we used the United States Department of Agriculture National Nutrient Database for Standard Reference release 25, the major source of food composition data in the United States [26]. When necessary, we contacted companies to obtain nutrient values of their product. Energy and nutrient intakes were compiled, particularly proteins, carbohydrates (CHO), lipids, saturated fatty acids (SFA), monounsaturated fatty acids (MUFA), polyunsaturated fatty acids (PUFA), cholesterol, dietary fiber, alcohol, calcium, iron, folate, and vitamins A, C, D and E.

3-day food record

The 3-DFRs were analysed with the application Nutrific® developed by the Department of Food Science and Nutrition, Université Laval (https://nutrific.fsaa.ulaval.ca). Nutrient values from this application are derived from the 2010 CNF and, when a specific food item was not available, its nutrient value was added to the database.

Mediterranean diet score

Using the FFQ, we calculated a Mediterranean diet score based on a validated short questionnaire developed by Martinez-Gonzalez et al. [27]. The questionnaire is composed of nine food groups and assesses the consumption of cardio protective elements included in the Mediterranean diet. We calculated the Mediterranean diet score using the FFQ by regrouping each food item corresponding to each category (Table 1).

Statistical analysis

Relative validity

Medians and interquartile ranges were calculated for energy and nutrient intakes for the FFQ and the 3-DFR. Wilcoxon signed-rank tests were used to compare values obtained from both tools, as the data were not normally distributed. We used Spearman correlations to assess the relationships for energy, nutrient intakes and energy-adjusted nutrient intakes. The residual method proposed by Willett et al. was used to calculate the energy-adjusted variables [28]. With this method, the nutrient intakes of each individual are regressed on their total energy intakes. The residual from the regression represent the differences between each individual's actual intake and the intake predicted by their total energy intake [28]. The following classification was utilized to interpret correlation coefficients: very well correlated (coefficient 0.7 to 0.9), well correlated (coefficient 0.5 to 0.7) [29] and moderately well correlated (coefficient 0.3 to 0.5). This classification was also used to interpret the correlation coefficients in one of the FFQ that was used to develop our questionnaire [21]. Bland Altman Plots were used to assess agreement between the two tools for intakes of energy, macronutrients and micronutrients (vitamins A, C, E and D, and calcium). The limits of agreements were calculated by using the mean and the standard deviation (SD) of the differences between the two measurements (mean difference ± 1.96 * SD) [12, 30–32]. Through a graph representation, the differences of the two-paired measurements were plotted against the mean of the two measurements [32].

Cross-classification analyses were completed to validate agreement between the two tools in terms of proportions of participants' energy and nutrient intakes, classified into the same or contiguous quartiles (same ±1 quartile) or in opposite quartile (misclassified). Crude values of nutrient intakes were used for these analyses. Cohen's quadratic weighted kappa values were calculated. To interpret the kappa values, we used the arbitrary cut-off points proposed by Flight et al. and Landis and Koch [33, 34]: less than 0.20 indicated poor agreement, 0.21–0.40 fair agreement, 0.41–0.60 moderate agreement, 0.61–0.80 good agreement, and 0.81–1.00 very good agreement.

Table 1 Calculation of the Mediterranean diet score

	Points if yes
Olive oil (≥1 spoon/day)	+1
Fruits (≥1 serving/day)	+1
Vegetables of salad (≥1 serving/day)	+1
Fruits (≥1 serving/day) *and* Vegetables or salad (≥1 serving/day)[a]	+1
Legumes (≥ 2 servings/week)	+1
Fish (≥ 3 servings/week)	+1
Wine (≥1 glass/day)	+1
Meat (< 1 serving/day)	+1
[White bread (< 1 slice/day) *and* rice (< 1 cup/week)] *or* whole-grain bread (> 5 slices/week)[b]	+ 1

[a]One point is added when ≥1 serving/day of both fruits and vegetables is consumed

[b]One point is added when either consumption of both white bread and rice is low or when consumption of whole-grain bread is high. Adapted from Martinez-Gonzalez et al. 2004. Development of a short dietary intake questionnaire for the quantitative estimation of adherence to a cardioprotective Mediterranean diet. European Journal of Clinical Nutrition 58: 1550–1552

Reproducibility

Medians and interquartile ranges were calculated for energy and nutrient intakes for the FFQs at visits 1 and 2. Wilcoxon signed-rank tests were also used to compare values obtained from both visits. To measure the FFQ reproducibility, we calculated intraclass correlation coefficients between crude values obtained at visits 1 and 2 using the two-way mixed model and computed the absolute agreement type [35]. Energy-adjusted values were not used to calculate intraclass correlation coefficients because, due to the small sample size ($n = 29$), any modification in the composition of diet would greatly impact the residual values and the correlation coefficients. Data on nutrient intake were log-transformed because they were not normally distributed. To assess the quality of reliability, we used the scale suggested by Koo et al. for intraclass correlation coefficients: less than 0.5 indicated poor reliability, 0.5 to 0.75 moderate, 0.75 to 0.9 good, and greater than 0.90 excellent reliability [35].

Intakes of energy, proteins, CHO, lipids, calcium, vitamins A, C, D, E and Mediterranean diet score derived from the FFQs at visits 1 and 2 were also classified into quartiles and cross-classification analyses were completed to validate agreement between the two FFQs. Crude values not adjusted for energy intake were used. Cohen's quadratic weighted kappa values were also calculated to measure the agreement between the two FFQs.

Statistical analyses were performed with IBM SPSS Statistics Version 24, and the extension bundle Stats weighted kappa.spe for SPSS was used.

Results

Descriptive characteristics of participants are summarized in Table 2. Each registered nutritionist interviewed 40 participants. All participants were Caucasian and French-speaking.

Relative validity

The response rate obtained was 75 and 45% for the 3-DFR in Phases 1 and 2, respectively. Therefore, on a total of 100 participants who were invited to both phases, 39 completed and handed two 3-DFRs. We evaluated the time difference between the administration of the FFQ and the completion of the 3-DFR. We found that 66 of 80 participants (82.5%) filled out the 3-DFR within a month following the administration of the FFQ. Four of 80 participants (5%) completed the food record after 1.5 to 3.5 months and 10 of 80 (12.5%) did not inscribe the date.

The median values of daily energy and nutrient intakes derived from the FFQ and the 3-DFR are reported in Table 3. Two of 3 macronutrients derived from the FFQ showed higher values compared to the 3-DFR (proteins + 12.7% and CHO + 20.0%), resulting in higher reported energy intake (+ 12.1%). Reported intakes of dietary fiber and micronutrients (vitamins A, C, E and D, calcium, iron and folate) were also higher with the FFQ, differences ranging between + 16.0% (iron) and + 52.6% (vitamin C). Similar trends were observed when children and adults were analyzed separately (Additional file 1: Tables S1 and S2). The variability of differences between the FFQ and the 3-DFR are illustrated in the Bland Altman plots (Fig. 2) for the intakes in energy, CHO, proteins, lipids, calcium and vitamins D, C, A and E.

Spearman correlations between nutrient intakes derived from the FFQs and the 3-DFRs are shown in Table 3. Crude analyses revealed very good correlations for lipids and good correlations for proteins, SFA, MUFA, PUFA, alcohol, vitamins C, D and E, and calcium. CHO, cholesterol, dietary fiber, vitamin A, iron and folate were moderately well correlated. After adjustment for energy intake, the quality of correlations remained unchanged for vitamins A C, D and E, calcium, iron and folate. A slight reduction in the coefficient for proteins and CHO adjusted for energy was observed. Adjusting for energy decreased the coefficients for all lipids: total lipids (0.28 vs. 0.74), SFA (0.33 vs. 0.69), MUFA (0.25 vs. 0.61), PUFA (0. 33 vs. 0.58) and cholesterol (0.24 vs. 0.46). No major differences in correlation coefficients were noticeable when children and adults were analysed separately (Additional file 1: Tables S1 and S2). However, when the analyses were performed separately for males and females, the correlation coefficients followed the same trend with the exception of the female children group (girls) in which coefficient correlations were lower. The nutrients for which we found lower coefficients in female group were energy, proteins, CHO, cholesterol, vitamin C and iron, coefficients ranging between 0.07 (cholesterol) and 0.48 (energy intake) (Additional file 1: Tables S3, S4, S5, S6, S7 and S8).

Bland-Altman plots show that the FFQ overestimated energy intake by an average of 251 kcal/day, CHO intake by 51 g/day and protein intake by 11 g/day (Fig. 2). Micronutrients were also overestimated by the FFQ (vitamin A: 231 µg, vitamin C: 72 mg, vitamin E: 2.5 mg, vitamin D: 47 IU and calcium: 248 mg) (Fig. 2). More than 93% of the points fell within the limits of agreement for energy intake, CHO, proteins, lipids, vitamin A, C, E and D, and calcium.

Over 82% of participants' energy intake, macronutrients- and lipid-related nutrients derived from FFQ and 3-DFR were classified into the same or adjacent quartile (Table 4). Weighted kappa values were above 0.41 for all nutrients indicating moderate to good agreement with the exception of iron (0.37, fair agreement).

Intraclass correlations assessing FFQ reproducibility between visits 1 and 2 are shown in Table 5. Coefficients for macronutrients ranged between 0.76 (lipids) and 0.81 (CHO), indicating good reliability, which translated into a 0.84 coefficient for energy intake demonstrating good reliability. For micronutrients, intraclass correlation coefficients ranged from 0.68 (vitamin A) to 0.88 (vitamin D) with the indication of moderate to good reliability. Coefficients were found lower for three nutrients: MUFA (0.62), PUFA (0.56) and dietary fiber (0.63), but still indicating moderate reliability. Classification into quartiles showed that more than 75% of macro- and micronutrients derived from FFQs visit 1 and visit 2 were classified into the same or adjacent quartile (Table 6). Notably, 86% of Mediterranean diet scores were classified into the same or adjacent quartile. Weighted kappa values

Table 2 Descriptive characteristic of participants

	Total *N* = 80	Adults *N* = 40	Children *N* = 40
Gender, *N* (%)			
Male	80 (50.0)	40 (50.0)	40 (50.0)
Age at visit, years			
Mean (SD)	21.9 (7.2)	27.8 (5.6)	16.0 (1.5)
Median (range)	18.0 (11.4–40.1)	26.7 (18.2–40.1)	16.2 (11.4–17.9)

Subjects were stratified according to age (adults: ≥ 18 years old and children: < 18 years old)

Table 3 Food frequency questionnaires and 3-day food records: Comparison of nutrient median (inter-quartile range) daily intake and correlation coefficients

	Median (IQR) daily intake			Correlations[c]	
	3-DFR	FFQ[b]	Difference % (IQR)[a]	Unadjusted	Energy-adjusted[d]
Energy (kcal)	2093 (1860–2518)	2439 (2020–2802)***	12.1 (−1.1–24.9)	0.72**	
Protein (g)	87.2 (78.4–106)	102 (82.9–122)***	12.7 (−3.2–32.0)	0.59**	0.47**
CHO (g)	248 (214–307)	295 (254–379)***	20.0 (1.75–43.0)	0.50**	0.39**
Lipids (g)	82.8 (68.3–103)	84.1 (74.8–103)	2.5 (− 12.9–16.5)	0.74**	0.28*
SFA (g)	28.9 (21.8–37.3)	28.3 (23.7–32.7)	−4.7 (− 17.9–18.7)	0.69**	0.33**
MUFA (g)	29.2 (23.1–35.6)	29.8 (25.8–36.8)	2,6 (−14.2–25.9)	0.61**	0.25*
PUFA (g)	15.0 (10.7–19.5)	15.8 (12.8–19.3)	3.2 (− 10.8–26.1)	0.58**	0.33**
Cholesterol (mg)	266 (195–351)	256 (197–332)	− 9.1 (− 31.1–32.0)	0.46**	0.24*
Dietary fiber (g)	17.3 (13.6–21.0)	23.8 (18.1–29.8)***	31.1 (0.4–60.0)	0.50**	0.58**
Alcohol (g)	0.0 (0.0–4.6)	1.1 (0.0–9.5)*	–	0.59**	0.47**
Vitamin A (μg)	720 (564–988)	950 (747–1171)***	34.3 (− 8.5–80.4)	0.47**	0.41**
Vitamin C (mg)	122 (74.9–183.2)	187 (139–257)***	52.6 (14.5–122)	0.55**	0.50**
Vitamin E (mg)	6.2 (4.6–8.4)	8.9 (7.35–10.6)***	50.6 (16.4–73.5)	0.54**	0.47**
Vitamin D (IU)	176 (114–255)	226 (157–296)**	24.3 (− 16.0–83.1)	0.58**	0.50**
Calcium (mg)	1080 (690–1407)	1307 (1002–1654)***	23.0 (2.5–49.6)	0.70**	0.52**
Iron (mg)	12.5 (11.0–16.3)	16.0 (13.2–19.0)***	16.0 (3.7–45.6)	0.49**	0.42**
Folate (mcg)	347 (296–437)	492 (388–620)***	39.6 (14.4–72.4)	0.46**	0.41**

Values are median (IQR), $N = 80$

IQR inter-quartile range, *3-DFR* 3-day food record, *FFQ* food frequency questionnaire, *CHO* carbohydrates, *SFA* saturated fatty acids; *MUFA* monounsaturated fatty acids, *PUFA* polyunsaturated fatty acids

Note: Data presented as means ± SD are available in Additional file 1: Table S9

$^{*}P \leq 0.05$; $^{**}P \leq 0.01$; $^{***}P \leq 0.0001$

[a](Daily intake as per FFQ − Daily intake as per 3-DFR)/(Daily intake as per 3-DFR) × 100

[b]Wilcoxon signed-rank tests were used to compare values obtained from both FFQ and 3-DFR

[c]Spearman correlations were used to assess the relationship of energy, nutrient intakes and energy-adjusted nutrient intakes between 3-DFR and FFQ

[d]The residual method was used to calculate the energy-adjusted variables

varied from 0.52 (lipid) to 0.66 (CHO) for energy intake and macronutrients and from 0.46 (vitamin C) to 0.66 (vitamin D) for micronutrients, indicating moderate to good agreement for both groups. Weighted kappa value coefficient for the Mediterranean score was 0.68 indicating good agreement. No statistical differences were found between the mean values of daily energy and nutrient intakes derived from the FFQs from both visits. The variability between FFQs visit 1 and 2 of the differences for energy, CHO, protein and lipids are shown in Bland Altman plots (Additional file 2: Figure S1).

Discussion

We have developed and relatively validated an interview-administrated FFQ specific for the cALL survivors from the Province of Quebec, Canada to assess habitual diet, Mediterranean score and nutrients promoting bone health and antioxidant defense.

We found good correlation coefficients between our FFQ and the 3-DFR for most of the nutrients. As previously stated, correlation coefficients are generally higher for interviewer–administered than for self-administered FFQs [36, 37]. The precise and comprehensive food list of our questionnaire and its adaptation to the population's dietary habits contributed to its good accuracy. Also, to limit bias based on seasonal variations of diets [38], our FFQ interrogated food consumption in the past 2 months.

Energy adjusted nutrient intakes were calculated for both tools to reduce the confounding impact of the total energy intake on specific nutrients. We found that, for CHO, proteins and micronutrients, correlations were slightly impacted by total energy intake, while lipids and lipid-related nutrient correlation coefficients were significantly decreased. The reduction of the correlation coefficient of the energy intake adjusted lipids reflects the variation in lipid consumption independently of total energy intake between the 3-DFR and the FFQ. Thereby, the contribution of lipids to total energy intake was lower in the FFQ compared to the 3-DFR. The correlation coefficients found between energy-adjusted nutrients derived from FFQs and 3-DFRs were similar to those reported in a literature review (range between 0.4 and 0.7) [39], with the exception of lipids and lipid-

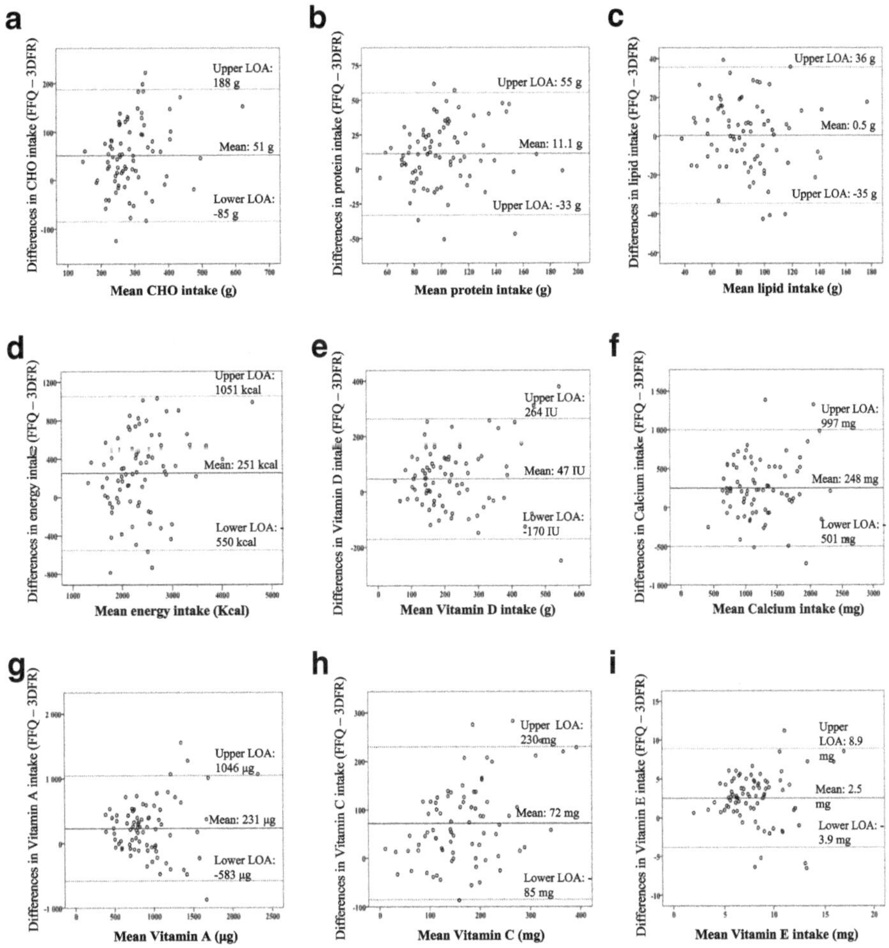

Fig. 2 Bland-Altman plot showing agreement between the average FFQ and the average 3-DFR for **a** carbohydrates, **b** proteins, **c** lipids, **d** energy intake, **e** vitamin D, **f** calcium, **g** vitamin A, **h** vitamin C, **i** and vitamin E. A mean of 0 indicates that the 2 methods are in perfect agreement. LOA, limit of agreement; IU, international unit

related nutrients for which coefficients were lower in our study.

Compared to 3-DFR, mean values for macro- and micronutrient intakes were overestimated by our FFQ with the exception of lipid-related nutrients. The differences were lower than 20% for all macronutrients. These results concur with many FFQ validation studies that have reported overestimations for energy and nutrient intakes compared to food records or 24-h recalls [30, 31, 40–48]. Still, other groups reported underestimation of energy and nutrient intakes [21, 37, 49, 50]. To our knowledge, only one other study aimed to validate a FFQ specifically for childhood cancer survivors [49]. Conversely to our findings, their FFQ revealed substantial underreporting of dietary intakes compared to repeated 24-h diet recalls. However, this comparison is flawed by the study smaller sample size (only 16 participants aged between 5 and 22 years), the different populations (Americans versus French Canadians) and inclusion criteria as well as the use of 24-h diet recalls as a reference tool [49].

We found larger differences between the FFQs and the 3-DFRs in micronutrients than in macronutrients, the latter being found in a wider range of food. Hence, if foods containing specific micronutrients were not consumed during the days covered by the 3-DFR, this will likely result in a poor correlation with the FFQ. Moreover, the detailed list of fruits and vegetables in the FFQ could explain the observed overestimations for vitamin A, vitamin C and dietary fiber. Of note, in the Province of Quebec, seasons have a considerable impact on the availability, variety and financial accessibility of several fruits and vegetables. Thereby, any delay in completing the 3-DFR could have impacted the reported consumption of fruits/vegetables and the abovementioned nutrients. However, in our study, most of the 3-DFR were filled out and returned within a month following the completion of the FFQ. Consequently,

Table 4 Food frequency questionnaires and 3-day food records: cross-classification analysis of energy and nutrient intakes

	% Classified into same quartile[1]	% Classified into same ±1 quartile[a]	% Misclassified[b]	Weighted[b] Kappa
Energy	47.5	40.0	12.5	0.64
Protein	45.0	37.5	17.5	0.52
CHO	45.0	32.5	22.5	0.46
Lipids	51.3	40.0	8.7	0.70
SFA	50.0	36.3	13.7	0.63
MUFA	35.0	51.3	13.7	0.55
PUFA	48.7	35.0	16.3	0.58
Cholesterol	30.0	51.3	18.7	0.42
Dietary fiber	46.3	30.0	23.7	0.43
Alcohol	57.5	28.7	13.8	0.67
Vitamin A	41.3	33.7	25.0	0.44
Vitamin C	38.7	43.8	17.5	0.47
Vitamin E	41.3	40.0	18.7	0.47
Vitamin D	40.0	41.3	18.7	0.51
Calcium	53.7	33.8	12.5	0.64
Iron	40.0	36.3	23.7	0.37
Folate	37.5	43.7	18.8	0.45

Values are expressed in percentage, $N = 80$

3-DFR 3-day food record, *FFQ* food frequency questionnaire, *CHO* carbohydrates, *SFA* saturated fatty acids, *MUFA* monounsaturated fatty acids, *PUFA* polyunsaturated fatty acids

[a]Cross-classification analyses were completed to validate agreement between FFQ and 3-DFR in terms of proportions of participants classified into the same or same ±1 quartile or misclassified

[b]Weighted kappa was used to measure the agreement between FFQ and 3-DFR. Analyses were completed on crude values not adjusted for energy intake

seasons probably did not influence the observed differences in micronutrients.

For our analyses, we used correlations in conjunction with the Bland-Altman method. While correlations quantify the degree to which two variables are related at an individual level [51], a high correlation does not automatically imply that there is good agreement between the two methods [32]. Bland-Altman plot is a method to assess the agreement between two quantitative measurements by constructing limits of agreement [32]. The plot illustrates the differences between the tools against the mean of the two tools. The closer the mean of differences is to zero and the narrower agreement interval is, the better the agreement between the two tools [32]. We consider the agreement interval, represented by the limits of agreement for energy intake and for macronutrients, sufficiently narrow to support the use of the FFQ. These agreement intervals were similar to those reported in an Italian study comparing a medium length FFQ (36 items) to 3-DFR [37].

It must be emphasised that one of the difficulties met by the interviewers was to obtain from the participants the diversity and quantity of oil and fat intakes in their diet. Furthermore, participants had a tendency to not report oil and fats used in homemade cooked meals in the 3-DFR. Consequently, it is difficult to determine whether our FFQ over- or underestimated lipid intakes and/or to what level they were underestimated by the participants in the 3-DFR, a limit that has been met in another FFQ validation study [21]. This might explain the equal plot distribution of differences in lipid intakes around the mean of differences (close to zero) between FFQ and 3-DFR shown in the Bland Altman plot. However, the low percentage of subjects misclassified in quartile for lipid-related nutrients (SFA, MUFA, PUFA and cholesterol) and the good agreement assessed by weighted kappa values support the use of the FFQ to rank lipid intakes inside a group.

As stated by Willet & Lenart, reproducibility refers to consistency of questionnaire measurements on more than one administration to the same person at different times, considering that conditions are never identical on repeated administration [29]. Intraclass correlation application assess consistency or reproducibility of measurements and coefficient reflects both degree of correlation and agreement between measurements [35]. While a minimum of 3 raters and a sample size of 30 have been suggested for reliability studies [35], the intraclass correlation coefficients obtained in our analyses were found moderate to good despite having two interviewers and a sample of 29 individuals. As stated by Cade et al., correlation coefficients of 0.5 to 0.7 between two administrations of an FFQ are common [36]. Our results surpassed 0.7 in most of the nutrients tested even though 1 year on average separated the administration of the two FFQs. It has been shown that repeating FFQ administration within 1 month leads to higher correlation coefficients than repeated administrations further apart [36]. In a Finnish study, reproducibility analysis of a 110-item FFQ tested as part as a breast cancer study led to intraclass correlation coefficients between 0.49 and 0.73 [52]. Similar results were found in a 112-item FFQ tested among Lebanese children (0.31 to 0.73) [30]. Furthermore, using quartile classification, we found that the percentage of participants misclassified was below 15% for most nutrients (with the exception of lipids and vitamins A and E) and for Mediterranean score. Further, the weighted kappa values showed moderate to good agreement for all nutrients and Mediterranean score. These results are comparable to a Lebanese study performed in children, although they have reported higher percentage of agreement in quartile classification [30].

Limits were identified to ensure proper usage of the validated FFQ and to avoid misleading conclusions. Accordingly, our FFQ should be utilized to rank individuals as per nutrient intakes rather than to assess their absolute

Table 5 Food frequency questionnaires at visits 1 and 2: Comparison of nutrient median (inter-quartile range) daily intake and intraclass correlation coefficients

	Median (IQR) daily intake			
	FFQ V1	FFQ V2[b]	Difference % (IQR)[a]	Correlations[c]
Energy (kcal)	2533 (2036–2892)	2416 (1941–3062)	4.9 (−16.6–18.7)	0.84***
Protein (g)	106 (92.3–127)	100 (88.4–140)	4.8 (− 15.9–12.8)	0.79***
CHO (g)	308 (254–380)	296 (226–368)	4.9 (− 10.9–24.7)	0.81***
Lipids (g)	91 (67.2–103)	85.7 (68.7–114)	−7.0 (− 15.4–13.0)	0.76***
SFA (g)	28.0 (19.0–31.6)	26.8 (22.8–37.0)	−4.3 (− 21.9–15.3)	0.81***
MUFA (g)	30.3 (24.3–39.0)	30.9 (24.4–43.5)	−6.8 (− 17.9–18.2)	0.62**
PUFA (g)	16.5 (12.2–20.1)	18.1 (13.9–21.9)	−12.4 (− 29.2–1.2)	0.56*
Cholesterol (mg)	265 (201–334)	319 (210–423)	−7.4 (− 24.2–6.7)	0.83***
Dietary fiber (g)	23.8 (15.9–29.9)	24.2 (16.2–31.4)	−4.4 (− 22.6–16.4)	0.63**
Alcohol (g)	2.8 (1.1–12.4)	3.3 (1.5–12.7)	− 6.2 (− 29.0–4.5)	0.92***
Vitamin A (µg)	904 (737–1158)	974 (775–1357)	−8.5 (− 19.3–15.0)	0.68**
Vitamin C (mg)	191 (131–254)	178 (121–214)	− 6.0 (− 16.1–19.9)	0.83***
Vitamin E (mg)	8.8 (6.7–12.9)	8.8 (6.9–12.7)	4.0 (−21.2–20.6)	0.86***
Vitamin D (IU)	224 (168–260)	237 (191–281)	−0.6 (− 13.4–18.6)	0.88***
Calcium (mg)	1220 (1045–1627)	1240 (1106–1552)	−3.6 (− 15.2–12.5)	0.87***
Iron (mg)	15.6 (13.7–19.1)	15.3 (12.8–19.1)	− 0.9 (− 14.0–19.6)	0.76***
Folate (mcg)	452 (398–684)	507 (387–664)	0.0 (−22.4–12.0)	0.76***

Values are median (IQR), $N = 29$

IQR inter-quartile range, *FFQ* food frequency questionnaire, *CHO* carbohydrates, *SFA* saturated fatty acids, *MUFA* monounsaturated fatty acids, *PUFA* polyunsaturated fatty acids

Note: Data presented as means ± SD are available in Additional file 1: Table S10

*$P \le 0.05$; **$P \le 0.01$; ***$P \le 0.0001$. V1, visit 1; V2, visit 2

[a](Daily intake as per FFQ V1 − Daily intake as per FFQ V2)/(Daily intake as per FFQ V2) × 100

[b]Wilcoxon signed-rank tests were used to compare values obtained from both FFQ V1 and FFQ V2. No statistical differences were found

[c]Intraclass correlations between FFQ V1 and FFQ V2 based on log transformed values. Analyses were completed on crude values not adjusted for energy intake

values. It is recognized that the 3-DFR is not a perfect tool to measure dietary intake [53], but there is no gold standard to validate FFQs [53]. One of the constraints of our study was that, to facilitate the analyses, we used two different calculation tools to evaluate nutrient intakes derived from the questionnaire and the food records. However, both tools were developed for a French-Canadian population using nutrient values derived from the 2010 Canadian Nutrient File. Another limitation was that teenagers constituted half the sample used for the FFQ validation. In general, the FFQ was administered to the adolescent with the help of the accompanying parent. When the precise information was difficult to obtain from the adolescent, parents were often able to complete the missing data for main meals. However, parents were not necessarily aware of what was eaten by their children outside the house or as snacks, which constitutes a possible source of imprecision. As stated previously, frequency and quantity of lipid intakes were difficult to capture using the FFQ, which could potentially under- or overestimates them. In addition, we observed that girls had a tendency to underestimate their intakes in the 3-DFR or/and to overestimate them in the FFQ. It has been previously shown in the literature that girls and women have a tendency to restrict their diet when using food records [54]. This limit has to be considered when analyzing data obtained in female participants.

The efforts invested to tailor the FFQ to our targeted population and the complementary nature of analyses completed to ensure the validity and reproducibility of the FFQ represent the main strengths of our study [51]. Few FFQs related to the Mediterranean diet and adapted to French-Canadian [21, 55] and European [56, 57] populations have been published in recent years. Other FFQs have targeted only the specific properties of food (e.g. antioxidant-rich foods) for North American [24, 58], European [13, 59] and Asian [60] populations. Also, while FFQs validated for populations at risk of cardiometabolic diseases were mostly developed in adult populations [24, 55, 57, 59], our FFQ was adapted to adolescents and young adults.

Conclusion

In conclusion, our results support the reproducibility and accuracy of the developed FFQ to correctly rank individuals according to their dietary intake. The validated

Table 6 Food frequency questionnaires visit 1 and 2: cross-classification analysis of energy intake, nutrient intake and Mediterranean diet score

	% Classified into same quartile[a]	% Classified into same ±1 quartile[a]	% Misclassified[a]	Weighted Kappa[b]
Energy	44.8	41.4	13.8	0.60
Protein	37.9	48.3	13.8	0.57
CHO	48.3	41.4	10.3	0.66
Lipids	44.8	34.5	20.7	0.52
Vitamin A	48.3	27.6	24.1	0.49
Vitamin C	44.8	41.4	13.8	0.46
Vitamin E	51.7	31.0	17.3	0.52
Vitamin D	51.7	37.9	10.4	0.66
Calcium	51.7	34.5	13.8	0.63
Mediterranean diet score	58.6	27.6	13.8	0.68

Values are expressed in percentage, $N = 29$

[a]Cross-classification analyses were completed to validate agreement between the two FFQs in terms of proportions of participants classified into the same or same ±1 quartile or misclassified

[b]Weighted kappa was used to measure the agreement between the two FFQs. Analyses were completed on crude values not adjusted for energy intake. CHO: carbohydrates

FFQ represents a valuable tool for future studies measuring the impact of nutrition in the development of long-term cardiometabolic and bone complications in cALL survivors from the Province of Quebec. This FFQ could further be adapted and validated for other adolescent and young adult French-speaking populations at risk of developing chronic diseases.

Additional files

Additional file 1: Table S1. Food frequency questionnaires and 3-day food records: Comparison of nutrient median (inter-quartile range) daily intake and correlation coefficients in adults, **Table S2.** Food frequency questionnaires and 3-day food records: Comparison of nutrient median (inter-quartile range) daily intake and correlation coefficients in adolescents, **Table S3.** Food frequency questionnaires and 3-day food records: Comparison of nutrient median (inter-quartile range) daily intake and correlation coefficients in males, **Table S4.** Food frequency questionnaires and 3-day food records: Comparison of nutrient median (inter-quartile range) daily intake and correlation coefficients in females, **Table S5.** Food frequency questionnaires and 3-day food records: Comparison of nutrient median (inter-quartile range) daily intake and correlation coefficients in boys, **Table S6.** Food frequency questionnaires and 3-day food records: Comparison of nutrient median (inter-quartile range) daily intake and correlation coefficients in men, **Table S7.** Food frequency questionnaires and 3-day food records: Comparison of nutrient median (inter-quartile range) daily intake and correlation coefficients in girls, **Table S8.** Food frequency questionnaires and 3-day food records: Comparison of nutrient median (inter-quartile range) daily intake and correlation coefficients in women, **Table S9.** Food frequency questionnaires and 3-day food records: Comparison of nutrient mean daily intake and correlation coefficients, **Table S10.** Food frequency questionnaires at visits 1 and 2: comparison of nutrient mean daily intake and intraclass correlation coefficients.

Additional file 2: Figure S1. Bland-Altman plots showing agreement between the average FFQ at visit 1 and 2 for (a) carbohydrates, (b) proteins, (c) lipids, (d) energy intake, (e) vitamin D and (f) calcium (g) vitamin A, (h) vitamin C, (i) vitamin E. A mean of 0 indicates that the 2 tools are in perfect agreement. LOA, limit of agreement; IU, international unit.

Abbreviations

3-DFR: 3-day food record; ALL: Acute lymphoblastic leukemia; cALL: childhood acute lymphoblastic leukemia; CHO: Carbohydrates; CNF: Canadian Nutrient File; FFQ: Food frequency questionnaire; MetS: Metabolic syndrome; MUFA: Monounsaturated fatty acids; PUFA: Polyunsaturated fatty acids; SFA: Saturated fatty acids

Funding

This work was supported by the Institute of Cancer Research (ICR) of the Canadian Institutes of Health Research (CIHR), in collaboration with C17 Council, Canadian Cancer Society (CCS), Cancer Research Society (CRS), Garron Family Cancer Centre at the Hospital for Sick Children, Ontario Institute for Cancer Research (OICR) and Pediatric Oncology Group of Ontario (POGO) (grant number: TCF 118694), by the J.A. DeSeve Research Chair in Nutrition, the Fonds de Recherche du Québec en Santé and by a Transition Grant from the Cole Foundation.

Authors' contributions

CL, MK, DS, EL and VM conceived the experiments and designed the study, SM, LB, CL and VM acquired the data, SM, OP, YC, JL, EL and VM analyzed and interpreted the data. SM, EL and VM drafted the article. All authors revised the manuscript and approved the final version.

Competing interests

The authors declare that they have no competing interests.

Author details

[1]Research Centre, Sainte-Justine University Health Center, Department of Nutrition, Université de Montréal, Montreal, QC H3T 1C5, Canada. [2]Research Centre, Sainte-Justine University Health Center, Department of Pediatrics, Université de Montréal, Montreal, QC H3T 1C5, Canada. [3]Institute of Nutrition and Functional Foods, Laval University, Quebec City, QC G1V 0A6, Canada.

References

1. Pui C-H, Mullighan CG, Evans WE, Relling MV. Pediatric acute lymphoblastic leukemia: where are we going and how do we get there? Blood. 2012;120:1165–74.
2. Essig S, Li Q, Chen Y, Hitzler J, Leisenring W, Greenberg M, Sklar C, Hudson MM, Armstrong GT, Krull KR, et al. Risk of late effects of treatment in children newly diagnosed with standard-risk acute lymphoblastic leukaemia: a report from the childhood Cancer survivor study cohort. Lancet Oncol. 2014;15:841–51.
3. Mody R, Li S, Dover DC, Sallan S, Leisenring W, Oeffinger KC, Yasui Y, Robison LL, Neglia JP. Twenty five year follow-up among survivors of childhood acute lymphoblastic leukemia: a report from the childhood Cancer survivor study. Blood. 2008;111(12):5515–23.
4. Janiszewski PM, Oeffinger KC, Church TS, Dunn AL, Eshelman DA, Victor RG, Brooks S, Turoff AJ, Sinclair E, Murray JC, et al. Abdominal obesity, liver fat,

and muscle composition in survivors of childhood acute lymphoblastic leukemia. J Clin Endocrinol Metab. 2007;92:3816–21.
5. Chow EJ, Pihoker C, Hunt K, Wilkinson K, Friedman DL. Obesity and hypertension among children after treatment for acute lymphoblastic leukemia. Cancer. 2007;110:2313–20.
6. Neville KA, Cohn RJ, Steinbeck KS, Johnston K, Walker JL. Hyperinsulinemia, impaired glucose tolerance, and diabetes mellitus in survivors of childhood cancer: prevalence and risk factors. J Clin Endocrinol Metab. 2006;91:4401–7.
7. Malhotra J, Tonorezos ES, Rozenberg M, Vega GL, Sklar CA, Chou J, Moskowitz CS, Eshelman-Kent DA, Janiszewski P, Ross R, Oeffinger KC. Atherogenic low density lipoprotein phenotype in long-term survivors of childhood acute lymphoblastic leukemia. J Lipid Res. 2012;53:2747–54.
8. Marcoux S, Drouin S, Laverdière C, Alos N, Andelfinger GU, Bertout L, Curnier D, Friedrich MG, Kritikou EA, Lefebvre G, Levy E, Lippé S, Marcil V, Raboisson MJ, Rauch F, Robaey P, Samoilenko M, Séguin C, Sultan S, Krajinovic M, Sinnett D. The PETALE study: Late adverse effects and biomarkers in childhood acute lymphoblastic leukemia survivors. Pediatr Blood Cancer. 2017;64(6). https://doi.org/10.1002/pbc.26361. Epub 2016 Dec 4.
9. Robien K, Ness KK, Klesges LM, Baker KS, Gurney JG. Poor adherence to dietary guidelines among adult survivors of childhood acute lymphoblastic leukemia. J Pediatr Hematol Oncol. 2008;30:815.
10. Tonorezos ES, Robien K, Eshelman-Kent D, Moskowitz CS, Church TS, Ross R, Oeffinger KC. Contribution of diet and physical activity to metabolic parameters among survivors of childhood leukemia. Cancer Causes Control. 2013;24:313–21.
11. Landy DC, Lipsitz SR, Kurtz JM, Hinkle AS, Constine LS, Adams MJ, Lipshultz SE, Miller TL. Dietary quality, caloric intake, and adiposity of childhood cancer survivors and their siblings: an analysis from the cardiac risk factors in childhood cancer survivors study. Nutr Cancer. 2013;65:547–55.
12. Perreault MRM, Xu VYB, Hamilton SRB, Wright DRM, Foster WP, Atkinson SAP. Validation of a food frequency questionnaire for bone nutrients in pregnant women. Can J Diet Pract Res. 2016;77:133–9.
13. Tovar J, Johansson M, Björck I. A multifunctional diet improves cardiometabolic-related biomarkers independently of weight changes: an 8-week randomized controlled intervention in healthy overweight and obese subjects. Eur J Nutr. 2016;55:2295–306.
14. Valtueña S, Pellegrini N, Franzini L, Bianchi MA, Ardigò D, Del Rio D, Piatti P, Scazzina F, Zavaroni I, Brighenti F. Food selection based on total antioxidant capacity can modify antioxidant intake, systemic inflammation, and liver function without altering markers of oxidative stress. Am J Clin Nutr. 2008; 87:1290–7.
15. Kaliora AC, Dedoussis GV. Natural antioxidant compounds in risk factors for CVD. Pharmacol Res. 2007;56:99–109.
16. Erlund I, Koli R, Alfthan G, Marniemi J, Puukka P, Mustonen P, Mattila P, Jula A. Favorable effects of berry consumption on platelet function, blood pressure, and HDL cholesterol. Am J Clin Nutr. 2008;87:323–31.
17. Bach A, Serra-Majem L, Carrasco JL, Roman B, Ngo J, Bertomeu I, Obrador B. The use of indexes evaluating the adherence to the Mediterranean diet in epidemiological studies: a review. Public Health Nutr. 2006;9:132.
18. Salas-Salvado J, Guasch-Ferre M, Lee CH, Estruch R, Clish CB, Ros E. Protective effects of the Mediterranean diet on type 2 diabetes and metabolic syndrome. J Nutr. 2016;
19. Dontas AS, Zerefos NS, Panagiotakos DB, Valis DA. Mediterranean diet and prevention of coronary heart disease in the elderly. Clin Interv Aging. 2007;2:109.
20. Jacobs DR Jr, Tapsell LC. What an anticardiovascular diet should be in 2015. Curr Opin Lipidol. 2015;26:270–5.
21. Goulet J, Nadeau G, Lapointe A, Lamarche B, Lemieux S. Validity and reproducibility of an interviewer-administered food frequency questionnaire for healthy French-Canadian men and women. Nutr J. 2004;3:13.
22. Molag ML, de Vries JH, Ocké MC, Dagnelie PC, van den Brandt PA, Jansen MC, van Staveren WA, van't Veer P. Design characteristics of food frequency questionnaires in relation to their validity. Am J Epidemiol. 2007;166:1468–78.
23. Pritchard JM, Seechurn T, Atkinson SA. A food frequency questionnaire for the assessment of calcium, vitamin D and vitamin K: a pilot validation study. Nutrients. 2010;2:805–19.
24. Satia JA, Watters JL, Galanko JA. Validation of an antioxidant nutrient questionnaire in whites and African Americans. J Am Diet Assoc. 2009;109: 502–8. 508 e501-506
25. Health Canada: Canadian Nutrient File (2010 version) [https://aliments-nutrition.canada.ca/cnf-fce/index-fra.jsp].
26. United States Department of Agriculture (USDA) 2. https://ndb.nal.usda.gov/ndb/.
27. Martinez-Gonzalez M, Fernandez-Jarne E, Serrano-Martinez M, Wright M, Gomez-Gracia E. Development of a short dietary intake questionnaire for the quantitative estimation of adherence to a cardioprotective Mediterranean diet. Eur J Clin Nutr. 2004;58:1550–2.
28. Willett WC, Howe GR, Kushi LH. Adjustment for total energy intake in epidemiologic studies. Am J Clin Nutr. 1997;65:1220S–8S. discussion 1229S-1231S
29. Willet W, Lenart E. Reproducibility and validity of food-frequency questionnaires. Monographs Epidemiol Biostat. 1998;1:101–47.
30. Moghames P, Hammami N, Hwalla N, Yazbeck N, Shoaib H, Nasreddine L, Naja F. Validity and reliability of a food frequency questionnaire to estimate dietary intake among Lebanese children. Nutr J. 2016;15:4.
31. Athanasiadou E, Kyrkou C, Fotiou M, Tsakoumaki F, Dimitropoulou A, Polychroniadou E, Menexes G, Athanasiadis AP, Biliaderis CG, Michaelidou AM. Development and validation of a Mediterranean oriented culture-specific semi-quantitative food frequency questionnaire. Nutrients. 2016;8
32. Bland JM, Altman D. Statistical methods for assessing agreement between two methods of clinical measurement. Lancet. 1986;327:307–10.
33. Hight L, Julious SA. The disagreeable behaviour of the kappa statistic. Pharm Stat. 2015;14:74–8.
34. Landis JR, Koch GG. The measurement of observer agreement for categorical data. Biometrics. 1977;33:159–74.
35. Koo TK, Li MY. A guideline of selecting and reporting Intraclass correlation coefficients for reliability research. J Chiropr Med. 2016;15:155–63.
36. Cade J, Burley V, Warm D, Thompson R, Margetts B. Food-frequency questionnaires: a review of their design, validation and utilisation. Nutr Res Rev. 2004;17:5–22.
37. Buscemi S, Rosafio G, Vasto S, Massenti FM, Grosso G, Galvano F, Rini N, Barile AM, Maniaci V, Cosentino L. Validation of a food frequency questionnaire for use in Italian adults living in Sicily. Int J Food Sci Nutr. 2015;66:426–38.
38. Shahar D, Yerushalmi N, Lubin F, Froom P, Shahar A, Kristal-Boneh E. Seasonal variations in dietary intake affect the consistency of dietary assessment. Eur J Epidemiol. 2001;17:129–33.
39. Willett WC. Future directions in the development of food-frequency questionnaires. Am J Clin Nutr. 1994;59:171S–4S.
40. Papazian T, Hout H, Sibai D, Helou N, Younes H, El Osta N, Khabbaz LR. Development, reproducibility and validity of a food frequency questionnaire among pregnant women adherent to the Mediterranean dietary pattern. Clin Nutr. 2016;35(6):1550–6.
41. Tayyem RF, Abu-Mweis SS, Bawadi HA, Agraib L, Bani-Hani K. Validation of a food frequency questionnaire to assess macronutrient and micronutrient intake among Jordanians. J Acad Nutr Diet. 2014;114:1046–52.
42. Rodriguez MM, Mendez H, Torun B, Schroeder D, Stein AD. Validation of a semi-quantitative food-frequency questionnaire for use among adults in Guatemala. Public Health Nutr. 2002;5:691–9.
43. Mouratidou T, Ford F, Fraser RB. Validation of a food-frequency questionnaire for use in pregnancy. Public Health Nutr. 2006;9:515–22.
44. Deschamps V, De Lauzon-Guillain B, Lafay L, Borys J-M, Charles M-A, Romon M. Reproducibility and relative validity of a food-frequency questionnaire among French adults and adolescents. Eur J Clin Nutr. 2009;63:282–91.
45. Erkkola M, Karppinen M, Javanainen J, Räsänen L, Knip M, Virtanen SM. Validity and reproducibility of a food frequency questionnaire for pregnant Finnish women. Am J Epidemiol. 2001;154:466–76.
46. Henn RL, Fuchs SC, Moreira LB, Fuchs FD. Development and validation of a food frequency questionnaire (FFQ-Porto Alegre) for adolescent, adult and elderly populations from southern Brazil. Cadernos de saude publica. 2010;26:2068–79.
47. Jaceldo-Siegl K, Knutsen SF, Sabaté J, Beeson WL, Chan J, Herring RP, Butler TL, Haddad E, Bennett H, Montgomery S. Validation of nutrient intake using an FFQ and repeated 24 h recalls in black and white subjects of the Adventist health Study-2 (AHS-2). Public Health Nutr. 2010;13:812–9.
48. Wen-Hua Z, Huang Z-P, Zhang X, Li H, Willett W, Jun-Ling W, Hasegawa K, Jun-Shi C. Reproducibility and validity of a chinese food frequency questionnaire. Biomed Environ Sci. 2010;23:1–38.
49. Zhang FF, Roberts SB, Must A, Wong WW, Gilhooly CH, Kelly MJ, Parsons SK, Saltzman E. Assessing dietary intake in childhood Cancer survivors: food frequency questionnaire versus 24-hour diet recalls. J Pediatr Gastroenterol Nutr. 2015;61:499–502.

50. Rimm EB, Giovannucci EL, Stampfer MJ, Colditz GA, Litin LB, Willett WC. Reproducibility and validity of an expanded self-administered semiquantitative food frequency questionnaire among male health professionals. Am J Epidemiol. 1992;135:1114–26.
51. Lombard MJ, Steyn NP, Charlton KE, Senekal M. Application and interpretation of multiple statistical tests to evaluate validity of dietary intake assessment methods. Nutr J. 2015;14:40.
52. Männistö S, Virtanen M, Mikkonen T, Pietinen P. Reproducibility and validity of a food frequency questionnaire in a case-control study on breast Cancer. J Clin Epidemiol. 1996;49:401–9.
53. Cade J, Thompson R, Burley V, Warm D. Development, validation and utilisation of food-frequency questionnaires–a review. Public Health Nutr. 2002;5:567–87.
54. Shim J-S, Oh K, Kim HC. Dietary assessment methods in epidemiologic studies. Epidemiol Health. 2014;36:e2014009.
55. Cantin J, Lacroix S, Latour É, Lambert J, Lalongé J, Faraj M, Nigam A. Validation of a Mediterranean food frequency questionnaire for the population of Québec. Can J Cardiol. 2014;30:S310.
56. Schröder H, Covas M, Marrugat J, Vila J, Pena A, Alcantara M, Masia R. Use of a three-day estimated food record, a 72-hour recall and a food-frequency questionnaire for dietary assessment in a Mediterranean Spanish population. Clin Nutr. 2001;20:429–37.
57. Fernández-Ballart JD, Piñol JL, Zazpe I, Corella D, Carrasco P, Toledo E, Perez-Bauer M, Martínez-González MÁ, Salas-Salvadó J, Martín-Moreno JM. Relative validity of a semi-quantitative food-frequency questionnaire in an elderly Mediterranean population of Spain. Br J Nutr. 2010;103:1808–16.
58. Turcot V, Brunet J, Daneault C, Tardif JC, Des Rosiers C, Lettre G. Validation of fatty acid intakes estimated by a food frequency questionnaire using erythrocyte fatty acid profiling in the Montreal heart institute biobank. J Hum Nutr Diet. 2015;28:646–58.
59. Sauvageot N, Guillaume M, Albert A. Validation of the food frequency questionnaire used to assess the association between dietary habits and cardiovascular risk factors in the NESCAV study. J Food Sci. 2013;3
60. Eng JY, Moy FM. Validation of a food frequency questionnaire to assess dietary cholesterol, total fat and different types of fat intakes among Malay adults. Asia Pac J Clin Nutr. 2011;20:639–45.

6

Hypothesis and data-driven dietary patterns and colorectal Cancer survival: findings from Newfoundland and Labrador colorectal Cancer cohort

Ishor Sharma[1], Barbara Roebothan[1], Yun Zhu[1], Jennifer Woodrow[1], Patrick S. Parfrey[2], John R. Mclaughlin[3] and Peter Peizhong Wang[1*]

Abstract

Background: Dietary patterns are commonly used in epidemiological research, yet there have been few studies assessing if and how research results may vary across dietary patterns. This study aimed to estimate the risk of mortality/recurrence/metastasis using different dietary patterns and comparison amongst the patterns.

Methods: Dietary patterns were identified by Cluster Analysis (CA), Principal Component Analysis (PCA), Alternate Mediterranean Diet score (altMED), Recommended Food Score (RFS) and Dietary Inflammatory Index (DII) scores using a 169-item food frequency questionnaire.

Five hundred thirty-two colorectal cancer patients diagnosed between 1999 and 2003 in Newfoundland were followed-up until 2010. Overall Mortality (OM) and combined Mortality, Recurrence or Metastasis (cMRM) were identified. Comparisons were made with adjusted Cox proportional Hazards Ratios (HRs), correlation coefficients and the distributions of individuals in defined clusters by quartiles of factor and index scores.

Results: One hundred and seventy cases died from all causes and 29 had a cancer recurrence/metastasis during follow-up. Processed meats as classified by PCA (HR 1.82; 95% confidence interval (CI) 1.07–3.09), clusters characterized by meat and dairy products (HR 2.19; 95% CI 1.03–4.67) and total grains, sugar, soft drinks (HR 1.95; 95% CI 1.13–3.37) were associated with a higher risk of cMRM. Poor adherence to AltMED increased the risk of all-cause OM (HR 1.62; 95% CI 1.04–2.56). Prudent vegetable, high sugar pattern, RFS and DII had no significant association with both OM and cMRM.

Conclusion: Estimation of OM and cMRM varied across dietary patterns which is attributed to the differences in the foundation of each pattern.

Keywords: Colorectal Cancer, Dietary patterns, Factor analysis, Cluster analysis, Index analysis

Background

Diet and behavioural factors have crucial roles in the risk and progression of several chronic diseases including colorectal cancer (CRC) [1]. Epidemiological studies on the role of a single nutrient or food items on disease outcome are often inconclusive, which may be in part due to dietary interactions, multi-collinearity [2' 3] and/ or inability to detect small effects [4]. Dietary patterns are advantageous in nutritional epidemiology to explore the combined effects of total diet on health and to some extent, overcome these limitations [5]. Dietary patterns not only represent total diet or key factors of diet [6] and the frequency by which foods are habitually consumed, but also reflect an individual's food preferences modulated by the combination of genetic, cultural, social, health, environmental, behavioural and economic determinants [7].

* Correspondence: pwang@mun.ca
[1]Division of Community Health and Humanities, Faculty of Medicine, Memorial University of Newfoundland, St. John's, NF, Canada

Data-driven and hypothesis-driven are two major approaches to identify dietary patterns [8]. Cluster and factor analysis are outcome independent empirical data-driven techniques used to determine dietary behaviour in the study population, while index/score-based are hypothesis-driven based on adherence to prior recommendations or guidelines [9].

Briefly, cluster analysis (CA) divides individuals into mutually exclusive, non-overlapping groups based on mean dietary intakes (gm) [10]. Food intake common to all contributes less to cluster formation. Optimal clusters are formed by the maximum ratio of variance across the cluster to within the cluster. No gradient is formed hence comparison is done with the reference cluster. Factorial analysis, specifically Principal Component Analysis (PCA), an exploratory approach, reduces a large set of correlated variables to smaller sets of non-correlated variables, which captures the majority of dietary variations within the study population. Linear combinations are created and each individual receives a score called factors [11]. A higher score represents higher adherence to the particular dietary pattern.

Recommended food score (RFS) [12] and alternate Mediterranean diet score (altMED) [13] are commonly used index-based dietary patterns for which scoring is based on the adherence to the US dietary guidelines and the Mediterranean diet, respectively. Dietary Inflammatory Index (DII) differs to other index-based scales as it doesn't directly measure the adherence to the established dietary guidelines; instead, it categorizes an individual's diet into pro- and anti-inflammatory diet based on their dietary response to six inflammatory biomarkers [14]. For such indexes, patterns are derived from gradients, which are then compared to reference quartiles.

Dietary patterns are commonly used in epidemiological research. Studies on how outcome estimation may vary across these different patterns are limited and comparing across the patterns are recommended to better understand disease diet association [15]; however, such studies are limited. This study aimed to use different approaches to identify pre-diagnostic dietary patterns and evaluate and compare their association with the CRC outcome (Overall Mortality (OM) and combined Mortality, Metastasis or Recurrence (cMRM)) using the Newfoundland and Labrador Familial Colorectal Cancer cohort.

Methods

Study population

This study used data from the Newfoundland Familial Colorectal Cancer Registry (NFCCR). Five hundred and thirty-two pathologically confirmed (ICD-9 codes: 153.0–153.9, 154.0–154.3, and 154.8 or ICD-10 codes: 18.0–18.9, 19.9, and 20.9) CRC patients diagnosed between 1999 and 2003 and residents of Newfoundland and Labrador, aged 20–75 years, were included in the study. A detailed description of the study population is published elsewhere [16]. Briefly, CRC cases were followed from the date of diagnosis until April 30th, 2010. Overall Mortality (OM; the time between the dates of diagnosis to end of follow-up, or the date of death from all causes until the end of follow-up) and combined Mortality, Metastasis or Recurrence (cMRM; the time between the dates of diagnosis to the end of follow-up, or date of death, recurrence, or metastasis, whichever came first) were calculated.

Individuals who were lost to follow up, still alive or who did not have a recurrence or metastasis by the end of the follow-up period were censored at the time of the last contact. We conducted follow-up questionnaires with participants and linked records to death certificates, pathology reports, autopsy records, physicians' notes, and surgical reports. Additional data were obtained from the Dr. H. Bliss Murphy Cancer Care Foundation [17]; many of the results can be mutually verified.

Data collection tools

Participants completing the consent were asked to complete validated food frequency questionnaire (FFQ) [18], personal history questionnaire (PHQ) and some further questions pertaining to family history and medical history. Briefly, the PHQ consisted of 74 questions including the history of bowel screening, medical conditions, use of medications, physical activity, intake of alcohol, tobacco use, socio-demographic information, and reproductive factors for females. Similarly, dietary intake data were collected using a 169-item FFQ retrospectively a year before the diagnosis. For each food item, subjects were asked the frequency of food consumption (daily, weekly, monthly and never scales). Nutrient content was calculated using the Canadian Nutrient File, 2005.

MSI (Microsatellite instability) and BRAF have been associated with cancer prognosis and survival [19, 20]. P V600E BRAF mutation and MSI for the tumour DNA have been determined in a previous study using standard protocol [21]. MSI status was defined as MS high if 30% or more of marker were unstable and MS-stable/MS-low if less than 30% showed instability [22].

Identifying dietary patterns

For CA, 169 food items were classified into 39 different food groups depending on the ways they are taken and nutrient profile. Food groupings are attached in the Additional file 1: Table S1. Clusters were identified by using K-means non-hierarchical method, an iterative technique which groups data into k clusters in such a way as to maximize the R2 ($R2 = 1 - W/T$), where W is the sum of squared Euclidean distances between each data point and its within-cluster mean, and T is the sum of squared distances between each data point and the overall mean. FASTCLUS procedure in SAS was applied. Clusters with less than five participants were temporarily removed while forming the stable cluster. A detailed description of cluster formation can be found elsewhere [23]. Overall, four stable clusters were identified. Characteristics of clusters are given in Additional file 1: Table S2.

Three patterns were identified using the PCA correlation matrix as the variables were on different scales. Briefly, exploratory principal component factor analysis was conducted using the same 39 predefined food groups. A varimax rotation (orthogonal) was applied to identify uncorrelated food groups. Factor Eigen-value greater than 1.15, the scree plot and proportion of variance explained were used to identify the number of factors. Patterns were labelled based on factor loading ≥0.5. The factor score of each participant was obtained by summing the intake of each food group multiplied by optimal weights and divided into quartiles. A higher factor score represents greater adherence to that particular dietary pattern. Factor loading and explained variances for three major dietary patterns are shown in Additional file 1: Table S3.

The RFS method developed by Kent, et al. [12] is based on fruits, vegetables, whole grains, lean meats or meat alternatives, and low-fat dairy products. Each individual is given 1 point for each recommended food consumed at least weekly. Based on the FFQ, the maximum score is 47. Total RFS score varies with the number of food items in the FFQ [24]. A higher score represents better adherence to RFS. Details are attached in Additional file 1: Table S4.

The altMED score is based on the Mediterranean diet scale [25]; scoring is based on 9 food groups. If the intake (servings/day) of a particular food group is greater than the median, then it is scored one (versus zero). For red and processed meat, reverse scoring is done. For alcohol, if intake is between 5 and 25 g/d, then it is scored as 1 (versus zero). The maximum altMED score is 9 with a higher score representing better adherence to the altMED diet. Details of the food groups are attached in Additional file 1: Table S5.

Detailed descriptions of the DII score are provided elsewhere [14, 26]. Briefly, a total of 29 nutrient parameters were scored based on their inflammatory response to six inflammatory biomarkers; IL-1β, IL-4, IL-6, IL-10, CRP and tumour necrosis factor (TNF-α). These included carbohydrate, protein, total fat, alcohol, onion, tea, tea (Herbal), pepper, β-carotene, Vitamin B-6, Vitamin B-12, caffeine, cholesterol, energy, fibre, folic acid, iron, Monounsaturated Fatty Acid (MUFA), Polyunsaturated Fatty Acid (PUFA), niacin, magnesium, riboflavin, saturated fatty acid, selenium, thiamine, Vitamin-E, Vitamin-D, vitamin C and zinc. Total DII score obtained is divided into quartiles; higher quartiles represents individuals having diets that are more inflammatory.

Statistical analysis

Adjusted hazards ratios were estimated using Cox proportional hazard analysis using SAS version 9.4 (SAS Institute, Inc. Cary). Comparisons across patterns were made with adjusted HRs, correlation coefficients and distributions of individuals in clusters by quartile of factor and index scores. Potential confounding factors include age; sex; body mass index (BMI) (classified as < 25, 25–29.99, ≥30 kg/m2); physical activity as measured by the Global Physical Activity Questionnaire (GPAQ) [27]; Metabolic equivalent hours/week (METs/Week, calculated and classified as < 10, 10–50, ≥50); and medical history including cholesterol level; triglycerides; family history of CRC; polyps; diabetes; history of screening; smoking (classified: Yes and No; Yes means smoke at least 1 cigarette/day for 3 months or more); alcohol drinking (classified: standard drink/week; not at all, < 15 and ≥ 15); and regular medication including non-steroidal anti-inflammatory drugs (NSAID), stage and grade of cancer, and reported hormone replacement therapy (HRT, females only). Energy adjustment was completed using the residual method wherever applicable.

The basis for assessing potential confounding factors included: existing evidence, biological plausibility, whether the regression coefficient of the primary variable of interest changed by 10% or more after addition of the potentially confounding variable for every covariate entered in the model at $P < 0.10$. Potential confounders were first selected based on the previous studies as well as a literature search. Initially, potential confounders were screened by the univariate test. Those variables that were statistically non-significant in the univariate test but have an important role in the etiology were included in the model selection step as default; those variables included marital status, the location of a tumor, smoking status, physical activity and reported chemotherapy. As there were too many variables, a stepwise procedure was employed in order to include potential confounding variables that have a detectable effect on the association of interest while retaining the above-mentioned variables in the model.

Results

Characteristics of the study population

Mean age of participants and mean age at diagnosis was 62.53 ± 9.06 years and 60.42 ± 9.02 years, respectively. A total of 170 cases died from all causes and 29 had a cancer recurrence or metastasis at the end of the follow-up. Mean time between the date of diagnosis to the end of follow up or date of death from all causes (OM) was 6.27± 1.98 years and mean time between the date of diagnosis to the end of follow up or the date of death, recurrence, or metastasis (CMRM) (whichever came first) was 5.70± 2.38 years). Almost 68% of the participants were censored for OM and 62.6% for cMRM during analysis.

Table 1 presents the characteristics of the study population with the log-rank test. In the univariate test, there is the significant difference in the OM across the age groups, gender, diagnosis stage and microsatellite instability status. The family history of CRC, reported screening status, history of co-morbidity including diabetes, higher blood cholesterol level, a location of a tumour, smoking status, physical activity and reported chemotherapy had no significant association with the survival.

Table 1 Characteristics of study participants with their overall survival status (Univariate); Newfoundland and Labrador Familial Colorectal Cancer Cohort (1999–2003)

Characteristic	No. of patients[a]	No. of deaths (%)	P log-rank
Age at diagnosis			
≤ 60	231	62 (26.83)	
> 60	301	108 (35.88)	0.04
Sex			
Female	211	57 (27.02)	
Male	321	113 (35.20)	0.02
Family history			
Yes	16	6 (37.5)	
No	516	164 (31.78)	0.61
Reported screening procedure			
Yes	68	15 (22.05)	
No	464	155 (33.4)	0.08
Stage at diagnosis			
I/II	311	74 (23.79)	
III/IV	221	96 (43.43)	< 0.001
Diabetes History			
Yes	115	42 (36.52)	0.22
No	417	128 (30.69)	
History of High Cholesterol			
Yes	153	44 (28.75)	
No	349	117 (33.52)	0.44
Tumour location			
Colon	349	105 (30.09)	
Rectum	183	65 (35.51)	0.25
Smoke			
No	139	34 (24.44)	0.07
Yes	393	136 (34.60)	
Physical Activity (Met-hrs/week)			
Low (< 10)	175	52 (29.71)	
Median (10–50)	163	56 (34.35)	0.27
High (50+)	193	62 (32.12)	
MSI status			
MSI-L	440	154 (35.0)	
MSI-H	61	6 (9.83)	< 0.002
Reported chemo Therapy			
Yes	108	42 (38.88)	
No	421	128 (30.40)	0.06

MSI Microsatellite instability, *MSI-L* Microsatellite instability low, *MSI-H* Microsatellite instability High [a]Column total varies due to missing values

Dietary patterns and survival outcome estimation

Table 2 shows the estimated adjusted hazards ratio corresponding to different dietary patterns with 95% confidence interval. Risk of mortality, recurrence and metastasises varied with the dietary pattern. Four different clusters were identified. When compared with the reference cluster characterized by higher intake of fruits, vegetables, whole grains and wine (Cluster I), the cluster characterized by high intake of meat and dairy products (Cluster II) had a higher risk of cMRM (HR 2.19, 95% 1.03–4.67). The cluster characterized by higher intake of refined grains, sugar/soft drinks (Cluster III) had a higher risk of both cMRM (HR 1.95, 95% 1.13–3.37) and OM (HR 2.05, 95% 1.18–3.57) outcomes. The cluster characterized by the many food groups (Cluster IV) had no significant relation with both OM and cMRM; this cluster was based on many foods as no specific distinguishing or dominating food item could be identified.

Three dietary patterns were identified using PCA: processed meat pattern, prudent vegetable pattern and high sugar pattern. Though the overall trend was not significant ($p = 0.09$), the highest quartile of processed meat pattern significantly increases the risk of cMRM (HR 1.82, 95% CI 1.07–3.09), however, there was no significant association with OM. Neither the prudent vegetable pattern nor the high sugar pattern showed a significant association with both cMRM and OM.

While using index-based patterns, DII and RFS showed no significant association with either OM or cMRM outcomes. The lowest quartile of the altMED score was significantly associated with the higher risk of OM (HR 1.62, 95% 1.04–2.56) but had no significant association with the cMRM.

Comparison amongst the dietary patterns

Spearman's correlation coefficients amongst the index-based scores are described in Table 3. Correlations were high and significant because of the similarity in the food items in scoring. A significant positive correlation was observed between RFS and the altMED score (0.60; $p = 0.001$). Significant negative correlations were found between the DII score and the altMED (– 0.601; $p = 0.001$) and RFS (– 0.602; $p = 0.001$) scores.

Table 2 Dietary patterns and Colorectal Cancer Survival (Multivariable adjusted analysis); Newfoundland and Labrador Familial Colorectal Cancer Cohort (1999–2003)

Dietary Pattern Identified by	Combined Mortality, Recurrence and Metastasis		Overall Mortality	
	HR[a] (95% CI)	P-trend	HR (95% CI)	p-trend
Factor Analysis				
Processed Meat pattern[a]	*1.82 (1.07–3.09)**	0.09	1.53 (0.85–2.27)	0.25
Prudent Vegetable Pattern[a]	1.12 (0.69–1.84)	0.62	1.03 (0.61–1.75)	0.90
High-sugar Pattern[a]	1.02 (0.62–1.69)	0.89	1.27 (0.72–2.23)	0.62
Cluster Analysis				
Fruit and Veg, Whole Grain, Fish, wine (Cluster I)	1[c]		1[c]	
Meat, dairy products(Cluster II),	*2.19 (1.03–4.67)**		2.04 (0.96–4.35)	
Refined grains, sugar soft Drinks (Cluster III)	*1.95 (1.13–3.37)**		*2.05 (1.18–3.57)**	
Many foods (Cluster IV)	1.55 (0.92–2.61)		1.50 (0.9–2.56)	
Index Based				
DII[a]	0.89 (0.56–1.42)	0.46	0.78 (0.47–1.25)	0.33
Alt. Mediterranean Diet Score[b]	1.44 (0.92–2.25)	0.08	*1.62 (1.04–2.56)**	0.03
Recommended Food Score[b]	1.51(0.92–2.48)	0.06	1.54 (0.92–2.56)	0.045

[a]Hazards Ratio while comparing with highest quartile to the lowest (reference quartile)
[b]Hazards Ratio while comparing with lowest quartile to highest (reference quartile)
[c]Reference group
*Statistically significant
HR ratios Adjusted for energy, stage of cancer, sex, age, marital status, tumour location, screening history, intake of alcohol, radiation and chemo therapy status, Microsatellite instability status wherever applicable
Events are defined as all-cause deaths for overall Mortality and death/recurrence/metastasis (which occurred earliest) for cMRM

Table 4 examines the percentage of individuals in the highest quartile of factor and index score in different clusters describing some level of similarity in the foundation of scale. Almost 92% of individuals from the processed meat pattern were in Cluster II characterized by meat and dairy products. Approximately 59% of individuals from the highest quartile of the prudent vegetable pattern were in Cluster I characterized by fruits and vegetables, whole grain, fish and wine. Around 35% of individuals in the highest quartile of high sugar pattern were in the many foods group. In all three index-based patterns, the lowest quartile of DII and highest quartile of altMED and RFS showed the higher proportion of individuals from Cluster I characterized by fruits and vegetables, whole grain, fish and wine (64.97, 36.31 and 57.32% respectively).

Table 3 Spearman's Correlation coefficients amongst the index-based score obtained from FFQ; Newfoundland and Labrador Familial Colorectal Cancer Cohort (1999–2003)

	RFS	DII	AltMED Score
RFS	1	−0.61[a]	0.60[a]
		< 0.001	< 0.001
DII		1	−0.61[a]
			< 0.001
AltMED			1

DII Dietary inflammatory Index, *AltMed Diet* Alternate Mediterranean diet, *RFS* Recommended Food Score [a]Significant at 0.05

Discussion

This study is a prospective analysis of mortality among CRC patients diagnosed between 1999 and 2003 from a Canadian population. Both data-driven and hypothesis-driven dietary patterns were determined and relation with CRC patient's mortality, recurrence and metastasises was estimated. The hypothesis-driven pattern showed how study population is adherent to dietary recommendation while data-driven pattern explains how whole population dietary practice can be classified into different categories. As each dietary pattern was designed to answer the different question, the discrepancy in the outcome estimation was expected despite some level of similarity in the foundation of dietary patterns.

In the current study as identified by CA, the meat and dairy product cluster was associated with increased risk of cMRM while the refined grains, sugar, soft drinks cluster was associated with increased risk of both cMRM and OM. A processed meat pattern as identified by PCA was associated with an increased risk of cMRM. Low adherence to the Mediterranean diet was associated with increased OM. RFS and DII had no significant association with the survival outcomes. The magnitude of estimated HR also varied accordingly.

Epidemiological studies reveal inconsistent results while assessing the relation between dietary patterns and disease outcome in the same population, which is in line with the current study. The study by Reedy J; et al. [15] showed that

Table 4 Percentage of individuals in each cluster in highest/lowest quartile of factor/index score; Newfoundland and Labrador Familial Colorectal Cancer Cohort (1999–2003)

	Cluster I	Cluster II	Cluster III	Cluster IV
Characteristics of Cluster	Fruits and Veg, whole grain, fish, wine	Meat, Dairy products, mixed dishes	Sugar/ drinks, total cereals and grains (refined included)	Many foods
Principle Component Analysis[a]				
Processed Meat pattern	15.29	91.89	38.38	16.21
Prudent vegetable pattern	58.60	24.32	6.06	11.46
High Sugar pattern	17.20	10.81	16.16	35.18
Index based				
DII[b]	64.97	13.51	10.1	7.91
AltMed Diet[a]	36.31	8.11	6.06	9.88
RFS[a]	57.32	35.14	13.13	11.86

DII Dietary inflammatory Index, *AltMed Diet* Alternate Mediterranean diet, *RFS* Recommended Food Score [a]Highest Quartile (reference) [b]Lowest Quartile (reference)

among male dietary patterns and clusters characterized by fruits, vegetables, lower fats foods, adherence to RFS and MED diet were associated with reduced risk of CRC. Among females, results were inconsistent: meat and potatoes pattern was associated with increased risk and neither MED nor RFS had a significant association.

In the Nurse's Health study [28] index-based score, AHEI (Alternate Healthy Eating Index) was associated with the lower levels of free oestradiol while no association was found with the patterns identified by factor analysis. In the Health Professionals Follow-up Study cohort, the risk of incident fatal or nonfatal myocardial infarction and stroke (CVD) in the highest quintile of the HEI, alternate HEI, and RFS, respectively, were 28, 39, and 23% lower [29] than the reference quartile, while the highest quintile of a prudent diet score from factor analysis was 30% [30]. While estimating the survival outcome using different dietary pattern, a prospective Danish observational study [31] showed that a prudent diet pattern obtained by PCA was associated with reduced mortality but index-based patterns had no significant association. In the SENECA study, the index based scales including Mediterranean Diet Score (MDS), the Mediterranean Adequacy Index (MDI) and the Healthy Diet Indicator (HDI) showed an inverse association with all-cause mortality [32].

The current study suggested good evidence of comparability between PCA and CA in identifying the dietary pattern as seen in other studies [33, 34] despite their different approach. Almost two-thirds of individuals in the fruit and vegetable cluster (Cluster I) were from the highest quartile of the prudent vegetable pattern identified by PCA having highest loading (> 0.50) for fruits, vegetables, greens, tomatoes and minimal loadings (< 0.15) for processed meat, red meat and refined foods. More than 90% of individuals in Cluster II, characterized by meat and dairy products, were from the highest quartile of the processed meat pattern identified by PCA having higher loading (> 0.5) for red meat, cured processed meat. Similar was the case with other clusters. Despite good evidence of comparability, they are not defined by the same foods, which is likely to be the reason for differential disease outcome estimates.

The hypothesis-driven dietary patterns give higher weight for fruits and vegetables, which is evident by having the majority of individuals in the lowest quartile of DII and the highest quartile of altMED and RFS in Cluster I, characterized by fruits and vegetables. Correlations between index scores were relatively strong and statistically significant as scores were based on similar food recommendations. An increasing score of altMED, RFS and a decrease in DII score are characterized by the higher amount of plant-based food [35].

Indexing systems vary in the definition of optimal diet quality and in their scoring which leads difference in their sensitivity to estimate the disease outcome. Differential classification of food leads to differential exposure. RFS accounts for intake of vegetables, fruits, healthy protein sources, grains and dairy products but does not differentiate between different types of fatty acids or penalize for consumption of foods that are not recommended. Alcohol, energy dense food items and meat products are associated with survival outcomes as seen from empirical approaches but are not considered in scoring. Hence, RFS is likely to underestimate the true association. Further, in the RFS approach, energy cannot be adjusted so the effect of body size, physical activity and higher basal metabolic rate cannot be taken into account for the analysis [36]. Energy adjustment may also help to reduce measurement error [37]. AltMED scoring is based on high consumption of fruits, vegetables, non-refined bread and cereals, legumes and nuts, and moderate consumption of fish, poultry and alcohol. High intake of red and processed meat and saturated fat is penalized during scoring [25]. DII score is based on the inflammatory potential of nutrient/food items in response to the six inflammatory biomarkers. DII is relevant among those diseases associated with chronic inflammation [14]. DII is not only limited to micro and macronutrients but also incorporates commonly used bioactive compounds including flavonoids, spices and tea. Since the current study was based on pre-diagnostic dietary pattern, dietary-induced inflammation may not have a significant role in the risk of mortality.

Multiple reasons could be suggested for the inconsistent results. First, several studies have suggested dietary guidelines have been more strongly related to coronary heart disease than to cancer mortality, even though guidelines are directed toward lowering cancer risk [38]. More extensive studies are done on diet-cardiovascular disease than cancer, and the role of dietary components in cancer causation is still unclear in many instances [29]. Second, dietary guidelines are more effective for cancer incidence than the survival (and therefore mortality) due to the other clinic-pathological factors in determining the cancer survival [38]. Third, the inconsistency might also be due to missing some important components, and some components in the scales may not have a significant association with the cancer risk and survival [29]. Also, our approximation of the three scales varied slightly than the original scale. Original RFS had 23 items and was developed for the all-cause mortality rather than cancer-specific mortality [12]. Likewise, altMED score was developed to assess the variations in the biomarkers level [39] and DII index was based on 45 different food parameters whilst the current study had only 28 parameters [14].

Each method has its own strengths and limitations [6]. Empirical methods are an initial approach and identify dietary patterns as they exist in the population [40] and form the basis for index-based patterns, but suffer certain limitations: (a) They are based on eating behaviour rather than the biological plausibility hence the diet pattern may not exactly reflect disease causation theory [40]; (b) Even though an association is detected, it may not represent beneficial or detrimental eating patterns [41]; (c) Lacks limited reproducibility across the studies [4]; and (d) Includes several arbitrary decisions including consolidation of food items into food groups, number of factors/clusters, method of rotations and labelling of the patterns/clusters [42]. Index-based patterns are based on adherence to the recommendation or guidelines and the foundation of each scale varies. Index-based patterns are generally considered better at estimating the disease outcome as compared to empirical patterns due to their inclusion of relevant and evidence-based components [43]. Results tend to be reproducible across studies. They are limited, however, in that they do not capture a full range of diets in scoring [40] and are difficult to use when scores do not vary considerably within the population [6] and results vary with the cut-offs defined.

Strengths and limitations of study

This is a prospective follow-up study. Detailed data for the variables (age; sex; marital status; Body Mass Index; screening history; use of medications; co-morbidity status; history of CRC; smoking; physical activity; dietary patterns; alcohol intake; stage and location of tumor; chemotherapy status; etc.) are available including the genetic data on MSI status. Multiple dietary patterns are used for comparison.

This study has a number of limitations. First, the sample is relatively small, which may not offer desirable statistical power and precision in multivariate analysis. Further, cases were followed until 2010 only. Recall error and possible bias are likely to exist as the cases were asked to remember their dietary patterns a year prior to their diagnosis. However, we believe the recall bias, if any, could be non-differential, which is likely to attenuate the observed association. Although bias may exist and sample size is less, it may have little impact on cross-comparison, which is the primary focus of the study. Some cases might have changed their dietary patterns, lifestyle and behaviour after diagnosis or even in the disease induction/latent period; this may lead to possible reverse causation bias, which should be explored in future studies.

Conclusions

The present study showed that the estimation of OM and cMRM amongst the CRC patients varied with the type of diet pattern used. Hazards ratios for cMRM varied from 1.82; 95% (CI- 1.07-3.09) for processed meat pattern identified by PCA to HR 2.19; 95% CI 1.03–4.67 for cluster characterized by meat and dairy products and HR 1.95; 95% CI 1.13–3.37 for cluster characterized by refined grains, sugar, soft drinks. Only cluster characterized by refined grains, sugar, soft drinks had higher risk of OM (HR 2.05; 95% CI 1.18–3.57). All the diet indices showed similar null associations with both cMRM and OM except Poor adherence to altMED increased the risk of all-cause OM (HR 1.62; 95% CI 1.04–2.56). On the average estimates were higher for data driven methods than hypothesis driven. The variations in the estimated hazards ratios is attributed to the foundation of each dietary pattern identified by various approaches.

Abbreviations

altMED: Alternative Mediterranean diet; BMI: Body mass index; CA: Cluster analysis; CI: Confidence interval; cMRM: Combined mortality, recurrence and metastasis; CRC: Colorectal cancer; DII: Dietary inflammatory index; FFQ: Food frequency questionnaire; FHQ: Family history questionnaire; HRT: Hormone replacement therapy; MUFA: Monounsaturated fatty acid; NFCCR: Newfoundland familial colorectal cancer registry; NL: Newfoundland and Labrador; NSAID: Non-steroidal anti-inflammatory drug; OM: Overall mortality; OR: Odds ratios; PCA: Principal Component analysis; PHQ: Personal history questionnaire; PUFA: Polyunsaturated fatty acid; RFS: Recommended food score

Acknowledgments
We are thankful to Dr. Meera Jain and all those who contributed to data collection and management for the Newfoundland and Labrador Familial Colorectal Cancer Study.

Financial support
The initial phase of data collection and management was supported by the Canadian Institutes of Health Research Team Grant [CIHR-CPT79845] and Canadian Institutes of Health Research Team in Interdisciplinary Research on Colorectal Cancer Studentship [205835]. Ishor Sharma was awarded by the Newfoundland and Labrador Healthy Aging Research Program (NL-HARP) and Translational and Personalized Medicine Initiative (TPMI, NL SUPPORT).

Authors' contributions
PPW and IS conceived and designed this study. IS analysed the data and drafted the manuscript. PPW, BR, YZ, JW, PSP and JRM revised the manuscript. All authors read and approved the final manuscript.

Competing interests
The authors declare that they have no competing interests.

Author details
[1]Division of Community Health and Humanities, Faculty of Medicine, Memorial University of Newfoundland, St. John's, NF, Canada. [2]Clinical Epidemiology Unit, Faculty of Medicine, Memorial University of Newfoundland, St. John's, NF, Canada. [3]Public Health Ontario, Toronto, ON, Canada.

References
1. World Cancer Research Fund/American Institute for Cancer Research: Chapter 7. Cancers. In food, nutrition, physical activity and the prevention of Cancer: a global perspective. Washington DC: AICR; 2007.
2. Shivappa N, Zucchetto A, Montella M, Serraino D, Steck SE, La Vecchia C, Hébert JR. Inflammatory potential of diet and risk of colorectal cancer: a case–control study from Italy. Br J Nutr. 2015;114(01):152–8.
3. Galas A, Kulig J. Low-grade dietary-related inflammation and survival after colorectal cancer surgery. J Cancer Res Clin Oncol. 2014;140(9):1517–25.
4. Miller PE, Lazarus P, Lesko SM, Muscat JE, Harper G, Cross AJ, Sinha R, Ryczak K, Escobar G, Mauger DT. Diet index-based and empirically derived dietary patterns are associated with colorectal cancer risk. J Nutr. 2010;140(7):1267–73.
5. Committee DGA. Report of the dietary guidelines advisory committee on the dietary guidelines for Americans, 2010, to the secretary of agriculture and the secretary of health and human services. Agric Res Serv. 2010;
6. Moeller SM, Reedy J, Millen AE, Dixon LB, Newby P, Tucker KL, Krebs-Smith SM, Guenther PM. Dietary patterns: challenges and opportunities in dietary patterns research: an experimental biology workshop, April 1, 2006. J Am Diet Assoc. 2007;107(7):1233–9.
7. van den Bree MB, Eaves LJ, Dwyer JT. Genetic and environmental influences on eating patterns of twins aged≥ 50 y. Am J Clin Nutr. 1999;70(4):456–65.
8. Previdelli ÁN, de Andrade SC, Fisberg RM, Marchioni DM. Using two different approaches to assess dietary patterns: hypothesis-driven and data-driven analysis. Nutrients. 2016;8(10):593.
9. Nettleton JA, Schulze MB, Jiang R, Jenny NS, Burke GL, Jacobs DR. A priori–defined dietary patterns and markers of cardiovascular disease risk in the multi-ethnic study of atherosclerosis (MESA). Am J Clin Nutr. 2008;88(1):185–94.
10. Quatromoni P, Copenhafer D, Demissie S, D'agostino R, O'horo C, Nam B, Millen B. The internal validity of a dietary pattern analysis. The Framingham nutrition studies. J Epidemiol Community Health. 2002;56(5):381–8.
11. Kleinbaum D, Kupper L, Muller K. Variable reduction and factor analysis. Applied regression analysis and other multivariable methods. 1988;24:605.
12. Kant AK, Schatzkin A, Graubard BI, Schairer C. A prospective study of diet quality and mortality in women. JAMA. 2000;283(16):2109–15.
13. Trichopoulou A, Costacou T, Bamia C, Trichopoulos D. Adherence to a Mediterranean diet and survival in a Greek population. N Engl J Med. 2003;348(26):2599–608.
14. Shivappa N, Steck SE, Hurley TG, Hussey JR, Hébert JR. Designing and developing a literature-derived, population-based dietary inflammatory index. Public Health Nutr. 2014;17(08):1689–96.
15. Reedy J, Wirfält E, Flood A, Mitrou PN, Krebs-Smith SM, Kipnis V, Midthune D, Leitzmann M, Hollenbeck A, Schatzkin A. Comparing 3 dietary pattern methods—cluster analysis, factor analysis, and index analysis—with colorectal cancer risk the NIH–AARP diet and health study. Am J Epidemiol. 2010;171(4):479–87.
16. Sun Z, Liu L, Wang PP, Roebothan B, Zhao J, Dicks E, Cotterchio M, Buehler S, Campbell PT, Mclaughlin JR. Association of total energy intake and macronutrient consumption with colorectal cancer risk: results from a large population-based case-control study in Newfoundland and Labrador and Ontario, Canada. Nutr J. 2012;11(1):18.
17. Lee H, Song M, Shin N, Shin CH, Min BS, Kim HS, Yoo JS, Kim H. Diagnostic significance of serum HMGB1 in colorectal carcinomas. PLoS One. 2012;7(4):e34318.
18. Liu L, Wang PP, Roebothan B, Ryan A, Tucker CS, Colbourne J, Baker N, Cotterchio M, Yi Y, Sun G. Assessing the validity of a self-administered food-frequency questionnaire (FFQ) in the adult population of Newfoundland and Labrador, Canada. Nutr J. 2013;12(1):49.
19. Guastadisegni C, Colafranceschi M, Ottini L, Dogliotti E. Microsatellite instability as a marker of prognosis and response to therapy: a meta-analysis of colorectal cancer survival data. Eur J Cancer. 2010;46(15):2788–98.
20. Shaukat A, Arain M, Thaygarajan B, Bond JH, Sawhney M. Is BRAF mutation associated with interval colorectal cancers? Dig Dis Sci. 2010;55(8):2352–6.
21. Raptis S, Mrkonjic M, Green RC, Pethe W, Monga N, Chan YM, Daftary D, Dicks E, Younghusband BH, Parfrey PS. MLH1–93G> a promoter polymorphism and the risk of microsatellite-unstable colorectal cancer. J Natl Cancer Inst. 2007;99(6):463–74.
22. Phipps AI, Baron J, Newcomb PA. Prediagnostic smoking history, alcohol consumption, and colorectal cancer survival. Cancer. 2011;117(21):4948–57.
23. SAS Institute Inc. SAS/STAT® 93 User's Guide. Cary: SAS Institute Inc.; 2011. pp. 2241–2266.
24. Reedy J, Mitrou P, Krebs-Smith S, Wirfalt E, Flood A, Kipnis V, Leitzmann M, Mouw T, Hollenbeck A, Schatzkin A, Subar AF. Index-based dietary patterns and risk of colorectal cancer: the NIH-AARP Diet and Health Study. Am J Epidemiol. 2008;168:38–48.
25. Trichopoulou A, Kouris-Blazos A, Wahlqvist ML, Gnardellis C, Lagiou P, Polychronopoulos E, Vassilakou T, Lipworth L, Trichopoulos D. Diet and overall survival in elderly people. BMJ. 1995;311(7018):1457–60.
26. Sharma I, Wang PP, Zhu Y, Woodrow JR, Mulay S, Parfrey PS, Mclaughlin JR, Hebert JR, Shivappa N, Li Y. Inflammatory diet and risk of colorectal cancer: a population based case-control study in Newfoundland, Canada. Nutrition. 2017;42:69–74.
27. Craig CL, Marshall AL, Sjorstrom M, Bauman AE, Booth ML, Ainsworth BE, Pratt M, Ekelund U, Yngve A, Sallis JF. International physical activity questionnaire: 12-country reliability and validity. Med Sci Sports Exerc. 2003;35(8):1381–95.
28. Fung TT, Willett WC, Stampfer MJ, Manson JE, Hu FB. Dietary patterns and the risk of coronary heart disease in women. Arch Intern Med. 2001;161(15):1857–62.
29. McCullough ML, Feskanich D, Rimm EB, Giovannucci EL, Ascherio A, Variyam JN, Spiegelman D, Stampfer MJ, Willett WC. Adherence to the dietary guidelines for Americans and risk of major chronic disease in men. Am J Clin Nutr. 2000;72(5):1223–31.
30. Menotti A, Kromhout D, Blackburn H, Fidanza F, Buzina R, Nissinen A. Food intake patterns and 25-year mortality from coronary heart disease: cross-cultural correlations in the seven countries study. Eur J Epidemiol. 1999;15(6):507–15.
31. Osler M, Heitmann BL, Gerdes LU, Jørgensen LM, Schroll M. Dietary patterns and mortality in Danish men and women: a prospective observational study. Br J Nutr. 2001;85(02):219–25.
32. Knoops K, Fidanza F, Alberti-Fidanza A, Kromhout D, Van Staveren W. Comparison of three different dietary scores in relation to 10-year mortality in elderly European subjects: the HALE project. Eur J Clin Nutr. 2006;60(6):746–55.

33. Hearty ÁP, Gibney MJ. Comparison of cluster and principal component analysis techniques to derive dietary patterns in Irish adults. Br J Nutr. 2008;101(4):598–608.
34. Smith AD, Emmett P, Newby P, Northstone K. A comparison of dietary patterns derived by cluster and principal components analysis in a UK cohort of children. Eur J Clin Nutr. 2011;65(10):1102–9.
35. Steck SE, Guinter M, Zheng J, Thomson CA. Index-based dietary patterns and colorectal cancer risk: a systematic review. Adv Nutr: An Int Rev J. 2015;6(6):763–73.
36. Willett W, Stampfer MJ. Total energy intake: implications for epidemiologic analyses. Am J Epidemiol. 1986;124(1):17–27.
37. Kipnis V, Subar AF, Midthune D, Freedman LS, Ballard-Barbash R, Troiano RP, Bingham S, Schoeller DA, Schatzkin A, Carroll RJ. Structure of dietary measurement error: results of the OPEN biomarker study. Am J Epidemiol. 2003;158(1):14–21.
38. Cerhan J, Potter J, Gilmore J, Janney C, Kushi L, Lazovich D, Anderson K, Sellers T, Folsom A. Adherence to AICR cancer prevention guidelines and subsequent morbidity and mortality in the Iowa women's health study cohort. In: CANCER EPIDEMIOLOGY BIOMARKERS & PREVENTION: 2001: AMER ASSOC cancer research PO box 11806, BIRMINGHAM, al 35202 USA; 2001. p. 158.
39. Fung TT, McCullough ML, Newby P, Manson JE, Meigs JB, Rifai N, Willett WC, Hu FB. Diet-quality scores and plasma concentrations of markers of inflammation and endothelial dysfunction. Am J Clin Nutr. 2005;82(1):163–73.
40. Hu FB. Dietary pattern analysis: a new direction in nutritional epidemiology. Curr Opin Lipidol. 2002;13(1):3–9.
41. Fung TT, Brown LS. Dietary patterns and the risk of colorectal cancer. Curr Nutr Rep. 2013;2(1):48–55.
42. Martinez ME, Marshall JR, Sechrest L. The arbitrary nature of the factor analytical process. Am J Epidemiol. 1998;148(1):17–9.
43. Schulze MB, Hoffmann K, Kroke A, Boeing H. Risk of hypertension among women in the EPIC-Potsdam study: comparison of relative risk estimates for exploratory and hypothesis-oriented dietary patterns. Am J Epidemiol. 2003;158(4):365–73.

Beverage consumption patterns among 4–19 y old children in 2009–14 NHANES show that the milk and 100% juice pattern is associated with better diets

Matthieu Maillot[1], Colin D. Rehm[2], Florent Vieux[1], Chelsea M. Rose[3] and Adam Drewnowski[3*]

Abstract

Background: Patterns of beverage consumption among children and adolescents can be indicative of food choices and total diet quality.

Methods: Analyses of beverage consumption patterns among 8119 children aged 4–19 y were based on the first 24-h recall of the National Health and Nutrition Examination Survey (2009–14 NHANES). Four pre-defined beverage patterns were: 1) milk pattern; 2) 100% juice pattern; 3) milk and 100% juice pattern; and 4) other caloric beverages. Food- and nutrient-based diet quality measures included the Healthy Eating Index 2010.

Results: Most children drank other caloric beverages, as opposed to milk (17.8%), 100% juice (5.6%), or milk and 100% juice (13.5%). Drinkers of milk and 100% juice had diets that did not differ from each other in total calories, total and added sugars, fiber, or vitamin E. Milk drinkers consumed more dairy and had higher intakes of calcium, potassium, vitamin A and vitamin D as compared to all other patterns. Juice drinkers consumed more total fruit, same amounts of whole fruit, and had higher intakes of vitamin C as compared to the other consumption patterns. Drinkers of both milk and 100% juice had the highest HEI 2010 scores of all the consumption patterns.

Conclusions: Beverage consumption patterns built around milk and/or 100% juice were relatively uncommon. Promoting the drinking of milk and 100% juice, in preference to other caloric beverages, may be an effective strategy to improve children's diet quality. Restricting milk and 100% juice consumption may encourage the selection of other caloric beverages.

Keywords: Milk, 100% juice, Beverage consumption, Children, Diet quality

Background

The place of milk and 100% fruit juice in U.S. children's diets continues to be a topic of debate [1]. The consumption of whole milk and 100% fruit juice by young children has been linked to higher body weight in some studies [2, 3], though not in others [4, 5]. To prevent excess weight gain, the American Academy of Pediatrics (AAP) recommends that children switch to low-fat or non-fat milk after the age of 2 y [6]. The AAP has also set limits on the consumption of 100% juices. The suggested amounts are 4–6 oz./d for children aged 4–6 y and up to 8 oz./d for children aged 7–18 y [7].

The current trend in nutritional epidemiology is to examine food and beverage patterns as opposed to individual nutrients, foods, or dietary ingredients [8–12]. Most published studies have explored children's beverage consumption, a dependent variable, by gender, age subgroup, household income, or race/ethnicity [13–15]. Classifying children by their beverage consumption patterns is a relatively novel approach.

The present analyses, based on the three most recent cycles of the National Health and Nutrition Examination Survey (NHANES 2009–2014), identified children aged

* Correspondence: adamdrew@uw.edu
[3]Center for Public Health Nutrition, University of Washington, Box 353410, Seattle, WA 98195, USA
Full list of author information is available at the end of the article

4–19 y whose beverage drinking patterns were built around 1) milk and milk beverages, 2) 100% juices, and 3) milk and 100% juices. Their diet quality was then compared to that of children who drank other caloric beverages in preference to milk or 100% juice.

The primary hypothesis was that beverage drinking patterns characterized by milk and/or 100% juice would be associated with better dietary choices and higher quality diets. The secondary hypothesis was that beverage patterns featuring both milk and 100% juice would be associated with best dietary nutritional profiles and with highest Healthy Eating Index (HEI 2010) scores, a composite measure of diet quality.

Methods

The 2009–14 NHANES sample

Dietary intake data came from 3 cycles of the National Health and Nutrition Examination Survey (2009–10, 2011–12 and 2013–14 NHANES). Data from 2013 to 2014 NHANES were released in October 2016. Data analyses, based on the first-day single 24-h recall, were conducted for the entire population (4–19 y, n = 8119) and separately by age group: 4–8 y, 9–13 y, and 14–19 y.

Dietary intake assessment

The NHANES 24-h recall multi-pass method, conducted by a trained interviewer [16, 17], captured types and amounts of all food and beverages consumed during the previous 24-h, along with the time and occasion for each food item. For children aged 4–5 y the dietary recall was completed by a proxy respondent (parent or guardian). For children 6–11 y, the child was the primary respondent, but a proxy respondent was present and able to assist. Children aged 12–19 y were the primary respondents, but could be assisted by an adult when needed.

Classification of beverages

Beverages were classified into 14 categories following the USDA coding scheme: milk and milk beverages, citrus juices, apple juices (including fruit juice blends), other non-citrus juices, soda (regular & diet), fruit drinks (regular & diet), sports and energy drinks (regular & diet), vegetable juice, water (bottled & tap), flavored and enhanced water, alcoholic beverages, coffee, tea, and meal replacement beverages (See Additional file 1: Table S1).

The milk category included whole milk, 2%, 1%, skim, flavored milk, and nutritionally equivalent milk alternatives, but excluded milkshakes, eggnog, and Yoo-Hoo type milk drinks. Milk consumers were defined as those consuming milk as a beverage, and not e.g. with cereal, using NHANES food combination codes.

The 100% juices included citrus juices, apple juice, and non-citrus juices, and vegetable juices. The 100% fruit juice blends (e.g. apple-cranberry) were included but sweetened fruit-based drinks with added sugars were not. All the remaining beverages were classified as "other." Drinking water (bottled and tap) was excluded, as were alcohol and meal replacements.

Classification of beverage consumption patterns

Children can consume multiple beverages within a 24-h period. Beverage consumption patterns were categorized into 4 groups 1) milk and milk beverages pattern (no 100% juice); 2) 100% juice pattern (no milk); 3) milk and 100% juice pattern; and 4) other beverages pattern. To be assigned to the milk and/or 100% juice patterns, the consumption of milk and/or 100% juice (separate or joint) had to exceed the consumption of all other caloric beverages. A similar method had been used to identify drinkers of regular and diet sodas [18]. The groups were characterized as 1) milk drinkers; 2) 100% juice drinkers; 3) milk and 100% juice drinkers and 4) drinkers of other caloric beverages. Given the widespread use of caloric beverages, we expected the milk and/or 100% juice beverage patterns to be relatively infrequent.

Analytic approach

Dietary outcomes of interest were: dietary energy (kcal), total sugars (grams), added sugars (teaspoon equivalents), calcium (mg), vitamin D (mcg), vitamin A (IU), vitamin E (mcg), vitamin C (mg), potassium (mg), and fiber (g). Food groups of interest were dairy products (milk, yogurts and cheese), total fruit (whole fruit and fruit juice) and whole fruit, and total vegetables. The Healthy Eating Index 2010 (HEI 2010) was the principal measure of diet quality. The HEI measures compliance with the Dietary Guidelines for Americans along a 100-point scale and food group components are represented as "cup-equivalents." For example, 1 cup-equivalent of milk or juice equals 1 cup (237 ml).

All analyses accounted for the complex survey design of NHANES data and are representative of the US population. Data analyses were conducted using Stata 13.1 (College Station, TX) and SAS 9.4 (SAS institute, Cary, NC).

Funding

Funding for these analyses of publicly available federal data was provided by the Dr. Pepper Snapple group.

Results

Four out of five children (82.0%) drank multiple beverages on the same day. Out of 8119 children, 1209 (17.8%) showed the milk pattern; 543 (5.6%) showed the 100% juice pattern, and 1081 (13.5%) showed the milk and 100% juice pattern. The majority of children (5286 or 63.2%) drank other caloric beverages, with smaller amounts of milk, juice, or both.

Beverage patterns

The NHANES sample was evenly split between boys (4160 or 51.0%) and girls (3959 or 49.0%). Beverage consumption patterns varied by gender ($p = 0.0008$) and age group ($p < 0.001$). The milk pattern was more common among boys than among girls (54.1 vs. 45.9%); the 100% juice pattern was more common among girls than among boys (57.7 vs. 42.3%), consistent with past studies [19–21]. Other caloric beverages were consumed equally by both boys and girls (49.6% male vs. 50.4% female). The prevalence of the milk and 100% juice pattern dropped precipitously with age (from 60.8 to 14.3%), whereas the consumption of other caloric beverages increased (21.4 to 48.0%), doubling from the 4–8 y to the 14–19 y age group.

Milk drinkers drank 511.4 g of milk (95% CI: 478.8, 544.1) and 151.2 g of other beverages (95% CI: 127.5, 174.9), but no 100% juice. Juice drinkers drank 404.3 g of juice (95% CI: 365.7, 442.9) and 102.8 g of other beverages (95% CI: 78.4, 127.1) but no milk. Milk and juice drinkers drank 376.5 g of milk (95% CI: 350.4, 402.5), 274.5 g of juice (95% CI: 258.2, 290.7) and 155.2 g of other beverages (95% CI: 135.9, 174.4). Most children (63%) drank large volumes of other beverages (758.7 g (95% CI:729.8, 787.6)) but negligible amounts of either milk (89.3 g (95% CI: 80.7, 98.0)) or 100% juice (38.2 g (95%CI: 31.4, 45.1)).

Milk drinkers derived 15.3% of energy from milk; juice drinkers derived 11.6% energy from 100% juice. Drinkers of milk and juice derived 17.6% energy from those two beverages combined. No significant relation with age was observed. By contrast the amounts of other caloric beverages increased sharply with age: from 11.8% energy in young children to 15.1% energy in adolescents. Children who drank 100% juice had energy intakes that were lower when compared to drinkers of other beverages.

Drinkers of milk and 100% juice consumed amounts of 100% juice that were close to AAP guidelines: 250 g for 4–8 y (95% CI: 231.4, 268.9), 270 g for 9–13 y (95% CI: 253.0, 285.6) and 386 g for 14–19 y (95% CI: 313.5, 460.1). The age-related increase in consumption was modest for milk drinkers (milk 457 to 610 g, p for trend < 0.001) and for 100% juice drinkers (FJ 346 to 477 g, p for trend $= 0.007$), but very sharp for other beverages (502 to 950 g, p for trend < 0.001).

Diet quality among the beverage patterns

Table 1 shows that children classified as milk drinkers had diets with 3.44 cup-eq/day of dairy, largely from milk (2.53 cup-eq). Their consumption of milk (but not yogurt or cheese) was higher compared to 100% juice drinkers (0.47 cup-eq, $p < 0.001$) or drinkers of other beverages (0.83 cup-eq, $p < 0.001$).

Children classified as 100% juice drinkers had diets with 2.31 cup-eq of total fruit (including 0.68 cup-eq whole fruit). Importantly, their diets were not reduced in whole fruit. Milk drinkers and juice drinkers ate comparable amounts of vegetables ($p = 0.999$).

Drinkers of milk and 100% juice had diets with 2.85 cup-eq of dairy, 2.02 cup-eq of total fruit, including 0.89 cup-eq of whole fruit. This group also had the highest HEI 2010 scores (55.70), compared to juice drinkers (52.44, $p = 0.005$), milk drinkers (49.65, $p < 0.001$) and to children who drank neither milk nor 100% juice (44.36, $p < 0.001$).

Figure 1 shows that comparable effects were observed across all age groups. Drinkers of milk, 100% juice or both had higher quality diets as compared to drinkers of other caloric beverages. Drinkers of both milk and 100% juice had the highest HEI 2010 scores.

Table 1 also shows that there were no significant differences between milk and 100% juice drinkers in terms of total energy (1924 vs. 1798 kcal/d, $p = 0.241$); total sugars (108.6 vs. 109.3 g, $p = 0.153$); added sugars (13.4 vs. 11.0 tsp-eq, $p = 0.250$), or fiber (14.8 vs. 14.5 g, $p = 0.999$). Milk drinkers consumed more calcium (1379 mg vs 920 mg), vitamin A (792 vs. 499 IU, $p < 0.001$) and vitamin D (9.1 vs. 3.9 mcg, $p < 0.001$) than did juice drinkers. Diets of juice drinkers were higher in vitamin C (144 vs. 47 mg, $p < 0.001$). There were no differences in vitamin E ($p = 0.999$).

Children classified as drinkers of milk and 100% juice had more nutrient-rich diets than did drinkers of either milk or 100% juice alone. Their potassium intakes were higher than for the other 3 beverage patterns ($p < 0.001$), calcium was higher than for juice ($p < 0.001$) or for other beverages ($p < 0.001$). Intakes of calcium ($p < 0.029$), vitamin A ($p < 0.001$), and vitamin D ($p < 0.001$) were higher than for milk drinkers. The diet's content of vitamin C (118 mg/d) was higher than for milk drinkers (47 mg/d, $p < 0.001$) but not as high as for juice (144 mg/d, $p < 0.001$). Drinkers of other beverages had the highest-energy diets with most added sugar.

HEI 2010 scores were highest for the milk and 100% juice pattern (55.70), followed by the juice pattern (52.44), and then by milk pattern (49.65) and other beverages (44.36).

Figure 2 shows that the drinkers of milk and 100% juice had the highest HEI 2010 scores. Whereas milk-based patterns provided more calcium, juice based patterns were associated with more vitamin C. Drinking both milk and juice was associated with higher levels of calcium and vitamin C. By contrast, beverage patterns built around other caloric beverages provided the most

Table 1 Food patterns, energy, and selected nutrients for drinkers of milk, 100% juice, milk and 100% juice, and other beverages NHANES 2011–2014: Ages 4-19 y [*n* = 8119]

	Milk Pattern			100% Juice Pattern			Milk and 100% Juice Pattern			Other Beverages Pattern			p^a	Ad^b
	n = 1209			*n* = 543			*n* = 1081			*n* = 5286				
	Mean	95% CI		Mean	95% CI		Mean	95% CI		Mean	95% CI			
Food groups and HEI														
Total Dairy (cup-eq)	3.44	3.25	3.63	1.30	1.13	1.48	2.85	2.69	3.01	1.76	1.70	1.83	*<.001*	*<.001*
Milk (cup-eq)	2.53	2.39	2.67	0.47	0.42	0.52	2.00	1.87	2.13	0.83	0.79	0.87	*<.001*	*<.001*
Yogurts (cup-eq)	0.05	0.03	0.06	0.04	0.02	0.06	0.09	0.06	0.12	0.04	0.03	0.05	*0.007*	*0.012*
Cheese (cup-eq)	0.84	0.74	0.94	0.78	0.62	0.94	0.75	0.65	0.84	0.88	0.83	0.93	*0.034*	*0.120*
Total Fruits (cup-eq)	0.72	0.65	0.80	2.31	2.15	2.48	2.02	1.92	2.12	0.82	0.74	0.89	*<.001*	*<.001*
Whole Fruits (cup-eq)	0.70	0.62	0.77	0.68	0.55	0.81	0.89	0.81	0.97	0.60	0.54	0.67	*<.001*	*0.001*
Total vegetable (cup-eq)	0.91	0.81	1.00	0.86	0.75	0.96	0.91	0.82	1.00	0.99	0.95	1.03	*0.034*	*0.33*
HEI 2010	49.65	48.79	50.51	52.44	51.09	53.79	55.70	54.36	57.04	44.36	43.69	45.02	*<.001*	*<.001*
Energy and nutrients														
Energy (kcal)	1924	1828	2020	1798	1718	1879	1998	1933	2063	2029	1991	2066	*<.001*	–
Total sugars (g)	109	104	113	109	103	115	133	129	137	130	127	134	*<.001*	*<.001*
Added sugars (teaspoon eq)	13	13	14	11	10	12	14	13	15	23	22	24	*<.001*	*<.001*
Fiber (g)	15	14	16	15	14	15	15	15	16	14	14	14	*0.008*	*<.001*
Calcium (mg)	1379	1308	1450	920	837	1004	1314	1262	1366	934	909	958	*<.001*	*<.001*
Potassium (mg)	2475	2339	2611	2182	2069	2295	2713	2629	2796	2100	2058	2142	*<.001*	*<.001*
Vitamin A (IU)	796	753	839	499	461	538	698	660	736	527	510	545	*<.001*	*<.001*
Vitamin C (mg)	47	40	54	144	130	158	118	111	124	70	66	75	*<.001*	*<.001*
Vitamin D (mcg)	9	9	10	4	3	4	8	8	9	4	4	4	*<.001*	*<.001*
Vitamin E (mcg)	7	6	8	7	6	7	7	6	7	7	7	8	*0.032*	*0.008*

[a]unadjusted regression models
[b]regression models adjusted for gender, poverty level and total dietary energy

added sugar, the consumption of which sharply increased with age.

Discussion

Stratifying NHANES participants by beverage drinking patterns is less common than exploring beverage consumption by gender, age group, or race/ethnicity [22–26]. The present analyses assigned children into four categories: milk drinkers, 100% juice drinkers, milk and 100% juice drinkers, and drinkers of other caloric beverages. For most children, other caloric beverages were the overwhelming beverage of choice; the milk and/or 100% juice drinking patterns were relatively infrequent. Furthermore, the consumption of other caloric beverages sharply increased with age, displacing both milk and 100% juice.

HEI 2010 scores for milk drinkers and 100% juice drinkers were comparable. Milk drinkers consumed more dairy products than did juice drinkers; juice drinkers consumed more total fruit and comparable amounts of whole fruit. Milk drinking did not reduce consumption of yogurt and cheese; juice drinking did not cut into the eating of whole fruit. Diets of milk drinkers and juice drinkers did not differ in terms of energy, total or added sugars, fiber, or vitamin E. Diets of milk drinkers were higher in calcium, potassium, vitamin A and vitamin D than those of juice drinkers. Diets of juice drinkers were higher in vitamin C than those of milk drinkers.

Children rarely limit their drinking choices to a single beverage. The present analyses identified children whose drinking patterns were built around milk and 100% juice, with smaller amounts of other caloric beverages. That group had diets that were close to the dietary recommendations for both dairy (2.85 servings) and for total fruit (2.0 servings). This composite beverage pattern featuring both milk and 100% juice was associated with higher intakes of calcium, potassium, vitamin A and vitamin D along with vitamin C and with the highest HEI 2010 scores. Importantly, drinkers of milk and 100% juice consumed amounts of 100% juice that were close to AAP guidelines: 250 g for 4-8 y, 270 g for 9–13 y and 386 g for 14-19 y. The 100% juice drinkers had

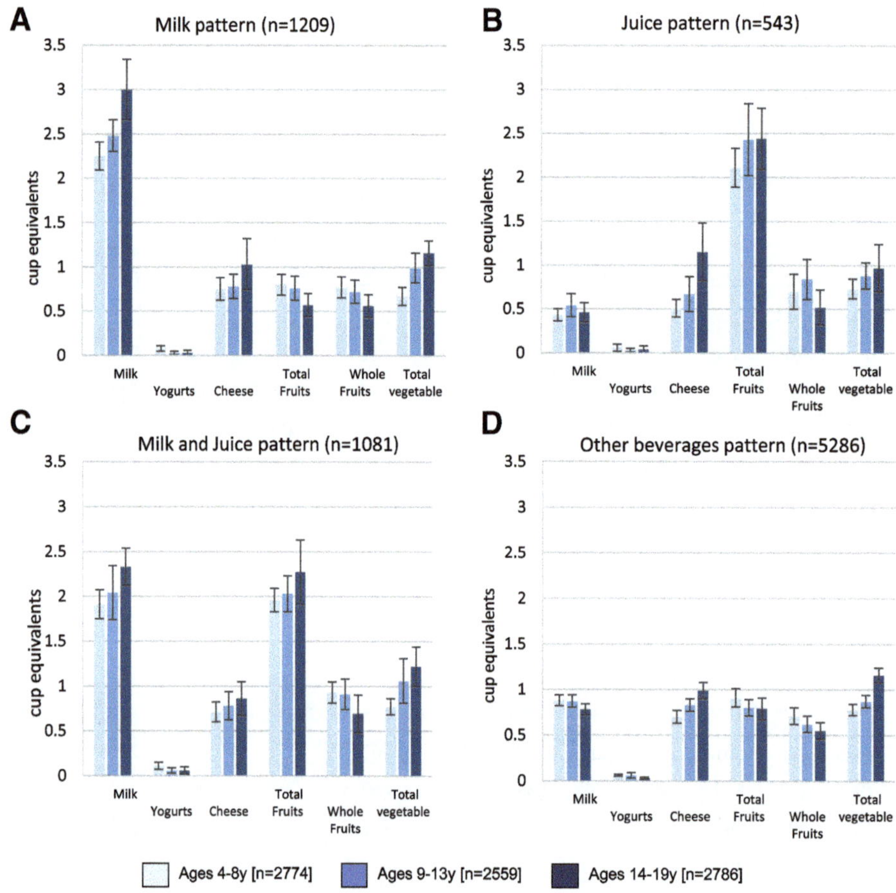

Fig. 1 a-d: Food group intake by beverage pattern and age group, NHANES 2011–2014

energy intakes that were actually lower when compared to drinkers of other beverages [6].

It should be noted that the milk pattern was strongly age-dependent; milk consumption typically decreases with age. The juice pattern showed less of an age dependence; typically 100% apple juice consumed in childhood is replaced by more citrus juices in adolescence. However, both patterns were vulnerable to a dramatic age-related increase in other beverages, with substantial amounts of added sugars.

The current dietary recommendations are for older children and teens to limit fruit juice to only one of the recommended 2 to 2 ½ cups of fruit servings per day. In the present analysis, the consumption of more than 2 fruit servings per day was only observed among exclusive or predominant 100% juice drinkers. There was no evidence in the present cross-sectional data that juice drinkers ate less whole fruit. In past studies, a combination of whole fruit and 100% juice was an effective way to address fruit shortfall, without increasing diet cost [27].

The current dietary recommendations are to replace whole milk with low fat or skim starting at age 2 y. It should be noted that milk drinking patterns follow a socioeconomic gradient. More whole milk is consumed by groups of lower socioeconomic status (SES); higher SES groups drink more low-fat and nonfat milk [19]. Lower SES groups also drink more 100% fruit juice, whereas higher SES groups eat more whole fruit. Higher SES groups drink more plain water (bottled and tap) [28]. Linking the consumption of selected beverages with health outcomes may not have adequately accounted for all the potential (and mostly unobserved) socioeconomic determinants of body weight and health [8].

The study had limitations. First, the data were based on self-report, including proxy report for younger children. However, that is a characteristic of the NHANES database, still the basis for food and nutrition policy in the US. Second, a single 24-h recall may not be sufficient to separate regular consumers from non-consumers; the database only provides beverage patterns on that particular day [21]. Third, the algorithm to identify

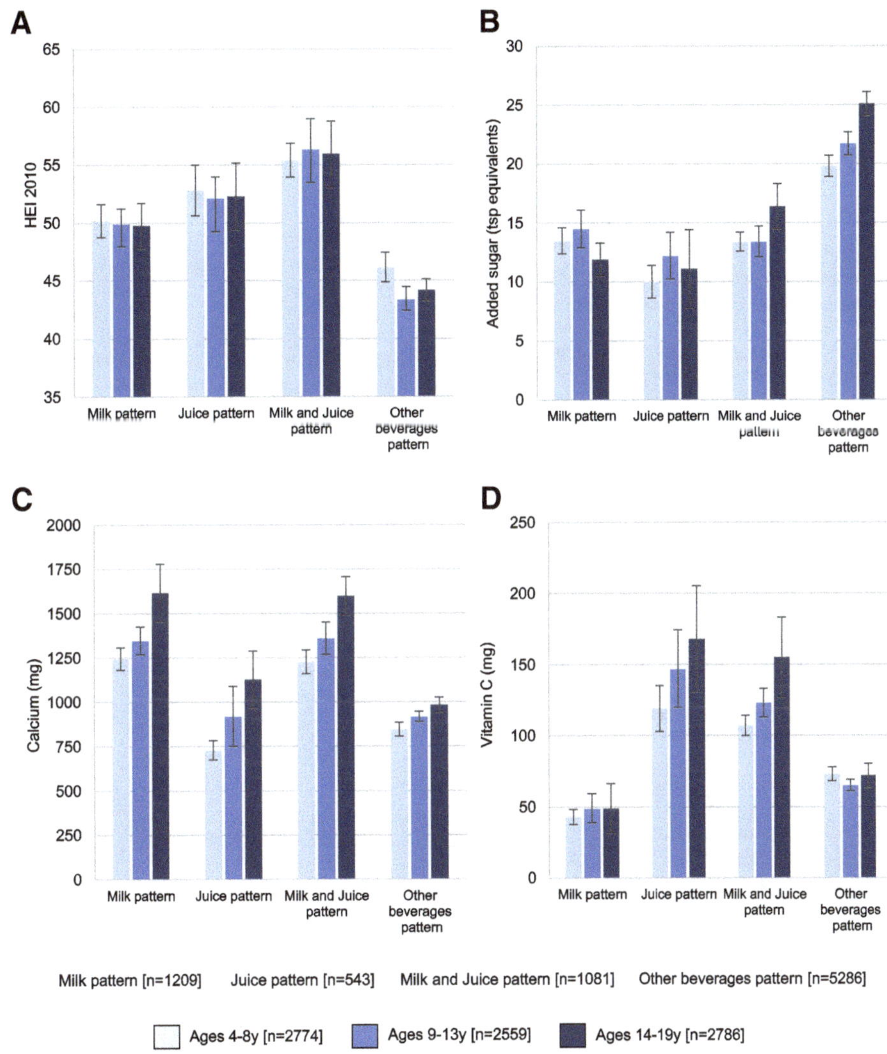

Fig. 2 a-d: HEI and nutrient intakes by beverage pattern and by age group, NHANES 2011–2014

predominant consumption of milk, 100% fruit juice or both was based on weight, as opposed to calories. However, most beverages other than diet beverages or skim milk, are of comparable energy density (< 1 kcal/g). Finally, the HEI 2010 score, technically a measure of compliance with the 2010 Dietary Guidelines, may not capture the multiple components of a healthy diet.

Conclusions

In summary, beverage patterns built around milk and/or 100% juice were relatively rare. Most US children drank other caloric beverages. Yet beverage drinking patterns built around milk and 100% juice were associated with better dietary choices and highest quality diets. Dietary intervention strategies ought to promote rather than restrict milk and 100% juice. Based on the current analyses, milk and 100% juice, along with plain, drinking water should be the main beverages of choice.

Abbreviations

AAP: American Academy of Pediatrics; HEI: Healthy Eating Index; NHANES: National Health and Nutrition Examination Survey

Funding

Funding for these analyses of publicly available federal data was provided by the Dr. Pepper Snapple group.

Author's contributions

MM, FV, CDR, FV, and AD designed the study. CDR developed the databases. MM and FV conducted the analyses. AD took the lead on writing the paper, along with CMR. All authors have responsibility for final contact. All authors read and approved the final manuscript.

Competing interests

AD: Has received grants, contracts, and honoraria from private industry, foundations, and public agencies on projects on nutrient profiling, diet and health.
FV and MM: are employed by MS-Nutrition.
CMR and CDR: have no competing interests to disclose.

Author details

[1]MS-Nutrition, 27 bld Jean Moulin Faculté de Médecine la Timone, Laboratoire NORT, 13385 Marseille cedex 5, France. [2]Albert Einstein College of Medicine, Montefiore Medical Center, New York, NY 10467, USA. [3]Center for Public Health Nutrition, University of Washington, Box 353410, Seattle, WA 98195, USA.

References

1. Heyman MB, Abrams SA. Fruit juice in infants, children, and adolescents: current recommendations. Pediatrics. 2017:e20170967.
2. Shefferly A, Scharf RJ, DeBoer MD. Longitudinal evaluation of 100% fruit juice consumption on BMI status in 2–5-year-old children. Pediatric obesity. 2016;11:221–7.
3. LaRowe TL, Moeller SM, Adams AK. Beverage patterns, diet quality, and body mass index of US preschool and school-aged children. J Am Diet Assoc. 2007;107:1124–33.
4. Auerbach BJ, Wolf FM, Hikida A, Vallila-Buchman P, Littman A, Thompson D, Louden D, Taber DR, Krieger J. Fruit juice and change in BMI: a meta-analysis. Pediatrics. 2017;139:e20162454.
5. Rolland-Cachera MF, Akrout M, Péneau S. Nutrient intakes in early life and risk of obesity. Int J Environ Res Public Health. 2016;13:564.
6. Gidding SS, Dennison BA, Birch LL, Daniels SR, Gilman MW, Lichtenstein AH, Rattay KT, Steinberger J, Stettler N, Van Horn L. Dietary recommendations for children and adolescents: a guide for practitioners. Pediatrics. 2006;117:544–59.
7. Baker SS, Cochran WJ, Greer FR, Heyman MB, Jacobson MS, Jaksic T, Krebs NF, Blum-kemelor D, Dietz W, Grave G. The use and misuse of fruit juice in pediatrics. Pediatrics. 2001;107:1210–3.
8. Aggarwal A, Monsivais P, Drewnowski A. Nutrient intakes linked to better health outcomes are associated with higher diet costs in the US. PLoS One. 2012;7:e37533.
9. Rose CM, Savage JS, Birch LL. Patterns of early dietary exposures have implications for maternal and child weight outcomes. Obesity. 2016;24:430–8.
10. Santos LP, Assunção MCF, Matijasevich A, Santos IS, Barros AJ. Dietary intake patterns of children aged 6 years and their association with socioeconomic and demographic characteristics, early feeding practices and body mass index. BMC Public Health. 2016;16:1055.
11. Hamner HC, Perrine CG, Gupta PM, Herrick KA, Cogswell ME. Dietary patterns among children birth to 23 months of age, NHANES 2009-2014. J Nutr Educ Behav. 2017;49:S1.
12. Mikkilä V, Vepsäläinen H, Saloheimo T, Gonzalez S, Meisel J, Hu G, Champagne CM, Chaput J-P, Church TS, Katzmarzyk PT. An international comparison of dietary patterns in 9–11-year-old children. International journal of obesity supplements. 2015;5:S17.
13. Mesirow MS, Welsh JA: Changing beverage consumption patterns have resulted in fewer liquid calories in the diets of US children: National Health and nutrition examination survey 2001-2010. J Acad Nutr Diet. 2015; 115: 559–566. e554.
14. Wang YC, Bleich SN, Gortmaker SL. Increasing caloric contribution from sugar-sweetened beverages and 100% fruit juices among US children and adolescents, 1988–2004. Pediatrics. 2008;121:e1604–14.
15. Ford CN, Ng SW, Popkin BM. Ten-year beverage intake trends among US preschool children: rapid declines between 2003 and 2010 but stagnancy in recent years. Pediatric obesity. 2016;11:47–53.
16. Blanton CA, Moshfegh AJ, Baer DJ, Kretsch MJ. The USDA automated multiple-pass method accurately estimates group total energy and nutrient intake. J Nutr. 2006;136:2594–9.
17. Moshfegh AJ, Rhodes DG, Baer DJ, Murayi T, Clemens JC, Rumpler WV, Paul DR, Sebastian RS, Kuczynski KJ, Ingwersen LA. The US Department of Agriculture Automated Multiple-Pass Method reduces bias in the collection of energy intakes. Am J Clin Nutr. 2008;88:324–32.
18. Drewnowski A, Rehm CD. Consumption of low-calorie sweeteners among US adults is associated with higher healthy eating index (HEI 2005) scores and more physical activity. Nutrients. 2014;6:4389–403.
19. Kit BK, Carroll MD, Ogden CL. Low-fat milk consumption among children and adolescents in the United States, 2007–2008. Centers for Disease Control and Prevention, National Center for Health Statistics: US Department of Health and Human Services; 2011.
20. Murphy MM, Douglass JS, Johnson RK, Spence LA. Drinking flavored or plain milk is positively associated with nutrient intake and is not associated with adverse effects on weight status in US children and adolescents. J Am Diet Assoc. 2008;108:631–9.
21. Ahluwalia N, Dwyer J, Terry A, Moshfegh A, Johnson C. Update on NHANES dietary data: focus on collection, release, analytical considerations, and uses to inform public policy. Advances in Nutrition: An International Review Journal. 2016;7:121–34.
22. Kant AK, Graubard BI. Energy density of diets reported by American adults: association with food group intake, nutrient intake, and body weight. Int J Obes. 2005;29:950.
23. Drewnowski A, Rehm CD. Consumption of added sugars among US children and adults by food purchase location and food source. Am J Clin Nutr. 2014;100:901–7.
24. Virudachalam S, Long JA, Harhay MO, Polsky DE, Feudtner C. Prevalence and patterns of cooking dinner at home in the USA: National Health and nutrition examination survey (NHANES) 2007–2008. Public Health Nutr. 2014; 17:1022–30.
25. Wang DD, Leung CW, Li Y, Ding EL, Chiuve SE, Hu FB, Willett WC. Trends in dietary quality among adults in the United States, 1999 through 2010. JAMA Intern Med. 2014;174:1587–95.
26. Ahluwalia N, Herrick KA, Rossen LM, Rhodes D, Kit B, Moshfegh A, Dodd KW. Usual nutrient intakes of us infants and toddlers generally meet or exceed dietary reference intakes: findings from NHANES 2009–2012. Am J Clin Nutr. 2016;104:1167–74.
27. Rehm CD, Drewnowski A. Dietary and economic effects of eliminating shortfall in fruit intake on nutrient intakes and diet cost. BMC Pediatr. 2016;16:83.
28. Dubowitz T, Heron M, Bird CE, Lurie N, Finch BK, Basurto-Dávila R, Hale L, Escarce JJ. Neighborhood socioeconomic status and fruit and vegetable intake among whites, blacks, and Mexican Americans in the United States. Am J Clin Nutr. 2008;87:1883–91.

8

Dietary vitamin A intake among Chinese adults: findings from CNTCS2015

Wenwen Du, Huijun Wang, Zhihong Wang, Jiguo Zhang, Chang Su, Xiaofang Jia, Ji Zhang, Hongru Jiang, Feifei Huang, Yifei Ouyang, Yun Wang, Li Li and Bing Zhang*

Abstract

Background: Vitamin A plays an important role in human functions, which mainly come from foods. This study aims to examine dietary vitamin A intake and major food sources of Chinese adults.

Methods: We analyzed the cross-sectional data from 12,246 adult aged 18 to 64 years old in 2015 China Nutritional Transition Cohort Study. Three consecutive 24-h dietary recalls combined with household weighing method were used to assess dietary vitamin A intake.

Results: The average dietary vitamin A intakes were 480.9 μg retinol equivalents (RE) or 307.2 μg retinol activity equivalents (RAE). The carotenes and retinol intake of subjects were 2084.7 μg/day and 133.5 μg/day, respectively. Approximately 87% of adults consumed less vitamin A than the Chinese Estimated Average Requirement (EAR), and only 6% of adults consumed more than Chinese Recommended Nutrient Intake (RNI). Chinese adults derived vitamin A mainly from plant source foods, which is supplied as carotenes (67.4% RE or 56.4% RAE). Dark- and light- vegetables and fruits were major contributors of carotenes (accounted for 84.2%). The most import food sources of retinol were egg, meats and meat products, poultry, fish and milk, representing 94.7% of retinol intake. The major four contributors of total vitamin A (as both RE and RAE) were dark vegetables, egg, light vegetables, and meats and meat products. In conclusion, dietary vitamin A remains a problem for Chinese adults.

Conclusions: Public health actions are needed to increase vitamin A intake in China.

Keywords: Vitamin A, Retinol, Carotenes, China

Background

Vitamin A is an essential fat-soluble nutrient for eye health, immune function, embryonic development, cell differentiation and growth hormone production [1]. Low vitamin A intake may lead to blindness and increased morbidity and mortality. Vitamin A deficiency remains a major public-health issue in developing countries, especially in low-income regions, such as south Asia and sub-Saharan Africa [2]. In China, vitamin A deficiency is now considered a moderate public-health problem. On the positive side, recent studies indicate that vitamin A status has been improved in the past decade for Chinese children and pregnant women [3, 4].

Vitamin A is a generic term comprising retinol and provitamin A carotenoids (β-carotene, α-carotene, and β-cryptoxanthin). People obtain dietary vitamin A either as retinol from animal foods or as provitamin A carotenoids from vegetables and fruits [5, 6]. With respect to the rentinol activity, the former equivalent of vitamin A intake is proposed by FAO/WHO (1988) as RE (retinol equivalent) = retinol+(β-carotene/6) + (α-carotene/12) + (β-cryptoxanthin/12) [7],while the present equivalent is introduced by IOM (2001) as RAE (retinol activity equivalent) = retinol + (β-carotene/12) + (α-carotene/24) + (β-cryptoxanthin/24) [1, 8]. Several countries have issued new dietary reference intakes (DRIs) of vitamin A as RAE, such as the United States, Canada, and Australia, where it recommended 900 μg for men and 700 μg for women [1, 9]. Chinese DRIs recommended 800 μg for men and 700 μg for women [10].

It is still unclear whether Chinese adults eat enough to meet the recent recommended dietary intakes of vitamin A as well as its food sources at the national level. In the

* Correspondence: zhangbing@chinacdc.cn; zzhangb327@aliyun.com
National Institute for Nutrition and Health, Chinese Center for Disease Control and Prevention, 29 Nanwei Rd, Beijing, China

present article, we examined the dietary vitamin A status (as retinol, carotenoids, RE and RAE) and its food sources among Chinese adults aged 18 to 64 years, using data from the most recent China Nutritional Transition Cohort Study (CNTCS, 2015).

Methods

CNTCS and sample

We used data from CNTCS 2015, which was conducted by National Institute for Nutrition and Health, Chinese Center for Disease Control and Prevention. CNTCS was an amplified survey based on the China Health and Nutrition Survey (CHNS), an ongoing and longitudinal study established in 1989 by the Chinese Center for Disease Control and Prevention, and the University of North Carolina at Chapel Hill. Detailed information on the rationale and methods of CHNS can be found on the project website and published papers [11, 12]. CNTCS was designed to provide a wide range of socio-demographic characteristics, diet, health, physical activity, behaviors and environment changes in China. The original sample was collected using a multistage random cluster sampling method from representative households in eight provinces (Liaoning, Shandong, Henan, Hubei, Hunan, Jiangsu, Guizhou and Guangxi) by economic levels, geographical areas, and public resources. During the past decades, more provinces joined the study using the consistent sampling method and protocol: Heilongjiang joined in 1997, three mega cities (Beijing, Shanghai and Chongqing) joined in2011, and three more provinces (Zhejiang, Shanxi and Yunnan) joined in2015.

All subjects gave their written informed consent before they participated in the study. The study was conducted in accordance with the Declaration of Helsinki, and the protocol was approved by the Ethics Committee of the National Institute for Nutrition and Health, China CDC (No.2015017).

The current paper analyzed data from 12,246 adults (5710 men and 6536 women), aged18 to 64 years old, who had complete dietary data on three consecutive days in 2015. The final sample came from 6018 households, residing in 361 communities from15 provinces in China.

Assessment of dietary carotenes, retinol and vitamin a (RE, RAE) intake

Personal dietary data were collected using 24-h recalls on three consecutive days (two weekdays and one weekend day) by face-to-face interview. The trained interviewers collected detailed information of all foods and beverages consumed at home and away from home in the past 24 h for each individual. Household edible oil and condiments consumption were weighed during the same days and divided among household members according to their dietary energy intake levels.

Dietary carotenes and vitamin A (RE) intake were calculated using the China Food Composition Table 2009 [13]. However, carotenes was tested using chromatography in the China Food Composition Dataset, which could not distinguish the subtypes, such as β-carotene, α-carotene, and β-cryptoxanthin. Other research showed thatβ-caroteneaccounts for 86% of provitamin A carotenoids intake [14]. Therefore, we used the conversion factor of β-carotene instead that of total carotenes in the calculation procedures. Retinol and vitamin A (RAE) were derived from the following simplified formulas:

$$\mu g\,RE = \mu g\,retinol + \mu g\,carotenes/6, \quad (1)$$

$$\mu g\,RAE = \mu g\,retinol + \mu g\,carotenes/12. \quad (2)$$

Food groups were defined according to the classification in China Food Composition Tables. Carotene was the major contributor to vitamin A intake in vegetables, which varied in different vegetable types. Thus, we defined vegetables with carotene more than 500μg/100 g as dark vegetables, which mainly were dark green, red or orange (such as spinach, broccoli, tomato, carrot and pumpkin); and those with carotene less than 500μg/100 g as light vegetables (such as eggplant, cucumber and cabbage).

Socio-demographic variables

Socio-demographic variables used in the present analysis include: age, gender, education and income level, and regions. Age (years) was categorized to 2 groups, 18–49 years, and 50–64 years. Highest level of education attained was categorized to 3 groups, primary school andbelow, junior middle school and senior middle school and above. Per capita annual household income was classified into 3 groups using tertile method, low (1^{st}tertile), middle (2ndtertile), and high (3rdtertile). Ethnic groups were divided into Han, Miao, Buyi, Man, and others. To explore region disparities on vitamin A intake, we included 3 variables, region1 (urban, rural), region2 (east: Being, Liaoning, Shanghai, Jiangsu, Zhejiang and Shandong; middle: Heilongjiang, Henan, Hubei and Hunan; west: Chongqing, Guizhou, Yunnan, Shanxi and Guangxi), and region3 (north: Beijing, Liaoning, Shandong, Heilongjiang, Henan and Shanxi; south: Shanghai, Jiangsu, Zhejiang, Hubei, Hunan, Chongqing, Guizhou, Yunnan and Guangxi).

Statistical methods

In our analysis, vitamin A was expressed as both retinol equivalent (RE) and retinol activity equivalent (RAE). The present paper reported dietary carotenes, retinol, vitamin A (RE), and vitamin A (RAE) intakes (mean of the three days for each adult) as mean (SD) and median by age, gender, region, education, income and ethnic groups. The intake levels of vitamin A (RAE) were assessed using estimated average requirement (EAR) and recommended nutrient intake (RNI) from Chinese Dietary Reference Intakes (DRIs) 2013 [15]. The proportions of retinol to total RE and RAE, as well as the main food sources contributing to each of the vitamin A components were also determined. Non-parametric statistical methods were used for difference test by each of the stratifications. Significance level was set at $p < 0.05$. All statistical analysis was conducted using SAS 9.4 (SAS Institute Inc., Cary, NC, USA).

Results

Dietary intake of vitamin a among Chinese adults

Table 1 reports the dietary intake of carotenes, retinol, and vitamin A (excluding supplements) by age, gender, region, education, income level and ethnic groups among Chinese adults. Mean total dietary intake of vitamin A was 480.9 μg RE/day (male: 499.4μg RE/day; female: 464.7μg RE/day) or 307.2 μg RAE/day (male: 321.3μg RAE/day; female: 294.8μg RAE/day), carotenes intake was 2084.7 μg/day (male: 2137.7 μg/day; female: 2038.4μg/day), and retinol was 133.5 μg/day (male: 143.2μg/day; female: 125.0μg/day).

Higher intake of carotenes was observed in western areas vs. middle and eastern areas, in rural areas vs. urban area, in southern areas vs. northern areas, in Buyi and Miao minorities VS. other ethnic groups. Lower carotenes intake was found in low subgroup compared with middle-high groups of education and income. No significant differences of carotenes intake were detected by age and gender.

Retinol intake was significantly higher in younger adults compared to older adults, and in males compared to females. Opposite to carotenes intake, the higher intake of retinol was observed in urban areas vs. rural areas, and in eastern areas vs. middle and western areas. Adults in southern areas tended to have significant higher retinol intake than those in northern areas. Similarly, retinol intake was found to increase with education and income level. Buyi minorities had the significant lowest retinol intake. Vitamin A intake (expressed in both RE and RAE) showed coincident trends with that of retinol in all stratifications, except for ethnic groups. The highest vitamin A intake level (both RE and RAE) was found in Han, followed by Miao and Buyi, while the lowest level was observed in Man minorities.

Proportion below EAR and above RNI among Chinese adults

In Chinese DRIs, the estimated average requirement (EAR) and the recommended nutrient intake (RNI) of vitamin A is set to 560 μg RAE/day and 800 μg RAE/day for males, 480 μg RAE/day and 700 μg RAE/day for females. The proportion of Chinese adults who consumed vitamin A less than EAR, as well as the proportion of adults who consumed vitamin A more than RNI is shown in Table 2. In general, the proportion below EAR was 88.3% in males and 87.0% in females; consumption above RNI was only 6.3% in males and 6.5% in females. Younger adults seemed to have a healthier vitamin A intake level than older adults, with a lower proportion below EAR and a higher proportion above RNI, whereas no remarkable gender difference in proportions was found for each age group.

Contribution of retinol to total vitamin a intake

Figure 1a and b shows the percentage of daily contribution of retinol to total vitamin A intake (RE and RAE). In terms of RE, retinol accounted for 32.6% of total vitamin A intake, which contributed 33.5% in males and 31.8% in females. 43.6% of vitamin A intake was attributed to retinol, when expressed in RAE (44.7% for males and 42.8% for females). Social-economic differences in the contribution of retinol to total vitamin A were detected. Retinol provided a higher proportion of vitamin A in young, male, urban, eastern, northern, higher education, and higher income groups.

Food sources to the daily vitamin a intake

Figure 2a shows the percentage contribution of the main food sources to the daily carotene intake in urban and rural adults. Overall, dark vegetables (54.6%) afforded more than half of carotene intake for the whole population, contributing to a higher percentage for urban groups vs. rural group. Light vegetables (23.6%) ranked second and fruit (6.0%) third; tubers contributed 3.8% and legumes 2.4%. Compared with rural adults, urban adults appeared to consume less carotene from light vegetables and tubers, more from fruit and legumes. All the listed food groups in Fig. 2a afforded more than 95% to the carotene intake.

Figure 2b shows the percentage contribution of the main food sources to the daily carotene intake in east, middle and west areas. Compared with adults in middle and east areas, west adults consumed more carotene from dark vegetables, and less from light vegetables, fruit and tubers.

As shown in Fig. 3a, eggs provided 44.6% of retinol intake, and were the major contributing food source. Meats and meat products provided 29.2% and poultry 9.9% of retinol intake. Finally, fish and milk afforded 6.5 and 4.5% to retinol intake, respectively. Urban adults seemed to consume more retinol from fish and milk, and less from meats and meat products and poultry than rural adults, with a roughly similar amount from eggs.

Table 1 Dietary daily intake of Vitamin A among Chinese adults aged 18 to 64 years*

Variables	N	%	Carotenes (μg/day)				Retinol (μg /day)				Vitamin A (μg RE/day)				Vitamin A (μg RAE/day)			
			Mean	SD	Median	P	Mean	SD	Median	P	Mean	SD	Median	P	Mean	SD	Median	P
Total	12,246	100.0	2084.7	3061.2	1175.0		133.5	264.4	76.3		480.9	583.5	307.6		307.2	374.3	202.0	
Age																		
18–49 years	6875	56.1	2099.2	3092.5	1175.4	0.7079	141.6	281.3	78.0	< 0.0001	491.4	598.1	311.8	0.0485	316.5	389.9	205.7	0.0179
50–64 years	5371	43.9	2066.0	3021.0	1172.9		123.1	240.6	74.2		467.4	564.1	302.8		295.2	353.0	198.8	
Gender																		
Male	5710	46.6	2137.7	3132.4	1194.7	0.0975	143.2	279.8	81.4	< 0.0001	499.4	600.4	318.5	< 0.0001	321.3	388.9	211.2	< 0.0001
Female	6536	53.4	2038.4	2997.2	1158.8		125.0	249.8	72.3		464.7	567.9	298.0		294.8	360.6	195.5	
Region 1																		
Urban	4781	39.0	2114.9	2985.9	1259.0	0.0001	147.4	268.6	91.2	< 0.0001	499.9	568.0	332.5	< 0.0001	323.6	368.1	224.2	< 0.0001
Rural	7465	61.0	2065.3	3108.6	1129.8		124.5	261.2	67.7		468.7	593.0	290.5		296.6	377.9	190.4	
Region 2[§]																		
East	4659	38.1	1695.4	2827.1	905.4^{a}	< 0.0001	149.9	268.4	94.9^{a}	< 0.0001	432.4	548.2	277.8^{a}	< 0.0001	291.2	361.6	193.1^{a}	< 0.0001
Middle	3239	26.5	1667.0	1911.6	1044.2^{b}		105.2	183.1	70.6^{b}		383.0	372.5	271.4^{a}		244.1	246.6	180.6^{b}	
West	4348	35.5	2812.9	3780.0	1675.6^{c}		136.9	306.2	63.6^{c}		605.8	713.1	383.9^{b}		371.3	449.3	238.2^{c}	
Region 3																		
North	4713	38.5	1357.7	1758.3	801.7	< 0.0001	108.0	191.4	71.9	< 0.0001	334.3	358.1	238.3	< 0.0001	221.1	246.9	162.2	< 0.0001
South	7533	61.5	2539.5	3572.6	1494.2		149.4	300.1	78.7		572.6	671.9	365.3		361.0	426.8	234.2	
Education level[§]																		
Primary school and below	3104	25.4	1906.0	2702.1	1062.3^{a}	< 0.0001	115.4	249.4	61.0^{a}	< 0.0001	433.1	519.6	274.8^{a}	< 0.0001	274.3	339.6	180.7^{a}	< 0.0001
Junior middle school	4268	34.9	2123.6	3187.4	1199.2^{b}		126.3	256.5	70.7^{b}		480.3	605.4	301.7^{b}		303.3	381.5	197.3^{b}	
Senior middle school and above	4874	39.8	2164.3	3158.3	1226.3^{b}		151.2	279.0	91.2^{c}		511.9	600.4	333.1^{c}		331.5	387.1	225.5^{c}	
Income level[§]																		
Low (1sttertile)	4081	33.3	1982.9	2913.0	1113.1^{a}	0.0001	133.5	297.0	65.0^{a}	< 0.0001	464.0	585.2	285.8^{a}	< 0.0001	298.8	395.5	188.0^{a}	< 0.0001
Middle (2ndtertile)	4079	33.3	2191.6	3172.7	1230.1^{b}		126.1	244.7	73.3^{b}		491.4	589.7	313.2^{b}		308.7	365.9	205.2^{b}	
High (3rdtertile)	4086	33.4	2079.6	3089.4	1198.5^{b}		140.8	248.0	90.0^{c}		487.3	575.4	317.7^{b}		314.0	360.5	214.2^{c}	
Ethnic groups[§]																		
Han	11,053	90.3	2078.9	3133.4	1150.0^{a}	< 0.0001	134.5	265.1	77.9^{a}	< 0.0001	481.0	594.3	305.2^{a}	< 0.0001	307.8	378.9	201.0^{a}	< 0.0001
Miao	221	1.8	2855.7	2514.2	2400.0^{b}		107.9	228.8	57.1^{b}		583.8	494.0	471.1^{b}		345.8	322.9	281.1^{b}	
Buyi	182	1.5	3117.7	2132.7	2683.3^{c}		100.5	243.4	51.5^{c}		620.1	476.4	503.9^{b}		360.3	334.0	277.6^{b}	
Man	225	1.8	994.1	1195.6	633.3^{d}		125.8	274.0	71.0^{a,b}		291.5	339.4	211.3^{c}		208.6	291.9	148.4^{c}	
Others	565	4.6	1997.3	2347.8	1351.2^{a}		136.3	264.4	67.4^{a,b}		469.1	482.3	328.0^{a}		302.7	336.1	205.4^{a}	

*Mean, standard error, and median were calculated for the values of vitamin A. Significant difference by socio-demographic factors was determined using nonparametric median test

[§]If the difference was significant among more than two groups, multiple-comparison was further conducted by Student-Newman-Keuls (SNK). The same characters (a,b,c,d) indicated non-significant difference between the two sub-groups, while the different characters indicated significant difference, $p < 0.05$

Table 2 Vitamin A intake and proportion below EAR and above RNI among Chinese adults by age and gender

Age		N	Vitamin A (μg RAE/day)		*P*	Below EAR[a]		*P*	Above RNI[b]		*P*
			Mean	Median		N	%		N	%	
18–49 Years	Male	3157	330.1	214.7	0.0008	2764	87.6	0.1744	222	7.0	0.9497
	Female	3718	305.0	198.6		3214	86.4		260	7.0	
50–64 Years	Male	2553	310.4	207.8	0.0003	2276	89.2	0.0946	139	5.4	0.4805
	Female	2818	281.5	191.0		2471	87.7		166	5.9	
Total	Male	5710	321.3	211.2	< 0.0001	5040	88.3	0.0313	361	6.3	0.6599
	Female	6536	294.8	195.5		5685	87.0		426	6.5	

[a]EAR, Estimated Average Requirement, 560μg for male, and 480μg for female; [b]RNI, Recommended Nutrient Intake, 800μg for male and 700μg for female

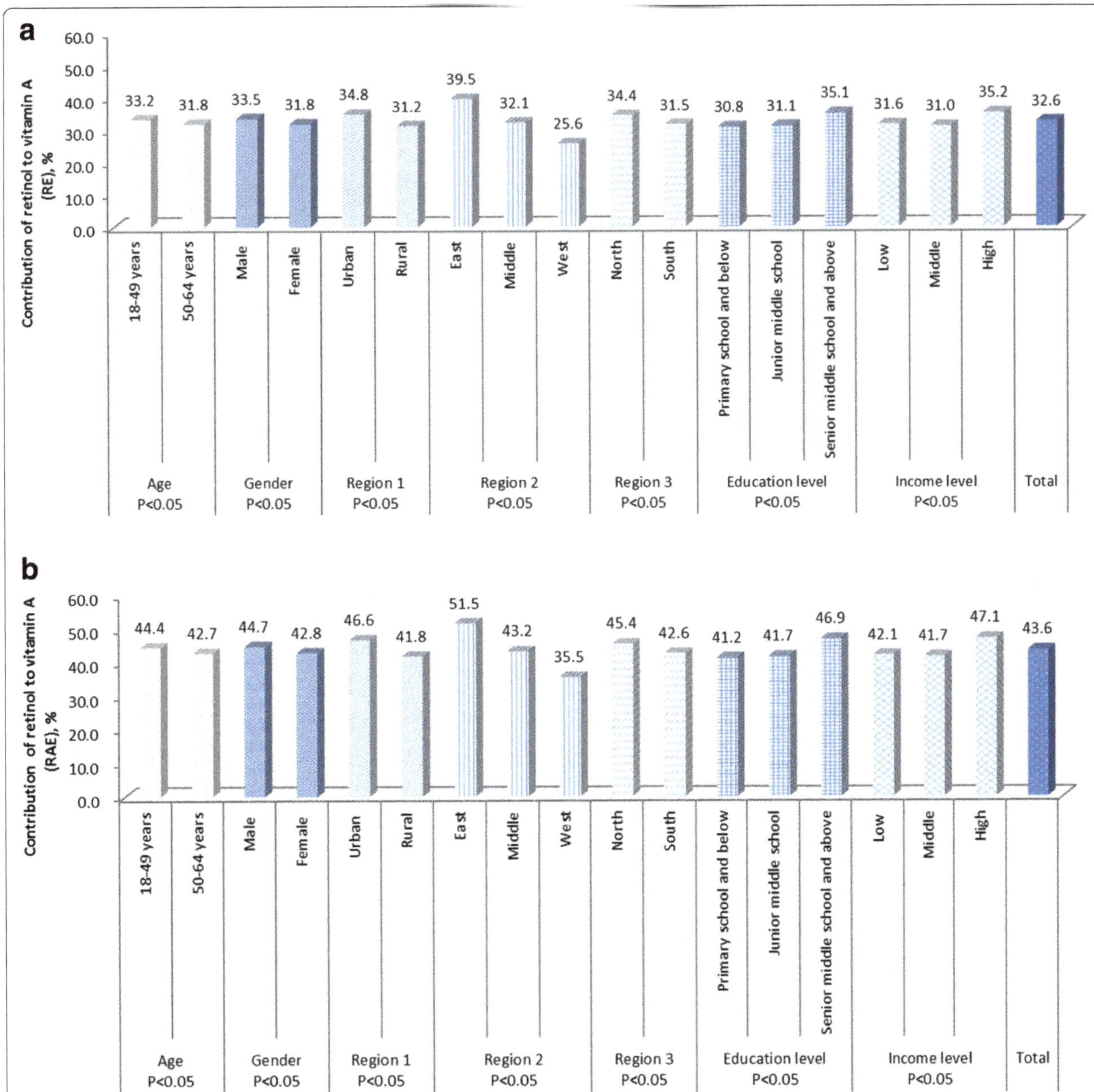

Fig. 1 Contribution of retinol to vitamin A among Chinese adults aged 18 to 64 years: (**a**) vitamin A expressed as RE; (**b**) vitamin A expressed as RAE

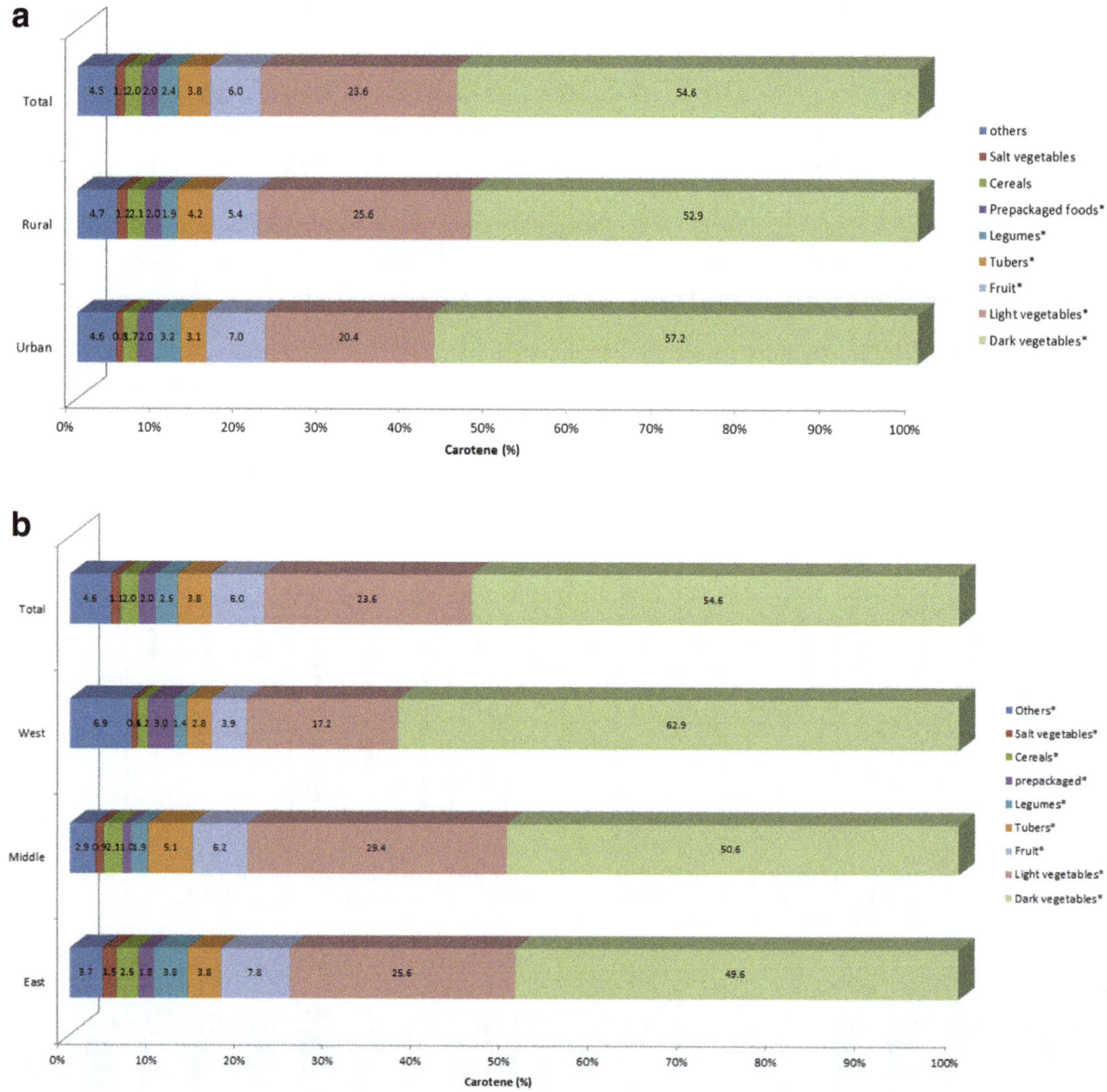

Fig. 2 Contribution of food sources to the daily carotene intake by regions among Chinese adults aged 18 to 64 years. $^{*}P < 0.05$. (**a**) by urban and rural; (**b**) by east, middle and west

All the food groups in Fig. 3 combined to provide more than 98% of retinol intake.

Figure 3b shows, unlike middle and east areas, meats and meat products were the major contributing food source in west area, providing 39.3% of retinol intake. Furthermore, west adults seemed to consume more retinol from poultry and animal oil, and less from egg and fish than middle and east adults. Noticeably, fish, milk and prepackaged foods afforded 10.2, 7.3 and 2.5% to retinol intake in east area, respectively, much higher than that in west and middle area.

Figures 4 and 5 shows that dark vegetables, eggs, light vegetables, meats and meat products, fruit and poultry are the major food sources ofvitamin A intake, contributing nearly 85% to RE and RAE for the whole population. Due to different conversion factors of carotene in RE and RAE calculation formulas, animal source foods contributed a higher proportion to vitamin A intake for RAE than RE. Urban adults consumed more vitamin A from egg and fruit, while less from light vegetables. Adults in west area consumed more vitamin A from dark vegetables, meats and meat products, and less from egg, light vegetables, fruit and fish, than those in middle

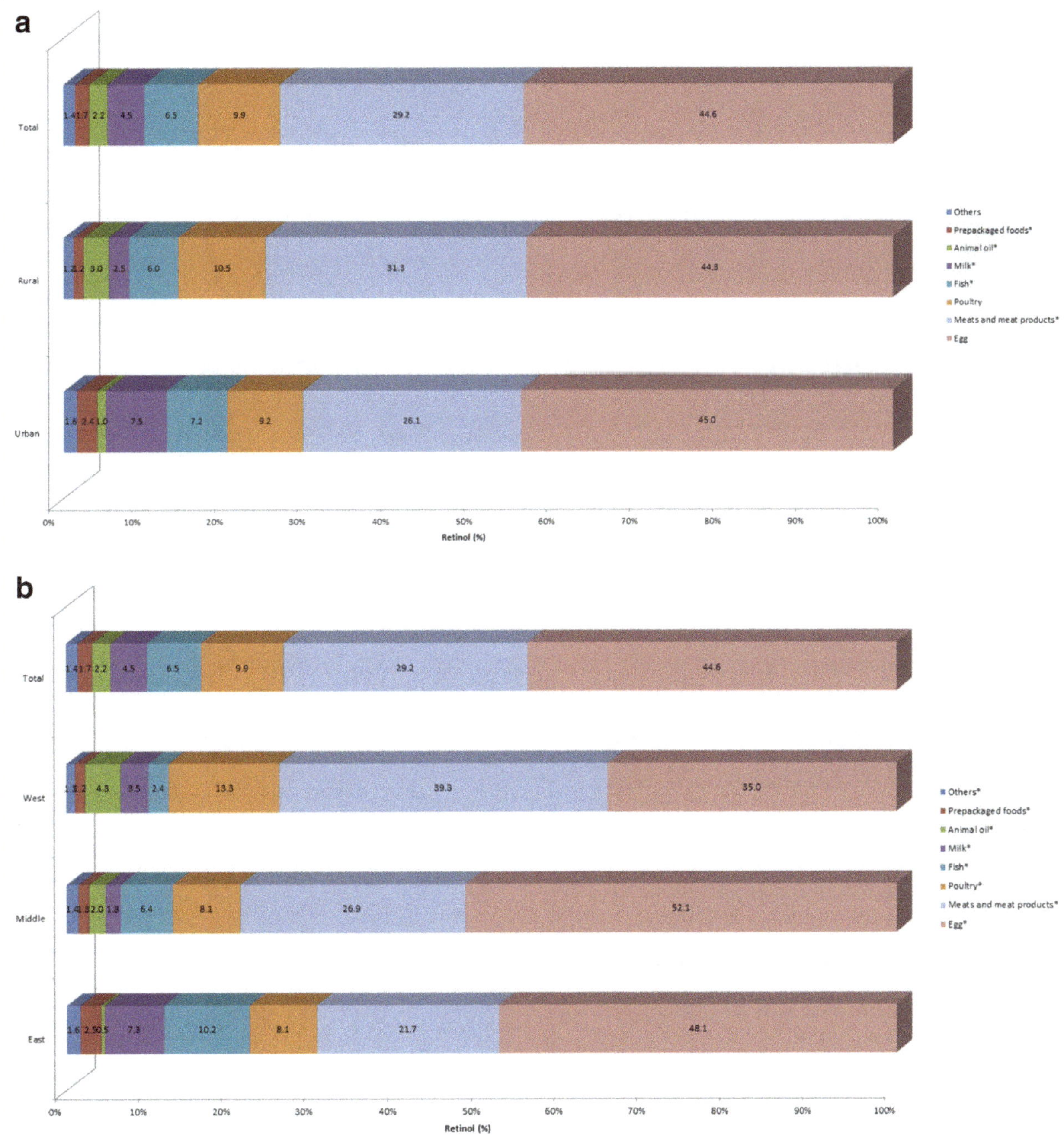

Fig. 3 Contribution of food sources to the daily retinol intake by regions among Chinese adults aged 18 to 64 years. $^*P < 0.05$. (**a**) by urban and rural; (**b**) by east, middle and west

and east areas. Interestingly, fish, milk and prepackaged foods combined to provide 8.8% of RE and 10.9% of RAE in east area, which were much higher than that in middle and west areas.

Discussion

The present article provides a snapshot of dietary intake of vitamin A among Chinese adults. The mean daily intake of vitamin A in this study (480.9 μg RE/day, and 307.2 μg RAE/day) was roughly in line with the findings from Chinese Nutrition and Health Surveillance (2010–2012) (441.9 μg RE/day, and 291.5 μg RAE/day) [16], and that from China National Nutrition and Health Survey 2002 (469.2 μg RE/day) [17]. The above two studies [16, 17] using the nationwide data, expressed the vitamin A intake at standard person level (60 kg adult men with light physical activity), which may overestimate the intake status. Take this into account, our results indicated

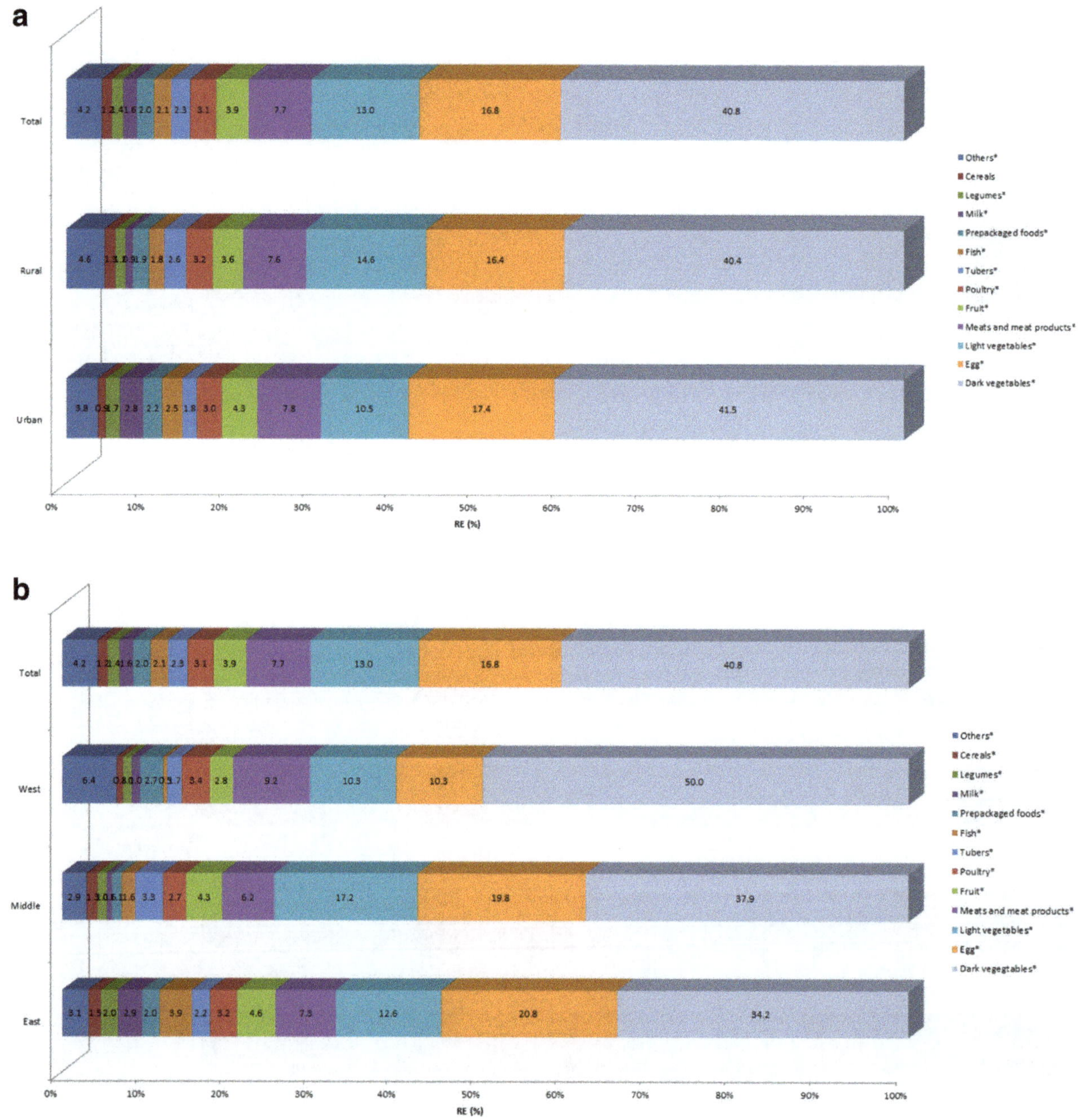

Fig. 4 Contribution of food sources to the daily vitamin A (RE) intake by regions among Chinese adults aged 18 to 64 years. *$P < 0.05$. (**a**) by urban and rural; (**b**) by east, middle and west

a mild growth of vitamin A intake among Chinese population during the past decade. Studies in other countries [18–22] usually showed vitamin A intake by gender/age groups for which DRIs have been established. Our research found that dietary vitamin A intake of adults in China was lower than that in Korea (887.8 μg RE/day, and 531.84 μg RAE/day) [18] and Japan (491 to 571 μg RE/day for men, and 603 to 609 μg RE/day for women) [19], and was much lower than that in other European and American countries, such as Italy (890 μg RE/day) [20], Spain (716.4 μg RE/day) [6], the United States(656 μg RAE/day for males, and 564 μg RAE/day for females) [21], and Mexico (547 μg RAE/day for men, and 536 μg RAE/day for women) [22]. When it comes to dietary intake of retinol and carotenes, Chinese adults consumed absolutely less retinol (133.5 μg/day) than those in European countries (835 μg/day), and less carotenes (2084.7μg/day) than most countries, excluding the Netherlands, Sweden, and Spain [5, 23]. Compared to other Asian countries, such as Japan and Korea, Chinese

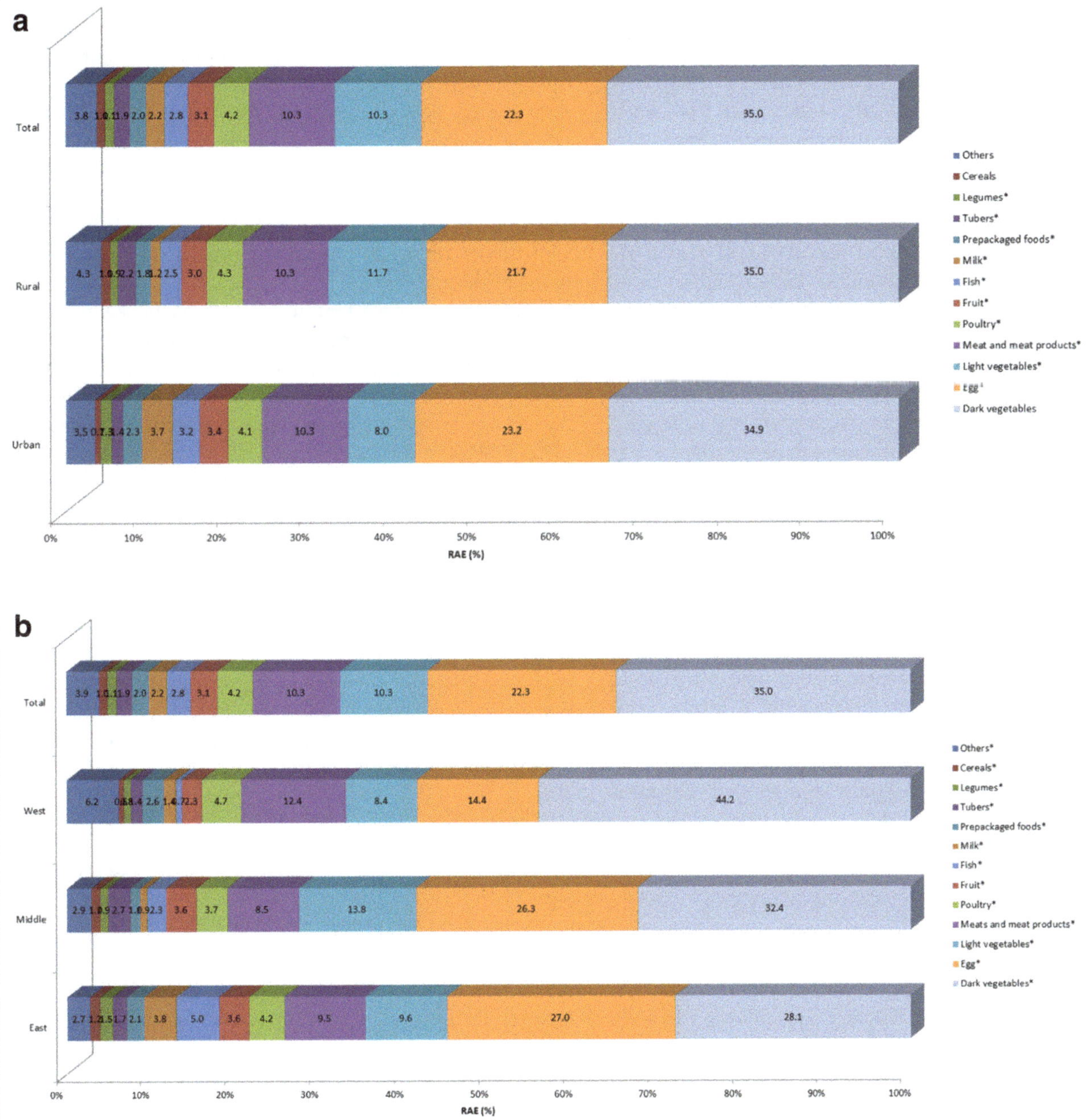

Fig. 5 Contribution of food sources to the daily vitamin A (RAE) intake by regions among Chinese adults aged 18 to 64 years. *$P < 0.05$. (**a**) by urban and rural; (**b**) by east, middle and west

adults had slightly lower retinol intake and much less carotenes intake [18, 19].

Data presented in the current study also shows some very interesting socioeconomic differences in the intake of vitamin A. Higher intake of vitamin A was found in younger, male, urban, western, southern, high education and income groups, and Miao and Buyi minorities. That finding may be explained by the fact that adults in those groups have better access to high quality and balanced foods.

Various countries have released different recommended dietary intake values for vitamin A, either as RE or RAE. These different recommendations lead to varying interpretations on the prevalence of inadequate intake. For example, the Korean vitamin A EARs for males and females (≥20 years) are 500 to 540 μg RE and 430 to 460 μg RE, respectively [24]. The US/Canadian vitamin A EARs are 625 μg RAE and 500 μg RAE for males and females (≥20 years), respectively [1]. The recent Chinese vitamin A EARs are 560 μg RAE and 480 μg RAE for males and females (≥18 years), respectively [15]. The reported inadequate proportions below EAR of vitamin A varied from 9.4 to 70.3% [18, 22, 25]. In our study, 88% of Chinese adults consumed less vitamin A than EAR, and only 6% of adults had higher intake than RNI, which meant an inadequate intake at the population level.

Both retinol and carotenes are the main sources of vitamin A intake. In industrialized, Western countries, retinol accounted for nearly 65% of total vitamin A intake, while carotenes made up only 35% [14]. Unlike the findings from developed countries, the current study indicated that retinol only accounted for 43.6% of total vitamin A intake (RAE) in China. The proportion even declined to 32.6%, when vitamin A intake was expressed as RE. The proportion of retinol to total vitamin A intake also showed a significant socio-economic difference. Adults in young, male, urban, eastern, northern, high education, and high income groups consumed more vitamin A from retinol.

Previous reports showed various food sources of vitamin A in different countries. ANIBES Study demonstrated that, among Spanish individuals, milk and products were the main source of retinol (38.7%), followed by eggs (22.6%) and fish (11.4%); vegetables afforded 52.7% of carotenes intake, and then fruits ranked second (13.5%).For total vitamin A intake, vegetables were the main source (31.3%); milk and products provided 21.7%; then eggs ranked third (11%) and fruits fourth (6.9%) [5]. EPIC Study showed that European adults obtained their retinol mainly from meats and meat products (51.7%); added fats and dairy products took the second and third place (18.5 and 15.6%, respectively); vegetables and fruit provided 67.8 and 7.8% of β-carotene intake [23].

Unlike the Western diet [26], dark vegetables and light vegetables were the major contributors of carotene in China (54.6 and 23.6%, respectively), followed by fruit (6.0%) and tubers (3.8%); egg provided 44.6% of retinol; meat and products afforded 29.2%; followed by poultry (9.9%) and fish (6.5%); milk only provided 4.5%. The current study also showed that when vitamin A was expressed as RE the order of the major contributors to vitamin A intake was dark vegetables, eggs, light vegetables, meats and meat products, fruit, poultry, tubers and fish; the order changed slightly when vitamin A was expressed as RAE, with animal source foods contributing more vitamin A and plant source foods less.

China has undergone dramatic socioeconomic changes in the past decades, as well as changes in food consumption and eating behaviors [27]. Although the consumption of animal source foods increased greatly during the past years [28], Chinese adults obtained vitamin A mainly from plant source foods.

It should be noted that there are some limitations in our study. First, vitamin A intake from supplements was not included in the analysis because of insufficient data of supplement use in CNTCS. However, unlike the common use of dietary supplements in the Western world [29, 30], supplement use was far lower in China [31], which leads to little bias of the results. Second, specific carotenes components, such as α-carotene, β-carotene, and β-cryptoxanthin, were not distinguished in the China food composition table and thus went beyond the scope of this paper.

Other study showed that adequate dairy intake greatly improved vitamin A intake, especially among women and older adults [25]. Meanwhile, in the recent Chinese Dietary Guidance (2016) [32], the Chinese Nutrition Society encourages people to consume plenty of vegetables, milk and soybeans, as well as an appropriate amount of fish, poultry, eggs and lean meant.

Conclusions

The present study highlights that, according to the current recommended values, there was a substantial percentage of Chinese adults who had low intakes of vitamin A. Compared with adults in developed countries, the intake of vitamin A, especially retinol intake, was much lower among Chinese adults. The findings illustrate the public health actions are needed to tackle the inadequate intake of vitamin A in China.

Abbreviations

CHNS: China Health and Nutrition Survey; CNTCS: China Nutritional Transition Cohort Study; DRIs: Dietary Reference Intakes; EAR: Estimated Average Requirement; RAE: Retinol Activity Equivalents; RE: Retinol Equivalents; RNI: Recommended Nutrient Intake

Funding

The "China Nutritional Transition Cohort Study" project received funding from Ministry of Finance of the People's Republic of China (NO. 13103110700015005). The present study is also sponsored by Carolina Population Center (P2C HD050924, T32 HD007168), the University of North Carolina at Chapel Hill, the NIH (R01-HD30880, DK056350, R24 HD050924, and R01-HD38700) and the NIH Fogarty International Center (D43 TW009077, D43 TW007709) for financial support for the CHNS data collection and analysis files from 1989 to 2011 and future surveys.

Authors' contributions

WWD analyzed and interpreted the data, and drafted the manuscript; HJW and ZHW contributed to data analysis; JGZ and CS contributed to statistical analysis and data interpretations; XFJ, JZ, HRJ, FFH, YYOY, YW and LL contributed to data interpretation; BZ supervised the study design, analysis and interpretation. All authors provided critical comments on the manuscript, read and approved the final manuscript.

Competing interests

The authors declare that they have no competing interests.

References

1. Panel on Micronutrients, Subcommittees on Upper Reference Levels of Nutrients and of Interpretation and Use of Dietary Reference Intakes, and the Standing Committee on the Scientific Evaluation of Dietary Reference Intakes. Dietary Reference Intakes for Vitamin A, Vitamin K, Arsenic, Boron, Chromium, Copper, Iodine, Iron, Manganese, Molybdenum, Nickel, Silicon, Vanadium, and Zinc. National Academy Press: Washington, D.C., the United States of America. 2001; p.82–146.
2. Stevens GA, Bennett JE, Hennocq Q, Lu Y, De-Reqil LM, Rogers L, Danaei G, Li G, White RA, Flaxman SR, Oehrle SP, Finucane MM, Guerrero R, Bhutta ZA, Then-Paulino A, Fawzi W, Black RE, Ezzati M. Trends and mortality effects of vitamin a deficiency in children in 138 low-income and middle-income countries between 1991 and 2013: a pooled analysis of population-based surveys. Lancet Glob Health. 2015;3(9):e528–36.
3. Yang C, Chen J, Liu Z, Yun C, Piao J, Yang X. Prevalence and influence factors of vitamin a deficiency of Chinese pregnant women. Nutr J. 2016;15:12.
4. Yang C, Chen J, Guo N, Liu Z, Yun C, Li Y, Piao J, Yang X. Comparison on the status of vitamin a in 6- to 13- year-old children between 2002 and 2012 in China. Nutr J. 2016;15(1):50.
5. Olza J, Aranceta-Bartrina J, Gonzalez-Gross M, Ortega RM, Serra-Majem L, Verela-Moreiras G, Gil A. Reported dietary intake and food sources of zinc, selenium, and vitamins a, E and C in the Spanish population: findings from the ANIBES study. Nutrients. 2017;9(7):E697.
6. Beltran-de-Miguel B, Estevez-Santiago R. Olmedilla-AlonsoB. Assessment of dietary vitamin a intake (retinol, alpha-carotene, beta-carotene, beta-cryptoxanthin) and its sources in the National Survey of dietary intake in Spain (2009-2010). Int J Food Sci Nutr. 2015;66(6):706–12.
7. FAO/WHO Joint Expert Consultation. Requirements of vitamin A, iron, folate and vitamin B12. In: FAO. FAO Food and Nutrition Series. Rome; 1988. No.23.
8. Trumbo P, Yates AA, Schlicker S, Poos M. Dietary reference intakes: vitamin a, vitamin K, arsenic, boron, chromium, copper, iodine, iron, manganese, molybdenum, nickel, silicon, vanadium, and zinc. J Am Diet Assoc. 2001; 101(3):294–301.
9. National Health and Medical Research Council, Australian Government Department of Health and Ageing, New Zealand Ministry of Health. Nutrient reference values for australia and new Zealand. 1.2 version. Canberra: National Health and Medical Research Council; 2006.
10. Cheng Y. The introduction fo Chinese dietary reference intakes 2013. Acta Nutriments Sinica. 2014;36(4):313–7.
11. Popkin BM, Du S, Zhai F, Zhang B. Cohort profile: the China health and nutrition survey–monitoring and understanding socio-economic and health change in China, 1989-2011. Int J Epidemiol. 2010;39(6):1435–40.
12. Zhang B, Zhai F, Du SF, Popkin BM. The China health and nutrition survey, 1989-2011. Obes Rev. 2014;15(Suppl 1):2–7.
13. Yang YX, Wang GY, Pan XC. China Food Composition, 2nd ed.;Peking University Medical Press: Beijing, China, 2009, ISBN: 9787811167276.
14. Weber D. GruneT. The contribution of beta-carotene to vitamin a supply of humans. Mol Nutr Food Res. 2012;56(2):251–8.
15. Chinese Nutrition Society. Chinese DRIs handbook. Beijing: Standards Press of China; 2014.
16. He YN, Wang Z, Zhao LY, Fang YH, Yang XG, Zhao WH. Dietary intake of vitamins in Chinese population from 2010 to 2012. Acta Nutrimenta Sinica. 2017;39(02):112–5.
17. Li Y, Zhai FY, He YN, Yu DM, Wang ZH, Zhao LY, Yu WT. Survey on the status of dietary vitamin a intakes in Chinese residents. Wei Sheng Yan Jiu. 2007;36(2): 200–2.
18. Kim S, Kim YN, Cho YO. Vitamin a status of 20- to 59-year-old adults living in Seoul and the metropolitan area. Korea Nutr Res Pract. 2012;6(1):45–50.
19. Kato Y, Ikehara S, Maruyama K, Inagawa M, Oshima M, Yokota K, Yamazaki T, Kishi M, Murai S, Umesawa M, Ma E, Yamagishi K, TanigawaT KM, Sato S, Shimamoto T, Iso H. Trends in dietary intakes of vitamins A, C and E among Japanese men and women from 1974 to 2001. Public Health Nutr. 2009; 12(9):1343–50.
20. Sette S, Le Donne C, Piccinelli R, Arcella D, Turrini A, Leclercq C, INRAN-SCAI 2005-6 Study Group. The third Italian National Food Consumption Survey, INRAN-SCAI 2005-06–part 1: nutrient intakes in Italy. Nutr Metab Cardiovasc Dis. 2011;21(12):922–32.
21. Moshfegh A, Goldman J, Cleveland L. What we eat in America, NHANES 2001–2002: usual nutrient intakes from food compared to dietary reference intakes. U.S. Department of Agriculture; 2005.
22. Pedroza-Tobias A, Hernández-Barrera L, López-Olmedo N, García-Guerra A, Rodríguez-Ramírez S, Ramírez-Silva I, Villalpando S, Carriquiry A, Rivera JA. Usual vitamin intakes by Mexican populations. J Nutr. 2016;146(9):1866S–73S.
23. Jenab M, Salvini S, van Gils CH, Brustad M, Shakya-Shrestha S, Buijsse B, Verhagen H, Touvier M, Biessy C, Wallström P, Bouckaert K, Lund E, Waaseth M, Roswall N, Joensen AM, Linseisen J, Boeing H, Vasilopoulou E, Dilis V, Sieri S, Sacerdote C, Ferrari P, Manjer J, Nilsson S, Welch AA, Travis R, Boutron-Ruault MC, Niravong M, Bueno-de-Mesquita HB, van der Schouw YT, Tormo MJ, Barricarte A, Riboli E, Bingham S, Slimani N. Dietary intakes of retinol, beta-carotene, vitamin D and vitamin E in the European Prospective Investigation into Cancer and Nutrition cohort. Eur J Clin Nutr. 2009; 63(Suppl 4):S150–78.
24. The Korean Nutrition Society. Dietary reference intakes for Koreans. Seoul: Kookjin Publishing Co; 2010.
25. Quann EE, Fulgoni VL 3rd, Auestad N. Consuming the daily recommended amounts of dairy products would reduce the prevalence of inadequate micronutrient intakes in the United States: diet modeling study based on NHANES 2007–2010. Nutr J. 2015;14:90.
26. Goldbohm RA, Brants HA, Hulshof KF, van den Brandt PA. The contribution of various foods to intake of vitamin a and carotenoids in the Netherlands. Int J Vitam Nutr Res. 1998;68(6):378–83.
27. Popkin BM. Synthesis and implications: China's nutrition transition in the context of changes across other low- and middle-income countries. Obes Rev. 2014;15(Suppl 1):60–7.
28. Zhai FY, Du SF, Wang ZH, Zhang JG, Du WW, Popkin BM. Dynamics of the Chinese diet and the role of urbanicity, 1991-2011. Obes Rev. 2014;15(Suppl 1): 16–26.
29. Beitz R, Mensink GB, Fischer B, Thamm M. Vitamins–dietary intake and intake from dietary supplements in Germany. Eur J Clin Nutr. 2002;56(6): 539–45.
30. Swan G. Findings from the latest National Diet and nutrition survey. Proc Nutr Soc. 2004;63(4):505–12.
31. He Y, Yang Z, Xu J, Sha YM, Ren ZY, Pang XH, Wang HJ, Zhai FY. Dietary supplement use in Beijing. Wei Sheng Yan Jiu. 2008;37(1):75–8.
32. Wang SS, Lay S, Yu HN, Shen SR. Dietary guidelines for Chinese residents (2016): comments and comparisons. J Zhejiang Univ Sci B. 2016;17(9):649–56.

9

Ramadan fasting alters food patterns, dietary diversity and body weight among Ghanaian adolescents

Zakari Ali and Abdul-Razak Abizari*

Abstract

Background: Ramadan is a monthlong fast for healthy adolescents and adult Muslims. The quality of foods eaten and eating patterns in Ramadan may be different from other months of the year. Food intake of adolescents is a concern as energy and nutrient requirements are higher and needed to support the growth spurt of this stage. The objective of the present study was to describe the food patterns, dietary diversity and body weight changes among adolescents during Ramadan.

Methods: A prospective cohort study design with four measurement points (baseline, midline, endline and post endline) was conducted among 366 adolescents in Junior High Schools. Food pattern was assessed with a food frequency questionnaire, a 24-h dietary recall was used to assess dietary diversity and body weight was measured using an electronic scale. A repeated measures ANOVA was used to compare changes in dietary diversity scores (DDS) and weight of pupils.

Results: Half of the pupils (50.3%) were female and average age was 15.9 ± 1.8 years. Pupils fasted for an average of 28.3 ± 4.0 days and 14.3 ± 0.5 h a day (dawn to dusk) during Ramadan. The number and types of dishes taken at meal times differed substantially between Ramadan periods and outside Ramadan. Consumption of vitamin A-rich fruits, other fruits, and milk and milk products increased markedly during Ramadan. However, fasting came with a reduction in consumption of foods from roots and tubers, legumes and nuts, and dark green leafy vegetables while other food groups remained unchanged. Mean DDS increased significantly during Ramadan (F (2.933, 1070.573) = 7. 152, $p < 0.001$) while mean daily meal frequency decreased (F (2.936, 1071.623) = 51.653, $p < 0.001$). There was significant body weight loss (-1.5 kg (95% CI: -1.1 kg to -1.6 kg)) among adolescents (F (2.656, 958.95) = 304.90, $p <$ 0. 001). Weight loss was short-lived; regained one month after Ramadan.

Conclusion: In this prospective cohort study among schooling Ghanaian adolescents who fast during Ramadan, fasting was characterised by marked changes in usual food patterns, increased dietary diversity and significant body weight loss.

Keywords: Ramadan, Fasting, Adolescents, Dietary diversity, Weight change, Ghana

* Correspondence: abizaria@yahoo.com
Department of Nutritional Sciences, School of Allied Health Sciences, University for Development Studies, P O Box 1883, Tamale, Ghana

Background

Ramadan is the ninth month of the Islamic lunar calendar and healthy adolescent and adult Muslims refrain from eating or drinking from dawn to dusk for 29 or 30 days [1]. During Ramadan, Muslims fast for an average period of 12 h during the day with a common practice of consuming one large meal after dusk and a lighter meal before dawn [2]. Although children who have not reached puberty are exempt from fasting [3], it is common to find some who practice fasting at 6 or 8 years of age [4] and by early adolescence many children participate fully in Ramadan fasting [5]. Meals taken during the day are normally reduced to two [6] and often little time is available for more meals before bedtime [4]. The quality of foods eaten and eating patterns are changed considerably [7]. The type of food eaten during the night in Ramadan may also be different from that usually consumed during the rest of the year [8]. Alterations in eating modes and infrequent meal schedules during Ramadan that lead to reduced food intake may affect important enzymatic and metabolic responses [9] and different aspects of human health [10]. The effect of fasting on human health has been the subject of a number of scientific investigations [2, 11]. However, mixed findings have been reported by studies on Ramadan fasting and health [12]. For instance, there have been mixed findings regarding body weight and important nutrient changes in response to Ramadan fasting [2]. There is, however, a general opinion that fasting has a potential non-pharmacological intervention for improving health and increasing longevity [2].

Adolescents have been reported to indulge in dietary behaviours that do not meet daily dietary recommendations [13] and a possible trigger of eating disorders [14] during Ramadan. This is a concern, as adolescence is a time of growth and development [15] and nutrient needs are higher than other periods of the life cycle [16]. Adequate nutrients and energy intake therefore, is critical to healthy growth and development at this stage of life [16].

Dietary diversity has proved to be an appropriate method to evaluate nutrient intake adequacy of individuals, including adolescents [17–19] and reflect specific nutrient adequacy [20].

There is, however, scarcity of data on the dietary diversity, food patterns and body weight changes of adolescents who fast during Ramadan. Present study, therefore aimed to fill this knowledge gap using adolescents in Junior High Schools in Northern Ghana, where majority of the people are Muslims.

Methods

Study area

The study was conducted in the Tamale Metropolis, one of the 26 districts of the Northern Region of Ghana. The Metropolis has a total estimated land size of 646.902 sqkm and located in the central part of the Region. The Metropolis has an estimated population of 233,252, comprising 49.7% males and 50.3% females with about 80.8% living in urban localities [21]. The Tamale Metropolis is dominated by Muslims; about 90.5% of the people practice Islamic religion. The population of the metropolis is youthful with about 36.4% aged below 15 years. About 60,000 of the children older than 3 years are enrolled in Primary Schools while 26,936 are enrolled in Junior High Schools (JHS) [22].

Study design

A prospective cohort study design was used in the present study with four measurement points: baseline (before Ramadan), two times during Ramadan (midline and end line) and one month after Ramadan. The 2017 Ramadan fast started on 27th of May for the majority of the people and ended on 24th or 25th of June, lasting for 29 or 30 days. The baseline survey was conducted one week before the start of fasting. Midline survey was conducted at the end of the second week of fast while the end line survey was conducted in the last week (fourth week) of fasting. The final follow up (post Ramadan survey) was conducted one month after the end of fasting.

Target population and sampling

The target population was adolescents aged 10 to 19 years enrolled in Junior High Schools within the Tamale metropolis. The Tamale Metropolis has 15 educational circuits with a total of 72 junior high schools. Half (7) of the circuits were selected using simple random sampling technique. The schools from the selected circuits were pooled together into a frame from which ten Junior High Schools (Anbariya Metropolitan Assembly (M/A) JHS Block 'A', Manhalia Islamic JHS, Datoyili T. I Ahmadiya JHS, Anbariya M/A JHS Block 'B', Lamashegu M/A JHS, Umar Al- Mukhtar JHS, Nahdah Islamic JHS, Zogbeli M/A JHS Block 'A', Kaladan Evangelical Presbyterian JHS and Wataniya Islamic JHS) were then selected by simple random sampling to form the participating schools. A total of 400 pupils in JHS 1 and 2 were then selected from the 10 schools using probability proportional to size (PPS) methodology. Pupils in their final year (JHS 3) were excluded from the study because they were falling out of follow up. Lists of pupils in JHS 1 and 2 of selected schools were compiled for each school using class registers to form the sampling frame. The required number of pupils for each school was selected from the sampling frame by simple random sampling technique using Excel generated random numbers.

Data collection

Data collection was done using a pretested semi-structured questionnaire through face-to-face interviews. The questionnaire elicited information on pupil, parental and household sociodemographic characteristics, fasting and dietary intake characteristics. A similar questionnaire was used for all the follow-up surveys. Data collection staff were first degree nutritionists and received training on questionnaire administration and anthropometric measurements before each assessment. Data collection field supervisors also provided on-site questionnaire checks for completeness and all wrong responses and measurements were repeated and corrected the same day.

Assessment of dietary diversity and dish variety scores

A qualitative 24-h dietary recall was used for dietary intake assessment of pupils. Pupils were asked to recall all foods they consumed at home and outside the home (including at school) the day preceding the survey. Foods recalled were classified into their respective food groups based on which the dietary diversity was determined. The Food and Agriculture Organization (FAO) defines dietary diversity as the number of food groups an individual consumes over the past 24-h [23]. The dietary diversity of participants was assessed following standard guidelines for measuring individual dietary diversity by the FAO [23]. Dietary diversity score was calculated based on consumption of fourteen food groups including: Cereals; white roots and tubers; vitamin a rich vegetables and tubers; dark green leafy vegetables; other vegetables; vitamin a rich fruits; other fruits; organ meat; flesh meats, eggs; fish and seafood; legumes, nuts and seeds; milk and milk products; and oils and fats. The dietary diversity score therefore ranged from 0 to 14, a score of 1 was assigned if one food group was consumed and 14 if all food groups were consumed. The dish variety score was calculated as the number of dishes consumed in an eating moment. Composite dishes such as *Waakye* (mixture of rice and beans) with stew and porridge with bread were given single scores. A pupil therefore had a dish variety score of 2 if they had both *Waakye* with stew and porridge with bread at an eating moment (For example: breakfast). The dish variety scores were then categorized into '1' when a pupil had a dish variety score of 1 and '2' if they had a score of 2 or more at an eating moment to give the dish variety of that eating moment.

Assessment of dietary patterns

Dietary pattern was assessed using a food frequency questionnaire. The seven day food frequency questionnaire included 60 foods commonly consumed in northern Ghana and was similar to the one used earlier in the same area [24]. Pupils were asked to recall how often they have on average had a particular food in the past one week preceding each assessment. The consumption scores ranged from 0 (when they had never or hardly ever taken a particular food for the past week) to 7 (if they had a particular food for more than six days in the past one week). Changes in dietary patterns were assessed using changes in food consumption frequency during Ramadan relative to the non-Ramadan periods.

Weight and height measurements

Weight and height measurements were taken following WHO standard anthropometry guidelines [25]. Electronic weighing scales (Seca 874) were used for all weight measurements. Weights were recorded to the nearest 0.1 kg. The scales were regularly checked for accuracy and precision using a standard weight. Data collection staff were also trained to minimize measurement errors. Weight measurements were taken around the same time of the day for all pupils and in all schools for the four surveys.

Data and statistical analysis

Data was entered, cleaned and analyzed using Statistical Package for Social Sciences (SPSS) for windows version 20. About 8.5% of the pupils had incomplete follow-up data. The a priori decision was to include only pupils who were available and completed all the four surveys. The analyses are therefore based on the remaining 91.5% (366) who completed all follow ups.

The data are presented as descriptive statistics in the form of frequencies and percentages for categorical variables and means and standard deviations for continuous variables. The association between mean dietary diversity scores, mean weight and sex of pupils at each assessment point was investigated using the independent student t-test. A repeated measures ANOVA was used to compare the changes in dietary diversity scores, daily meal frequency, and weight of pupils across the assessments. Differences were considered statistically significant at $p < 0.05$.

Results

Background characteristics of participating pupils in junior high schools in Tamale

Half of the pupils (50.3%) were female and average age was 15.9 ± 1.8 years. More than five in ten pupils (51.4%) were in JHS 1, belonged to the Dagomba ethnic group (87.2%) and were normal by BMI-for-age classification (87.7%). More than three-quarters of the pupils lived with their parents and almost all (92.6%) were given pocket money to school.

Though educational level of parents of pupils was generally low, 16.6% more of mothers had no formal education than fathers. While fathers (32.8%) mostly engaged in farming, the majority of mothers were traders (71.6%). Majority of fathers had more than one wife (57.4%) and

Table 1 Background characteristics of participating pupils in JHS

Characteristic	Summary values (*n* = 366)
Pupil characteristics	
Sex, n (%)	
Female	184 (50.3)
Age in years, (mean ± SD)	15.9 ± 1.8
Class of pupil, n (%)	
JHS 1	188 (51.4)
JHS 2	178 (48.6)
Ethnicity, n (%)	
Dagomba	319 (87.2)
Gonja	26 (7.1)
Others	21 (5.7)
Nutritional status (BMI-for-age classification), n (%)	
Underweight	23 (6.3)
Normal	321 (87.7)
Overweight/obese	22 (6.0)
Live with parents, n (%)	
Yes	286 (78.1)
Pocket money to school	
Yes	339 (92.6)
Parent characteristics	
Father's educational level, n (%)	
None	195 (53.3)
Primary/JHS	98 (26.8)
SHS/Tertiary	73 (19.9)
Father's occupation, n (%)	
Farmer	120 (32.8)
Trader	74 (20.2)
Civil servant	33 (9.0)
Others	139 (38.0)
Wives of father, n (%)	
At least two wives	210 (57.4)
Mother's educational level, n (%)	
None	256 (69.9)
Primary/JHS	83 (22.7)
SHS/Tertiary	27 (7.4)
Mother's occupation, n (%)	
Farmer	34 (9.3)
Trader	262 (71.6)
Civil servant	6 (1.6)
Others	64 (17.5)
Mother's position, n (%)	
First wife	277 (75.7)
Other	89 (24.3)
Household characteristics	
Family type, n (%)	
Extended	214 (58.5)
Nuclear	152 (41.5)
Family head, n (%)	
Father	216 (59.0)
Grandfather	61 (16.7)
Mother	15 (4.1)
Grandmother	24 (6.6)
Others	50 (13.7)
Household size, n (%)	
At least 10 members	240 (65.6)
Number of household members below 20 years, mean ± SD	6.2 ± 4.1

mothers of participating pupils were the first wives (75.7%) of the fathers. Majority of pupils lived with extended families (58.5%) which were headed by their father (59.0%). More than six in ten (65.6%) of the pupils belonged to families of at least ten members (Table 1).

Fasting characteristics of pupils in participating junior high schools

The average age pupils started fasting was 11.2 ± 2.5 years. The pupils endured fasting for almost the whole month of Ramadan (28.3 ± 3.6 days) for an average of 14.3 ± 0.54 h each day (dawn to dusk). Almost all parents (98.1%) were also fasting and provided encouragement (80.34%) to their children; fathers (40.5%) encouraged pupils a little more than mothers (39.9%) to fast. Pupils fasted for a number of reasons including: spiritual growth (43.1%), compulsion by family (24.0%), parents fasting (8.1%) and for good health (3.0%).

Most pupils missed fast mainly due to menstruation (49.5%) and sickness (40.0%). Some pupils (39.9%) also fasted some number of days (5.4 ± 1.6) after Ramadan. Most pupils (63.1%) did not experience any sickness during fasting. However, those who reported some sickness mainly experienced diarrhoea (25.9%) and malaria (22.2%). Foods used for fasting were mainly obtained from home (64.5% at midline and 66.4% at endline). While foods obtained as gifts increased by about 2% between midline and endline assessments, bought foods decreased by nearly 4% between midline and endline assessments (Table 2).

Table 2 Fasting characteristics of participating pupils in JHS

Characteristic	Summary values
Age started fasting ($n = 366$), mean ± SD	11.2 ± 2.5[a]
Days fasted during Ramadan ($n = 366$), mean ± SD	28.3 ± 3.6[d]
Fasting duration within a day (hours) ($n = 366$), mean ± SD	14.3 ± 0.54[b]
Days missed fasting (mean ± SD)	1.73 ± 3.59[d]
Reasons for missing fasting, n (%)	
Could not wake up in good time	7 (6.7)[c]
Was sick	42 (40.0)[c]
Menstruation (girls)	52 (49.5)[c]
Others	4 (3.8)[c]
Parents fasting? ($n = 363$), n (%)	
Yes	356 (98.1)
Encouragement to fast ($n = 351$), n (%)	
Father	142 (40.5)[b]
Mother	140 (39.9)[b]
Sibling	15 (4.3)[b]
Uncle	13 (3.7)[b]
Spiritual leader	3 (0.9)[b]
Others	38 (10.8)[b]
Reasons for fasting ($n = 334$), n (%)	
Spiritual growth (blessing)	144 (43.1)[b]
It is compulsory	80 (24.0)[b]
Parents fasting	27 (8.1)[b]
For good health	10 (3.0)[b]
Other reasons	73 (21.9)[b]
Continued fasting after Ramadan ($n = 366$), n (%)	
No	220 (60.1)[d]
Days fasted after Ramadan ($n = 146$), mean ± SD	5.38 ± 1.55[d]
Reasons for fasting after Ramadan ($n = 146$), n (%)	
Obeying religious recommendation	83 (56.8)[d]
Replacing missed days	52 (35.6)[d]
Others	11 (7.5)[d]
Sickness during Ramadan? ($n = 366$), n (%)	
No	231 (63.1)[c]
Type of sickness during Ramadan ($n = 135$), n (%)	
Malaria	30 (22.2)[c]
Diarrhoea	35 (25.9)[c]
Others	70 (51.9)[c]
Source of midline fasting food ($n = 366$), n (%)	
Gifts	35 (9.6)
Purchase	87 (23.8)
Home	236 (64.5)
others	8 (2.2)
Source of end line fasting food ($n = 366$), n (%)	
Gifts	42 (11.5)
Buying	74 (20.2)
Home	243 (66.4)
Others	7 (1.9)

[a]measured at baseline [b]measured at midline [c]measured at endline [d]measured at post Ramadan

Changes in daily meal frequency among participating pupils in junior high schools during fasting

A repeated measure ANOVA with a Greenhouse-Geisser correction showed that the mean feeding frequency changed significantly across the assessment stages (F (2.936, 1071.623) = 51.653, $p < 0.001$). Post hoc test using Bonferroni correction revealed that mean feeding frequency decreased significantly between baseline and midline assessments (3.1 vs 2.7, $p < 0.001$) and between baseline and endline assessments (3.1 vs 2.7, $p < 0.001$) but not between baseline and post Ramadan (3.1 vs 3.1, $p > 0.05$) (Table 3).

Daily meal composition and variations during Ramadan among participating pupils in junior high schools

We assessed the number of dishes taken at meal times as well as the main dishes taken at meal times and their variation during Ramadan. Majority of pupils (98.3%) had one main dish at breakfast before the start of Ramadan but more dishes at dawn (breakfast) during Ramadan. For instance, while only 2 % of the pupils consumed two or more dishes at breakfast before Ramadan, more than four in ten pupils (46%) had two or more dishes at dawn two weeks into fasting which increased to nearly 50% during the last week of fasting and reduced to baseline value (2%) a month after Ramadan. Before Ramadan, pupils would have tea with bread (37%) or porridge with bread/roasted groundnut/beancake (36%) for breakfast. During Ramadan however, pupils would have tea with bread (62% and 57% for midline and endline respectively) as well as rice with stew (20% and 27% for midline and endline respectively) or *tuo zaafi* with soup (30% and 26% for midline and endline respectively). A month after Ramadan the pupils had returned to taking breakfast as either tea with bread (45.4%) or porridge with bread/roasted groundnut/beancake (33%) (Table 4).

Foods usually taken before dinner which were used to break the fast during fasting doubled with Ramadan. For example, while majority (92% and 91%, respectively for baseline and post Ramadan) of the pupils had one dish outside Ramadan, they would have two or more dishes (68.4% and 71%, respectively for midline and endline) during Ramadan. Before Ramadan, pupils would have

Table 3 Pairwise comparisons of changes in feeding frequency of participating pupils in JHS before, during and aftrer Ramadan (Repeated measures ANOVA)

(I) feed frequency (mean ± SD)	(J) feed frequency (mean ± SD)	Mean Difference (I-J)	Std. Error	Sig.[b]	95% Confidence Interval for Difference[b]	
					Lower Bound	Upper Bound
Baseline frequency (3.1 ± 0.6)	Midline frequency (2.7 ± 0.8)	0.437[a]	0.048	< 0.001	0.311	0.564
	End line frequency (2.7 ± 0.7)	0.423[a]	0.044	< 0.001	0.308	0.539
	Post Ramadan frequency (3.1 ± 0.7)	0.052	0.042	1.000	−0.061	0.164
Midline frequency (2.7 ± 0.8)	End line frequency (2.7 ± 0.7)	− 0.014	0.048	1.000	−0.140	00.113
	Post Ramadan frequency (3.1 ± 0.7)	−0.385[a]	0.048	< 0.001	−0.513	−0.257
End line frequency (2.7 ± 0.7)	Post Ramadan frequency (3.1 ± 0.7)	−0.372[a]	0.047	< 0.001	−0.496	− 0.247

Based on estimated marginal means, [a]. The mean difference is significant at the .05 level, [b]Adjustment for multiple comparisons: Bonferroni

Table 4 Changes in breakfast/dawn and lunch meals in Ramadan among participating pupils in JHS

	Baseline n/N (%)	Midline n/N (%)	Endline n/N (%)	Post Ramadan n/N (%)
Dish variety score of breakfast/dawn meals, mean ± SD	1.0 ± 0.13	1.5 ± 0.51	1.5 ± 0.52	1.0 ± 0.14
Dish variety at breakfast/dawn				
One dish	341/347 (98.3)	196/361 (54.3)	181/357 (50.7)	352/359 (98.1)
Two or more dishes	6/347 (1.7)	165/361 (45.7)	176/357 (49.3)	7/359 (1.9)
Breakfast/dawn meals				
Tea/tea and bread	128/347 (36.9)	223/361 (61.8)	202/357 (56.6)	163/359 (45.4)
Porridge (with kose/groundnut/bread)	124/347 (35.7)	11/361 (3.0)	11/357 (3.1)	119/359 (33.1)
Rice and stew (plain rice/jollof/fried rice/riceballs)	20/347 (5.8)	71/361 (19.7)	97/357 (27.2)	20/359 (5.6)
Rice and beans with stew	20/347 (5.8)	31/361 (8.6)	43/357 (12.0)	14/359 (3.9)
Tuo zaafi with soup	5/347 (1.4)	107/361 (29.6)	92/357 (25.8)	8/359 (2.2)
Banku with soup	2/347 (0.6)	20/361 (3.8)	16/357 (4.5)	2/359 (0.6)
Cocoa drink with bread	25/347 (7.2)	27/361 (7.5)	18/357 (5.0)	18/359 (5.0)
Fufu with soup	0/347 (0.0)	7/361 (1.9)	2/357 (0.6)	0/359 (0)
Fruits	0/347 (0.0)	2/361 (0.6)	1/357 (0.3)	0/359 (0)
Other foods	26/347 (7.5)	30/361 (8.3)	19/357 (5.3)	20/359 (5.6)
Dish variety score of lunch meals, mean ± SD	1.0 ± 0.15	1.2 ± 0.38	1.1 ± 0.29	1.01 ± 0.11
Dish variety at lunch				
One dish	326/334 (97.6)	11/13 (84.6)	11/12 (92)	334/338 (98.8)
Two or more dishes	8/334 (2.4)	2/13 (15.4)	1/12 (8)	4/338 (1.2)
Lunch meals				
Rice and stew (plain rice/jollof/fried rice/riceballs)	108/334 (32.3)	6/13 (46.2)	3/12 (25)	92/338 (27.2)
Rice and beans with stew	71/334 (21.3)	0/13 (0)	3/12 (25)	103/338 (30.5)
Tuo zaafi with soup	69/334 (20.7)	2/13 (15.4)	5/12 (42)	58/338 (17.2)
Banku with soup	16/334 (4.8)	1/13 (7.7)	0/12 (0)	12/338 (3.6)
Kenkey with stew	11/334 (3.3)	0/13 (0)	0/12 (0)	10/338 (3.0)
Yam meal (Wasawasa)	14/334 (4.2)	0/13 (0)	0/12 (0)	9/338 (2.7)
Fufu with soup (pounded yams and/cassava)	4/334 (1.2)	0/13 (0)	0/12 (0)	0/338 (0)
Fruits	1/334 (0.3)	0/13 (0)	0/12 (0)	0/338 (0)
Other foods	46/334 (13.8)	4/13 (30.8)	1/12 (8.3)	56/338 (16.6)

Table 5 Changes in foods taken before dinner/foods for breaking fast and dinner meals in Ramadan among participating pupils in JHS

	Baseline n/N (%)	Midline n/N (%)	Endline n/N (%)	Post Ramadan n/N (%)
Dish variety score of taken before dinner meals/ foods for breaking fast, mean ± SD	1.1 ± 0.3	2.1 ± 1.0	2.1 ± 0.9	1.1 ± 0.3
Dish variety of foods taken before dinner/foods for breaking fast				
One dish	103/112 (92.0)	99/312 (31.6)	98/339 (28.9)	96/106 (90.6)
Two or more dishes	9/112 (8.0)	214/312 (68.4)	241 (71.1)	10/106 (9.4)
Before dinner meals/ foods at *Iftar*				
Dates	0/112 (0.0)	187/312 (59.9)	209/339 (61.4)	0/106 (0.0)
Watermelon	1/112 (0.9)	61/312 (19.6)	97/339 (28.6)	25/106 (23.6)
Mango	16/112 (14.3)	62/312 (19.9)	64/339 (18.9)	0/106 (23.6)
Banana	3/112 (2.7)	19/312 (6.1)	15/339 (4.4)	1/106 (0.9)
Orange	1/112 (0.9)	12/312 (3.8)	6/339 (1.6)	1/106 (0.9)
Other fruits	3/112 (2.7)	6/312 (1.9)	6/339 (1.6)	1/106 (0.9)
Mashed kenkey	16/112 (14.3)	169/312 (54.2)	188/339 (55.5)	11/106 (10.4)
Porridge	7/112 (6.2)	58/312 (18.6)	59/339 (17.4)	7/106 (6.6)
Tea	1/112 (0.9)	11/312 (3.5)	6/339 (1.8)	3/106 (2.8)
Roselle drink (*Sobolo*)	13/112 (11.6)	6/312 (1.9)	9/339 (2.7)	7/106 (6.6)
Tuo zaafi/ Rice and stew	26/112 (23.2)	6/312 (1.9)	5/339 (1.5)	19/106 (17.9)
Other foods	36/112 (32.1)	49/312 (15.7)	30/339 (8.8)	36/106 (34.0)
Dish variety score of dinner meals, mean ± SD	1.0 ± 0.0	1.1 ± 0.4	1.1 ± 0.3	1.0 ± 0.1
Dish variety at dinner				
One dish	340/340 (100)	317/349 (90.8)	313/352 (88.9)	330/336 (98.2)
Two or more dishes	0/340 (0.0)	32/349 (9.2)	39/352 (11.1)	6/336 (1.8)
Dinner meals				
Rice and stew	57/340 (16.8)	128/349 (36.7)	123/352 (34.9)	47/336 (14.0)
Rice and beans	17/340 (5.0)	48/349 (13.8)	60/352 (17.0)	27/336 (8.0)
Tuo zaafi and soup	216/340 (63.5)	125/349 (35.8)	121/352 (34.4)	216/336 (64.3)
Banku and soup/stew	16/340 (4.7)	27/349 (7.7)	28/352 (8.0)	23/336 (6.8)
Fufu with soup	0/340 (0.0)	4/349 (1.1)	4/352 (1.1)	4/336 (1.2)
Fruits	0/340 (0.0)	5/349 (1.4)	3/352 (0.9)	0/336 (0.0)
Other foods	27/340 (7.9)	45/349 (12.9)	41/352 (11.6)	24/336 (7.1)
Foods after dinner				
Fruits	31/61 (50.8)	29/78 (37.2)	11/45 (24.4)	10/41 (24.4)

tuo zaafi with soup (23%) or mangoes (14.3%) or mashed kenkey (14.3%) before dinner time. Pupils however, had dates (60% and 61%, respectively for midline and endline) and mashed kenkey (54% and 56%, respectively for midline and endline) at *Iftar* (period to "breakfast") during Ramadan. Fasting also came with a marked increase in the intake of watermelons and mangoes. One month after Ramadan, the pupils had one of the following; mangoes (24%) or watermelons (24%) or *tuo zaafi* with soup (18%) before dinner time.

The number of dishes taken at dinner remained unchanged during Ramadan at one dish. There were however, marked changes in the type of dishes taken. For example, while *tuo zaafi* was taken by the majority of the pupils (64% at baseline and post Ramadan) outside Ramadan, they had either rice with stew (36% and 35%, respectively for midline and endline) or *tuo zaafi* with soup (36% and 34%, respectively for midline and endline) for dinner during Ramadan (Table 5).

Patterns of food groups and local dish consumption among participating pupils in junior high schools during Ramadan

The consumption from various food groups varied greatly in some food groups while others hardly changed during Ramadan. Consumption from cereals, other

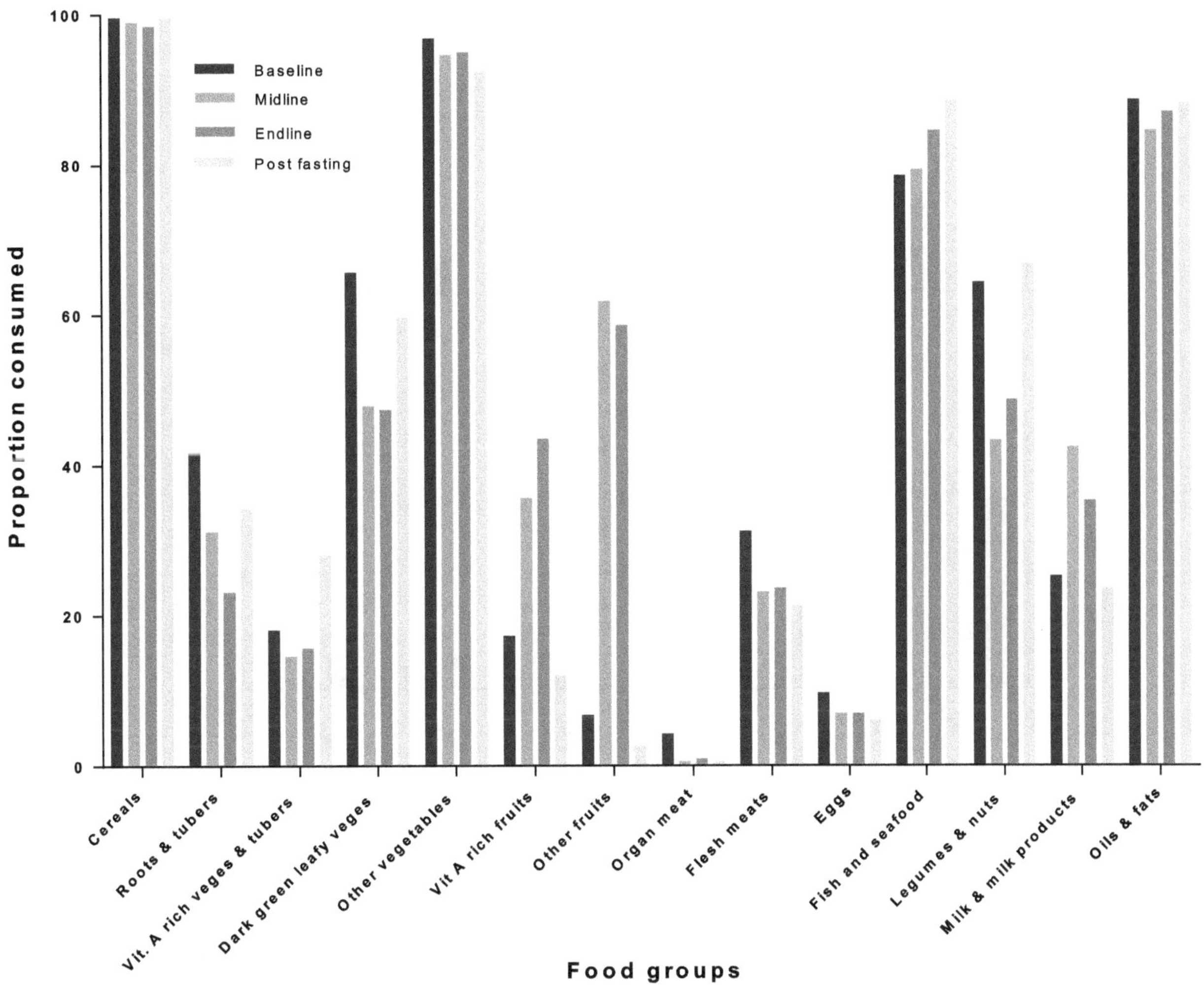

Fig. 1 Proportion of food group consumption among participating pupils in JHS

vegetables and fats and oils groups remained high without much changes with Ramadan. There was an increase in the consumption of vitamin A- rich fruits, other fruits, and milk and milk products during Ramadan. Fasting however, came with a reduction in consumption of foods from roots and tubers, legumes and nuts, vitamin A-rich vegetables and tubers and dark green leafy vegetables (Fig. 1).

Consumption patterns of vitamin A-rich fruits (watermelon, mango and shea fruit) generally increased during fasting except pawpaw which decreased during Ramadan. Intake of watermelons increased from about a day's frequency to nearly three days a week during Ramadan. Mango intake was high, averaging nearly three days in a week before Ramadan and reduced slightly during Ramadan and further to a day's frequency a month after Ramadan (Fig. 2a). Other fruits including pineapples, apples, bananas and oranges remained below a two day consumption frequency and almost unchanged with Ramadan. However, consumption of dates increased from below a two day frequency to nearly every day during Ramadan (Fig. 2b). Consumption of local vegetables (bra leaves (*Hibiscus sabdariffa*), *ayoyo* leaves (*Corchorus olitorius*), *aleefu* (*Amarantus sp.*), tomato, red hot pepper, onions, baobab leaves (dry), okro (fresh fruits, fruit powder)) remained high and almost unchanged while exotic vegetables (cabbage, lettuce, carrots, cucumber, green pepper) consumption fell slightly during Ramadan (Fig. 2c). Milk consumption increased from below two days in a week to above two days during Ramadan. Consumption frequency of other dairy foods such as yoghurt and local cheese remained below two days with no marked changes during Ramadan (Fig. 2d).

Commonly consumed cereal based staples maintained a daily consumption pattern (Fig. 3a). Such staples as *tuo zaafi*, plain rice, rice and beans, bread and porridge remained highly consumed, taken almost every day and unchanged during Ramadan. Tuber based foods were however, less frequently consumed before Ramadan and further reduced during Ramadan. For example, the consumption

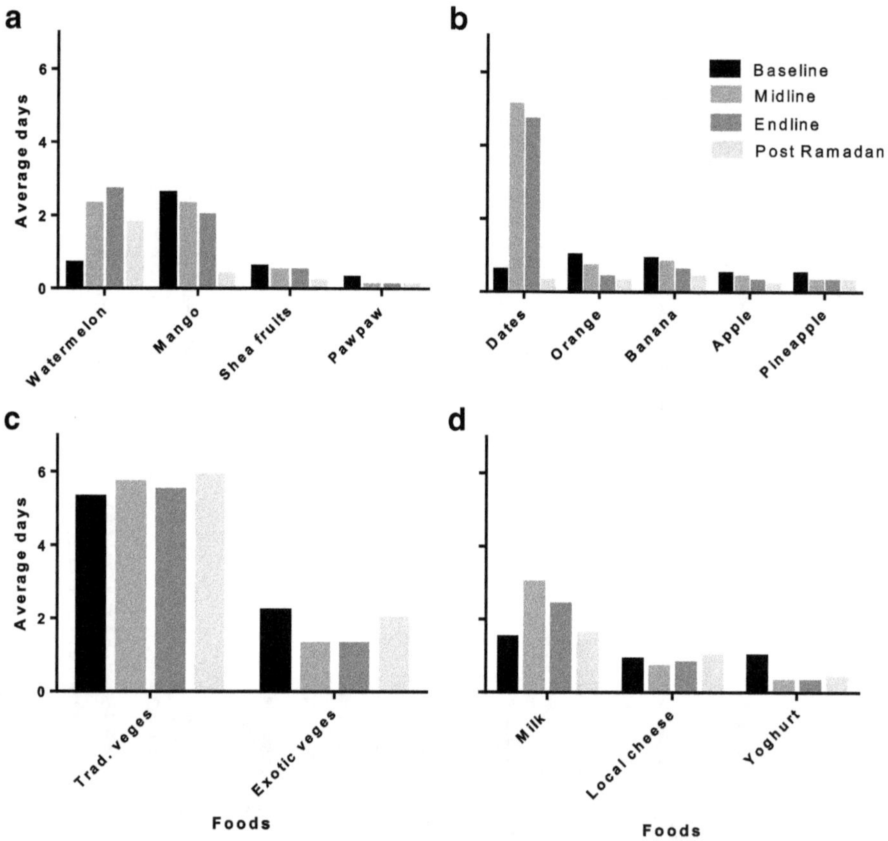

Fig. 2 Patterns of consumption of vitamin A rich fruits (**a**), other fruits (**b**), vegetables (**c**) and dairy products (**d**) among participating pupils in JHS

of *fufu* (made from pounded cassava and/or yams), boiled yams and sweet potatoes decreased during fasting and began to rise one month after fasting (Fig. 3b). There was a reduction in the consumption of leguminous foods such as soya beans (usually eaten as soya kebab), pigeon pea, groundnuts, and cowpea with varying patterns. While frequency of groundnut intake fell to below three days in a week during Ramadan and rose to baseline frequency a month after Ramadan, intake of cowpeas remained similar to baseline frequency of a little above three days at midline assessment and reduced thereafter at endline and post Ramadan assessments. Pattern of soya bean and pigeon pea consumption were similar with a little above two days weekly consumption frequency at baseline assessment which reduced steeply to below a day's frequency during Ramadan and began to rise to baseline frequency at post Ramadan assessment (Fig. 3c). Tea intake increased from a little below four days to almost six days in a week during Ramadan. Mashed *kenkey* (made from fermented corn dough with added sugar) consumption increased markedly from about once a week to nearly four times during Ramadan and reduced thereafter. Further, fasting came with a marked decrease in intake of sweets (toffees, gums). Before Ramadan, pupils would have sweets for about three times in a week but had sweets for less than a day in a week during Ramadan (Fig. 3d).

Meat (beef, mutton and chevon) consumption patterns remained relatively the same averaging three days in a week while poultry (chicken, guinea fowl, turkey) intake experienced a marginal decrease during Ramadan. There was nearly a one day increase in consumption of fish and sea foods during Ramadan which increased further after fasting. Intake of fats and oils remained high and relatively unchanged during the first half of Ramadan but reduced in the second half of Ramadan. There was lower consumption frequency of chocolates, fried rice (largely a fast food), energy drinks, coffee, yoghurt, soft drinks, and packed fruit drinks across assessment points which further reduced during Ramadan or remained unchanged (soft drinks and packed fruit juice) with frequencies of once or less in a week (See Additional file 1).

Changes in dietary diversity among participating pupils in junior high schools during Ramadan

Using a repeated measure ANOVA with a Greenhouse-Geisser correction, it was found that the differences in mean dietary diversity were statistically significant across the assessment stages (F (2.933,

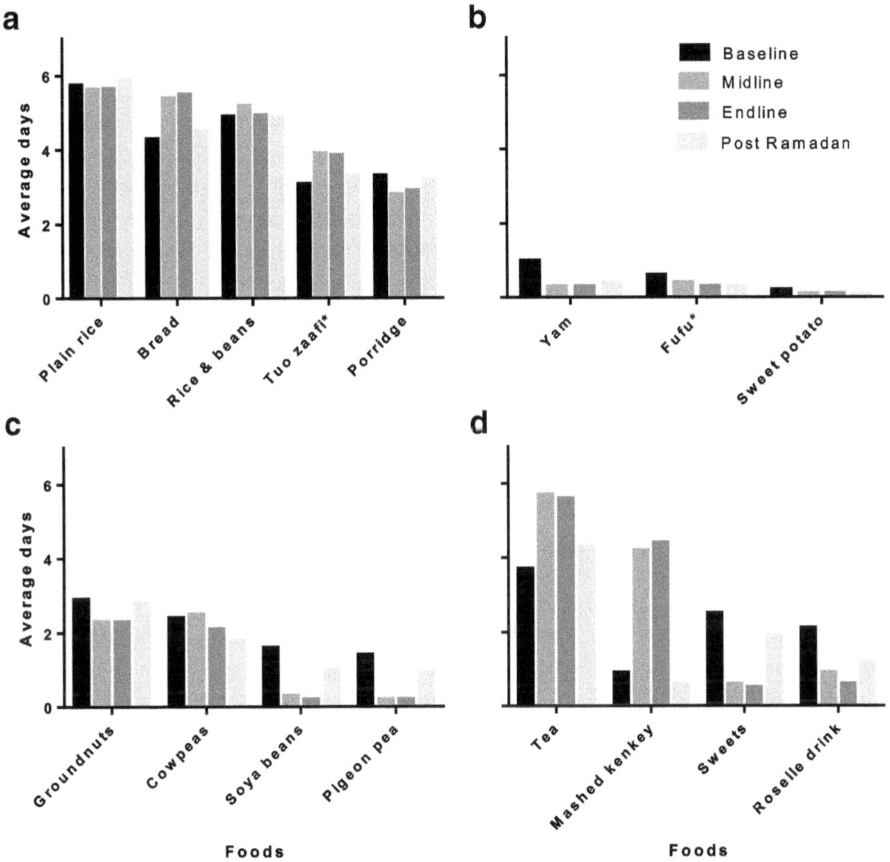

Fig. 3 Patterns of consumption of cereal based foods (**a**), tuber based foods (**b**), legumes (**c**) and sugar sweetened beverages and sweets (**d**). *Tuo zaafi: made from maize/millet flour. *Fufu: Made from pounded yams and/or cassava

1070.573) = 7.152, $p < 0.001$). There was a marginal increase in mean dietary diversity score from baseline (6.5 ± 1.6), midline (6.6 ± 1.8) through to the endline (6.7 ± 1.7) and decreased thereafter at post Ramadan (6.2 ± 1.4). Post hoc test using Bonferroni correction revealed a significant decrease in mean dietary diversity scores between midline and post Ramadan assessments ($p < 0.001$) and between endline and post Ramadan assessments ($p < 0.001$). There was however, no statistically significant mean difference between baseline and midline; baseline and endline; and baseline and post Ramadan assessments ($p > 0.05$) (Table 6). Differences in mean dietary

Table 6 Pairwise comparisons of changes in dietary diversity among participating pupils in JHS (Repeated measures ANOVA)

(I) Dietary diversity (mean ± SD)	(J) dietary diversity (mean ± SD)	Mean Difference (I-J)	Std. Error	Sig.[b]	95% Confidence Interval for Difference[b]	
					Lower Bound	Upper Bound
Baseline diversity (6.5 ± 1.6)	Midline diversity (6.6 ± 1.8)	−0.175	0.113	0.734	−0.474	0.125
	Endline diversity (6.7 ± 1.7)	−0.210	0.116	0.418	−0.517	0.096
	Post Ramadan diversity (6.2 ± 1.4)	0.235	0.102	0.127	−0.034	0.504
Midline diversity (6.6 ± 1.8)	Endline diversity (6.7 ± 1.7)	− 0.036	0.108	1.000	− 0.322	0.251
	Post Ramadan diversity (6.2 ± 1.4)	0.410[a]	0.105	0.001	0.132	0.688
Endline diversity (6.7 ± 1.7)	Post Ramadan diversity (6.2 ± 1.4)	0.445[a]	0.102	< 0.001	0.174	0.717

Based on estimated marginal means, [a]. The mean difference is significant at the .05 level, [b]Adjustment for multiple comparisons: Bonferroni diversity scores between males and females across assessment points were investigated using t- test. Females generally had higher dietary diversity scores outside Ramadan (baseline and post Ramadan) but lower during Ramadan (midline and endline), while the males had lower dietary diversity scores outside Ramadan but higher during Ramadan. Mean dietary diversity scores however, did not differ significantly between males and females at baseline (6.4 vs 6.5, $p > 0.05$), endline (6.7 vs 6.6, $p > 0.05$) and post Ramadan (6.2 vs 6.3, $p > 0.05$) but at midline (6.9 vs 6.4, $p = 0.002$) (Results not shown).

Weight changes among participating pupils in junior high schools during Ramadan

Our data showed statistically significant weight changes across the assessment points in a repeated measure ANOVA using Greenhouse-Geisser correction (F (2.656, 958.95) = 304.90, $p < 0.001$). Fasting explained about 46% of weight changes (Partial Eta Squared = 0.458) in pupils during Ramadan. There were significant weight loses from baseline through to midline and endline assessments ($p < 0.001$). For example, pupils lost an average of 1.1 kg of weight between baseline and midline assessments and 1.5 kg (95% CI: -1.1 kg to – 1.6 kg) by endline assessment. Overall weight loss during Ramadan was significantly higher among females (– 1.7 kg, 95% CI: -1.6 kg to – 1.9 kg) than males (– 1.2 kg, 95% CI: -1.0 kg to – 1.3 kg) ($p < 0.001$). Weight loss did not differ by age of pupil ($p > 0.05$) (Results not shown). Pupils had however, recovered their lost weight one month after Ramadan, evident in the lack of significant difference ($p = 0.233$) between mean baseline weight (51.1 ± 8.9) and post fasting weight (51.0 ± 8.8) (Table 7). In a t-test, it was revealed that mean weight of pupils did not differ by sex across all assessment points ($p > 0.05$) (Results not shown).

Discussion

This study sought to describe the food patterns, dietary diversity and weight changes among Ghanaian adolescents during Ramadan. The main findings were that daily meal frequency reduced significantly during Ramadan. There were marked changes in the number and types of dishes taken at meal times during Ramadan. In addition, dietary diversity increased significantly during Ramadan. Consumption of some food groups varied greatly while others hardly changed during Ramadan. Adolescent food intake during Ramadan was largely characterised by increases in fruit and vegetable consumption, dish variety, dietary diversity, reduced intakes of fast foods (such as fried rice), energy and soft drink, sweets, fats and oils and high intake of cereal based foods. Further, there was statistically significant body weight loss of 1.5 kg over the Ramadan period.

The significant reduction in the number of eating moments during Ramadan is not surprising because the whole daytime is typically spent without food during Ramadan. Daytime eating moments are therefore essentially lost. Significant decrease in daily meal frequency during Ramadan has been reported earlier [26].

The increased dish variety at dawn during Ramadan could be explained by the temptation to combine usual breakfast and lunch to provide sustenance for the day's fast. Pupils therefore, took a lighter meal (tea with/out bread) similar to their usual breakfast outside Ramadan in addition to a heavy meal (rice with stew or *tuo zaafi* with soup) similar to what they would normally have for lunch. Energy and nutrient intake from the increased dishes at dawn is however, not expected to be similar to energy and nutrient intakes from a combined usual breakfast and lunch outside Ramadan as increasing dishes at meal times could mean reduced portion sizes for both dishes [27]. In addition, appetite is likely to be suppressed at dawn due to the nocturnal rise in leptin

Table 7 Pairwise comparisons of changes in body weight among participating pupils in JHS (Repeated measures ANOVA)

(I) Weight changes (mean ± SD)	(J) Weight changes (mean ± SD)	Mean Difference (I-J)	Std. Error	Sig.[b]	95% Confidence Interval for Difference[b]	
					Lower Bound	Upper Bound
Baseline weight (51.1 ± 8.9)	Midline weight (50.0 ± 8.9)	1.085[a]	0.054	< 0.001	0.942	1.229
	Endline weight (49.6 ± 8.8)	1.452[a]	0.057	< 0.001	1.301	1.602
	Post Ramadan weight (51.0 ± 8.8)	0.140	0.068	0.233	−0.039	0.319
Midline weight (50.00 ± 8.87)	Endline weight (49.6 ± 8.8)	0.366[a]	0.045	< 0.001	0.248	0.485
	Post Ramadan weight (51.0 ± 8.8)	−0.945[a]	0.063	< 0.001	−1.113	−0.778
Endline weight (49.63 ± 8.81)	Post Ramadan weight (51.0 ± 8.8)	−1.312[a]	0.056	< 0.001	− 1.460	− 1.163

Based on estimated marginal means, [a]. The mean difference is significant at the .05 level, [b]Adjustment for multiple comparisons: Bonferroni levels among non-fasting people [28] and those fasting in Ramadan [29]. The increase in dish variety during *Iftar* may be due to the usual practice of taking fruits at *Iftar*.

The significant increase in dietary diversity during Ramadan could be due to increase in specific food groups such as other fruits, vitamin A rich fruits, and milk and milk products. The increase in fruits consumption were largely due to the marked increase in intake of dates, mangoes and watermelons normally taken at *Iftar* during Ramadan. The increase in milk and milk products intake is understandable as there was marked increase in tea intake which is served with milk. This increase could also be due to the increase in mashed *kenkey* which could be served with milk. The decrease in consumption from the legumes and nuts, and dark green leafy vegetables food groups may mean that these foods are normally taken at school as lunch. Rice and cowpeas (*Waakye*), and pigeon peas which are major legume based foods are normally served with assorted vegetables including cabbage, lettuce and carrots at school for lunch [30]. The marginally higher dietary diversity scores during Ramadan among males compared to females could be explained by the higher tendency of males to have other foods as gifts at *Iftar* usually provided at the Mosque in addition to family-provided meals. In addition, girls are likely to be home helping prepare meals while boys are outside grabbing whatever may be available.

Generally, we find adolescent food intakes during Ramadan to follow a relatively healthy diet pattern. Dietary intake was characterised by increase in fruit and vegetable consumption, increased dish variety, increased dietary diversity, reduced intake of fast foods (such as fried rice), reduced energy drink and soft drink intake, reduced intake of sweets, reduced fats and oils intake and high intake of cereal based foods. Healthy diet recommendations for adolescents stress the importance of fruits and vegetables, whole grains, fish, low fat dairy and lean meat intake [31, 32]. Increased dietary diversity has also been linked to specific nutrient adequacy [20] and represents an appropriate approach to measuring nutrient adequacy among adolescents [17] including those in resource poor settings [18]. This notwithstanding, nutrition education for adolescents during Ramadan should encourage reduction of table sugar in sugar sweetened beverages such as tea and mashed *kenkey* which are increased considerably during Ramadan.

Findings have been mixed regarding weight changes during Ramadan. Self-reported weight gain has been reported among a cohort of Saudi families [33], while other studies report unchanged weight during Ramadan [26, 34]. Conflicting results regarding weight changes among people who fast during Ramadan in different settings could be due to differences in dietary behaviours in different cultures, differences in fast duration and variations in climatic conditions. The significant weight loss among adolescents in present study is consistent with previous studies where a little above 1 kg of body weight was lost during Ramadan and regained shortly afterwards [35–37]. A recent study suggested that weight changes during Ramadan are more likely the result of differences in food intake [38]. Reduced nutrient intakes in adolescents have been reported earlier [13]. Smaller portion sizes may be consumed at dinner due to high intake of water following a prolonged thirst, increased intake of less energy dense fluids and fruits at *Iftar* as well as the shorter time between *Iftar* and dinner meals. In addition, daytime food quantities may be smaller due to lower appetite at dawn as well as a non-consumption of lunch meals and other lunch snacks during Ramadan. The significantly high loss in body weight among female adolescents is contrary to earlier findings reported among Malaysian adolescents [13] and among adults elsewhere [35]. Differences in activity level and food intake among males and females could account for the disparity in weight loss. Energy intake was more likely to be higher among males as they had multiple eating points – at home and as gifts at the Mosque during Ramadan. Males are also more likely to spend more time sleeping after school than females who are usually active at home assisting with food preparations and other household chores. The significant weight losses among adolescent females may have some important implications. Weight losses during Ramadan therefore mean a trade-off of nutrients for weight regain at the expense of growth and preparation towards future reproductive functions. Yearly weight losses among female adolescents over the period of adolescence could have cumulative important implications on their nutrition and health. It seems reasonable therefore, for female adolescents preparing for Ramadan to receive nutrition education on dietary practices essential in maintaining nutrient stores and optimal weight.

The strengths of this study include the use of a longitudinal design and a relatively large sample. Our study is however, constrained by the use of qualitative dietary assessment methods (food frequency questionnaire and 24-h dietary recall) which do not allow us to make quantitative estimates of food intake. It is important to note however, that the food frequency questionnaire is shown to be a useful tool in assessing eating habits of older children and adolescents [39]. It is also a practical tool for assessing usual intake of subjects, is relatively easy to complete and useful in prospective studies involving large numbers of subjects [40, 41]. Obviously quantitative diet assessments are useful, but may not always be feasible (due to high cost, logistics and poor adherence by subjects) especially in a prospective study involving large numbers of subjects [40]. Even though the 24-h recall method has an inherent limitation of relying on respondent's memory and respondents might not always be entirely truthful, the method has been thought to provide data which represent the population due to lower respondent burden compared with the diet record method [40].

Further, compensatory feeding is more likely in fasting conditions, but present study did not measure this behaviour. However, the increased number of dishes at major eating moments during Ramadan is suggestive of the behaviour. If more foods and fluids were taken at dawn to compensate for the absence of lunch meals and the day's thirst, then pupils were more likely to be heavier around the time (morning) of weight measurement during Ramadan than they would be outside Ramadan where breakfast meals could even be skipped with no much worries as pupils still have the chance to have lunch meals during the day. This could have led to an under estimation of weight loss. In spite of these limitations, the present study has shed much light on the food patterns, dietary diversity and weight changes among adolescents who fast during Ramadan in Ghana.

Conclusion

In this prospective cohort study among schooling Ghanaian adolescents who fast during Ramadan, fasting was characterised by marked changes in usual food patterns, increased dietary diversity and significant body weight loss.

Abbreviations

ANOVA: Analysis of variance; DDS: Dietary diversity score; JHS: Junior High School

Acknowledgements

We thank the pupils for their participation and patience in completing all surveys. We are grateful to the Northern regional Metropolitan Director of Ghana Education Service for giving the approval to conduct the study in Junior High Schools in the Metropolis. We also appreciate the head teachers, assistant head teachers and teachers of selected schools for their unflinching support during data collection in their schools. We are grateful to Mr. Emmanuel Kofi-Obeng Jnr for his assistance with field data collection and organising pupils in the schools. Further, we thank our data collection staff and team leaders for their dedication.

Funding

We did not receive external funding for this study.

Authors' contributions

ZA conceived the study idea. ARA and ZA designed the study and were responsible for field data collection and supervision. ZA and ARA analyzed and interpreted the data. ZA drafted the manuscript and ARA reviewed it critically for important intellectual content. ZA and ARA have responsibility for the final content. Both authors read and approved the final manuscript.

Competing interests

The authors declare that they have no competing interests.

References

1. Erol A, Baylan G, Yazici F. Do Ramadan fasting restrictions alter eating behaviours? Eur Eat Disord Rev. 2008;16(4):297–301.
2. Trepanowski JF, Bloomer RJ. The impact of religious fasting on human health. Nutr J. 2010;9:57.
3. Sakr AH. Fasting in Islam. J Am Diet Assoc. 1975;67(1):17–21.
4. Farooq A, Herrera CP, Almudahka F, Mansour R. A prospective study of the physiological and neurobehavioral effects of ramadan fasting in preteen and teenage boys. J Acad Nutr Diet. 2015;115(6):889–97.
5. Fenneni MA, Latiri I, Aloui A, Rouatbi S, Saafi MA, Bougmiza I, Chamari K, Saad HB. Effects of Ramadan on physical capacities of North African boys fasting for the first time. *Libyan J Med.* 2014;9 https://doi.org/10.3402/ljm.v3409.25391.
6. Ramadan J. Does fasting during Ramadan alter body composition, blood constituents and physical performance? Med Princ Pract. 2002;11(Suppl. 2):41–6.
7. Nematy M, Alinezhad-Namaghi M, Rashed MM, Mozhdehifard M, Sajjadi SS, Akhlaghi S, Sabery M, Mohajeri SAR, Shalaey N, Moohebati M, et al. Effects of Ramadan fasting on cardiovascular risk factors: a prospective observational study. Nutr J. 2012;11:69.
8. Leiper J, Molla A. Effects on health of fluid restriction during fasting in Ramadan. Eur J Clin Nutr. 2003;57:S30–8.
9. Akrami Mohajeri F, Ahmadi Z, Hassanshahi G, Akrami Mohajeri E, Ravari A, Ghalebi SR. Dose Ramadan fasting affects inflammatory responses: evidences for modulatory roles of this unique nutritional status via chemokine network. Iranian J Basic Med Sci. 2013;16(12):1217–22.
10. Al-Hourani H, Atoum M. Body composition, nutrient intake and physical activity patterns in young women during Ramadan. Singap Med J. 2007; 48(10):906.
11. Azizi F. Islamic fasting and health. Ann Nutr Metab. 2010;56(4):273–82.
12. Toda M, Morimoto K. Effects of Ramadan fasting on the health of Muslims. Nihon eiseigaku zasshi Japanese j hygiene. 2000;54(4):592–6.
13. Poh B, Zawiah H, Ismail M, Henry C. Changes in body weight, dietary intake and activity pattern of adolescents during Ramadan. Malays J Nutr. 1996; 2(1):1–10.
14. Akgül S, Derman O, Kanbur NÖ. Fasting during ramadan: a religious factor as a possible trigger or exacerbator for eating disorders in adolescents. Int J Eat Disord. 2014;47(8):905–10.
15. World Health Organization: Health for the world's adolescents: a second chance in the second decade: summary. 2014.
16. Croll JK, Neumark-Sztainer D, Story M. Healthy eating: what does it mean to adolescents? J Nutr Educ. 2001;33(4):193–8.
17. Mirmiran P, Azadbakht L, Esmaillzadeh A, Azizi F. Dietary diversity score in adolescents-a good indicator of the nutritional adequacy of diets: Tehran lipid and glucose study. Asia Pac J Clin Nutr. 2004;13(1):56–60.
18. Steyn N, Nel J, Nantel G, Kennedy G, Labadarios D. Food variety and dietary diversity scores in children: are they good indicators of dietary adequacy? Public Health Nutr. 2006;9(05):644–50.
19. Arimond M, Wiesmann D, Becquey E, Carriquiry A, Daniels MC, Deitchler M, Fanou-Fogny N, Joseph ML, Kennedy G, Martin-Prevel Y. Simple food group diversity indicators predict micronutrient adequacy of women's diets in 5 diverse, resource-poor settings. J Nutr. 2010;140(11):2059S–69S.
20. Mirmiran P, Azadbakht L, Azizi F. Dietary diversity within food groups: an indicator of specific nutrient adequacy in Tehranian women. J Am Coll Nutr. 2006;25(4):354–61.
21. Ghana Statistical Service. 2010 Population and Housing Census summary report of final results. Accra: Ghana Statistical Service; 2012.
22. Ghana Statistical Service. 2010 Population and Housing Census Distric analytical report Tamale Metropolis. Accra: Ghana Statistical Service; 2014.
23. Kennedy G, Ballard T, Dop MC: Guidelines for measuring household and individual dietary diversity: food and agriculture Organization of the United Nations; 2011.
24. Abubakari A, Jahn A. Maternal dietary patterns and practices and birth weight in northern Ghana. PLoS One. 2016;11(9):e0162285.
25. WHO: Physical status: The use of and interpretation of anthropometry, Report of a WHO Expert Committee. 1995.

26. Frost G, Pirani S. Meal frequency and nutritional intake during Ramadan: a pilot study. Human nutrition Applied nutrition. 1987;41(1):47–50.
27. Vermeer WM, Steenhuis IH, Leeuwis FH, Heymans MW, Seidell JC. Small portion sizes in worksite cafeterias: do they help consumers to reduce their food intake? Int J Obes. 2011;35(9):1200.
28. Sinha MK, Ohannesian JP, Heiman ML, Kriauciunas A, Stephens TW, Magosin S, Marco C, Caro JF. Nocturnal rise of leptin in lean, obese, and non-insulin-dependent diabetes mellitus subjects. J Clin Invest. 1996;97(5):1344–7.
29. Ajabnoor GM, Bahijri S, Borai A, Abdulkhaliq AA, Al-Aama JY, Chrousos GP. Health impact of fasting in Saudi Arabia during Ramadan: association with disturbed circadian rhythm and metabolic and sleeping patterns. PLoS One. 2014;9(5):e96500.
30. Abizari A-R, Buxton C, Kwara L, Mensah-Homiah J, Armar-Klemesu M, Brouwer ID. School feeding contributes to micronutrient adequacy of Ghanaian schoolchildren. Br J Nutr. 2014;112(6):1019–33.
31. Gidding SS, Dennison BA, Birch LL, Daniels SR, Gilman MW, Lichtenstein AH, Rattay KT, Steinberger J, Stettler N, Van Horn L. Dietary recommendations for children and adolescents: a guide for practitioners: consensus statement from the American Heart Association. Circulation. 2005;112(13):2061–75.
32. Hussein L, Gouda M, Fouad M, Labib E, Bassyouni R, Mohammad M. Dietary intervention with yoghurt, Synbiotic yogurt or traditional fermented Sobya: bio-potency among male adolescents using five bio-markers of relevance to colonic metabolic activities. Food Nutr Sci. 2014;5(12):1131.
33. Bakhotmah BA. The puzzle of self-reported weight gain in a month of fasting (Ramadan) among a cohort of Saudi families in Jeddah, western Saudi Arabia. Nutr J. 2011;10:84.
34. Lamine F, Bouguerra R, Jabrane J, Marrakchi Z, Ben MR, Ben CS, Gaigi S. Food intake and high density lipoprotein cholesterol levels changes during ramadan fasting in healthy young subjects. La Tunisie Médicale. 2006;84(10): 647–50.
35. Sadeghirad B, Motaghipisheh S, Kolahdooz F, Zahedi MJ, Haghdoost AA. Islamic fasting and weight loss: a systematic review and meta-analysis. Public Health Nutr. 2012;17(02):396–406.
36. Hajek P, Myers K, Dhanji A-R, West O, McRobbie H. Weight change during and after Ramadan fasting. J Pub Health. 2011;34(3):377–81.
37. Syam AF, Sobur CS, Abdullah M, Makmun D. Ramadan fasting decreases body fat but not protein mass. Int j endocrinol metabol. 2016;14(1):167–8.
38. Lessan N, Saadane I, Alkaf B, Hambly C, Buckley AJ, Finer N, Speakman JR, Barakat MT. The effects of Ramadan fasting on activity and energy expenditure. Am J Clin Nutr. 2018;107(1):54–61.
39. Rockett HR, Wolf AM, Colditz GA. Development and reproducibility of a food frequency questionnaire to assess diets of older children and adolescents. J Acad Nutr Diet. 1995;95(3):336–40.
40. Thompson FE, Subar AF. Dietary assessment methodology. In: *Nutrition in the Prevention and Treatment of Disease (Third Edition)*. New York: Elsevier; 2013. p. 5–46.
41. Willett W. Nutritional epidemiology. New York: Oxford University Press; 1998.

10

Dietary patterns are associated with blood lipids at 18-year-olds: a cross-sectional analysis nested in the 1993 Pelotas (Brazil) birth cohort

Juliana dos Santos Vaz[1*], Romina Buffarini[2], Gilberto Kac[3], Renata Moraes Bielemann[1], Isabel Oliveira[4], Ana Baptista Menezes[2] and Maria Cecilia Formoso Assunção[2]

Abstract

Background: Evidence regarding the deleterious effects of diet on blood lipids in adolescence has been inconsistent, and few studies have investigated this association using a dietary pattern approach. We examined whether dietary pattern of adolescents are associated with blood lipid concentrations.

Methods: Cross-sectional analysis of 3524 18-year-old participants in the 1993 Pelotas (Brazil) Birth Cohort Study. A semi-quantitative food frequency questionnaire was administered. Dietary patterns were established using principal component analysis and analysed as tertiles of factor scores. Independent associations between each dietary pattern tertile and blood lipid values (total cholesterol, LDL-cholesterol, HDL-cholesterol and triglycerides) were tested using adjusted linear regression models stratified by sex. Triglycerides were log-transformed due to their skewed distribution, and the beta coefficients should be interpreted as the % change (increase or decrease).

Results: Four dietary patterns were derived: Meat Products and Fast Foods; Fruits and Vegetables; Candies, Sodas and Dairy Products; and Common Brazilian Foods. In the adjusted models, which compared the highest and lowest tertiles of dietary pattern scores, we observed that among girls: 1) the third tertile of the Meat Products and Fast Foods pattern was associated with 1.5 mg/dL (95% CI -3.05; −0.04) lower HDL-cholesterol; 2) the second and third tertile of the Candies, Sodas and Dairy Products pattern was associated with 5% and 10% higher triglycerides (β 1.05, 95% CI 1.01; 1.09, β 1.10, 95% CI 1.05; 1.16), respectively; 3) the second and third tertiles of the Common Brazilian Foods pattern were associated with 4 mg/dL (β − 4.30, 95% CI -7.75; −0.85, β − 4.95, 95% CI -8.53; −1.36, respectively) lower total cholesterol and 6% lower triglycerides (β 0.94, 95% CI 0.90; 0.99, β 0.93, 95% CI 0.89; 0.98, respectively). For boys, 4) the third tertile of the Common Brazilian Foods was associated with 4.6 mg/dL (95% CI -7.91; −1.37) lower total cholesterol and 3.8 mg/dL (95% CI -6.51; − 1.13) lower LDL-cholesterol.

Conclusions: Dietary patterns were more closely associated with blood lipids among girls than boys at age 18. Higher scores for the Common Brazilian Foods pattern were associated with lower total cholesterol in both sexes.

Keywords: Dietary patterns, Food consumption, Adolescents, Lipoproteins, Cross-sectional studies

* Correspondence: juliana.vaz@gmail.com
[1]Faculty of Nutrition, Federal University of Pelotas, Rua Gomes Carneiro, 1, 2° andar, Pelotas, RS 96010-610, Brazil
Full list of author information is available at the end of the article

Background

The measurement and surveillance of blood lipids have become standard medical and public health practices for the early detection of cardiovascular disease risk [1, 2]. Blood lipid profiles in childhood are strongly related to adult values [3, 4]. The occurrence of dyslipidaemia in youth populations highlights the need to understand the influencing factors and the need to initiate prevention measures [1, 5]. Serum cholesterol fractions and triglycerides are determined by genetics and lifestyle factors [6–8], including eating habits [9]. A variety of dietary components, e.g., the solubility of dietary fibre, quality of carbohydrate, types of fats and antioxidant consumption, affect serum lipoproteins and triglycerides [9]. All these dietary components are determined by the source and the degree of industrial food processing of cereals, fruits and vegetables, dairy products, meats, and oils, e.g. the degree of refined grains and cereals affect the content of fibre and the availability of the carbohydrate [10].

Brazil has recently issued a new dietary guidelines focused on traditional eating habits to promote the consumption of traditional or minimally processed foods (e.g. fruits, seeds, leaves, roots, meats, eggs, milk, and any other natural foods altered by minimal processes such as removal of inedible parts, drying, boiling, pasteurisation). This is in lieu of processed (e.g. products made by adding sugar, oil, salt to increase durability of natural foods) and ultra-processed ones (e.g. snacks, drinks, ready to eat meals and many other products which often contain flavours, colours and other additives that imitate or intensify the sensory qualities) [11]. The guideline considers evidences of the increased ultra-processed food availability and intake [12] with obesity [13]. The most prevalent lipid alterations reported in a recent school-based study of Brazilian adolescents were low HDL-cholesterol and hypercholesterolaemia [5]. Studies of adolescents have shown that high saturated fat, sodium, and sugar consumption and low fruit and vegetable consumption is associated with dyslipidaemia [14, 15].

Dietary pattern analysis has emerged as a practical way to deliver information to the public and to implement policies in contrast to investigations of dietary risk factors focused on food groups or nutrients [16]. Evidence regarding the deleterious effects of diet on blood lipids in adolescence has been inconsistent [9, 17], and few studies have investigated this association using a dietary pattern approach [18, 19].

Thus, the present study sought to establish the dietary patterns of 18-year-old adolescents and to examine the possible associations of these patterns with blood lipids concentrations (total cholesterol, LDL-cholesterol, HDL-cholesterol and triglycerides) using data from the 1993 Pelotas Birth Cohort Study birth cohort study conducted in Pelotas, a city in southern Brazil. We hypothesized that higher scores on a dietary pattern characterized by traditional or minimally processed foods would be associated with a better lipid profile (i.e. lower total and LDL-cholesterol, triglycerides, and higher HDL-cholesterol), and higher scores on a pattern characterized by sweets and processed/ultraprocessed foods would be associated with a worse lipid profile (i.e. higher triglycerides, total and LDL-cholesterol and lower HDL-cholesterol).

Methods

1993 Pelotas birth cohort

The present study uses data from the 1993 Pelotas Birth Cohort, a prospective population-based study carried out with all newborns in Pelotas. This cohort includes all hospital births to mothers living in the urban area of the city from January 1 to December 31, 1993 ($n = 5265$) [20]. The initial cohort comprised 5249 eligible newborns (the mothers of 16 newborns declined to participate). Periodic follow-ups were conducted beginning at 3 months of age to assess several socioeconomic, health and nutritional features. The 18-year follow-up visit started in September 2011 and finished in April 2012. Of the original cohort of 5249 subjects, 4106 were interviewed and 979 were considered losses. Those who completed the interviews, added to those known to have died ($n = 164$), represented a retention rate of 81.3%. At a visit to the research clinic unit, participants provided informed consent and underwent a series of assessments that consisted of questionnaires, anthropometric measures, and blood sample collection. Those who refused to provide blood samples ($n = 180$) or reported being pregnant ($n = 57$) were excluded from blood collection, reported the use of medication for glucose or lipid control [insulin ($n = 9$), metformin ($n = 2$), statins ($n = 2$)], had haemoglobin A1c ≥6.5% ($n = 12$), were breastfeeding ($n = 92$), did not complete the food frequency questionnaire ($n = 22$), provided implausible dietary reports ($n = 205$; see the *Statistical analysis* section), were excluded from this study. Additionally, one case of hypertriglyceridaemia (triglycerides> 8000 mg/dL) was excluded. The final sample consisted of 3524 adolescents (67.1% of the original sample) (Fig. 1). More details about the cohort can be found elsewhere [20, 21].

Dietary assessment

A semi-quantitative food frequency questionnaire (FFQ) was administered in an electronic format [22]. Participants filled out the FFQ in a room with computers at the research clinic. A trained research assistant explained verbally and individually how subjects should use the platform before the FFQ was administered, even though the initial part of the platform presents the instructions on how to fill out the questionnaire. This aimed to minimize data entry errors and to maximize the quality of the data. For each food item, the participant was first asked about the frequency of intake

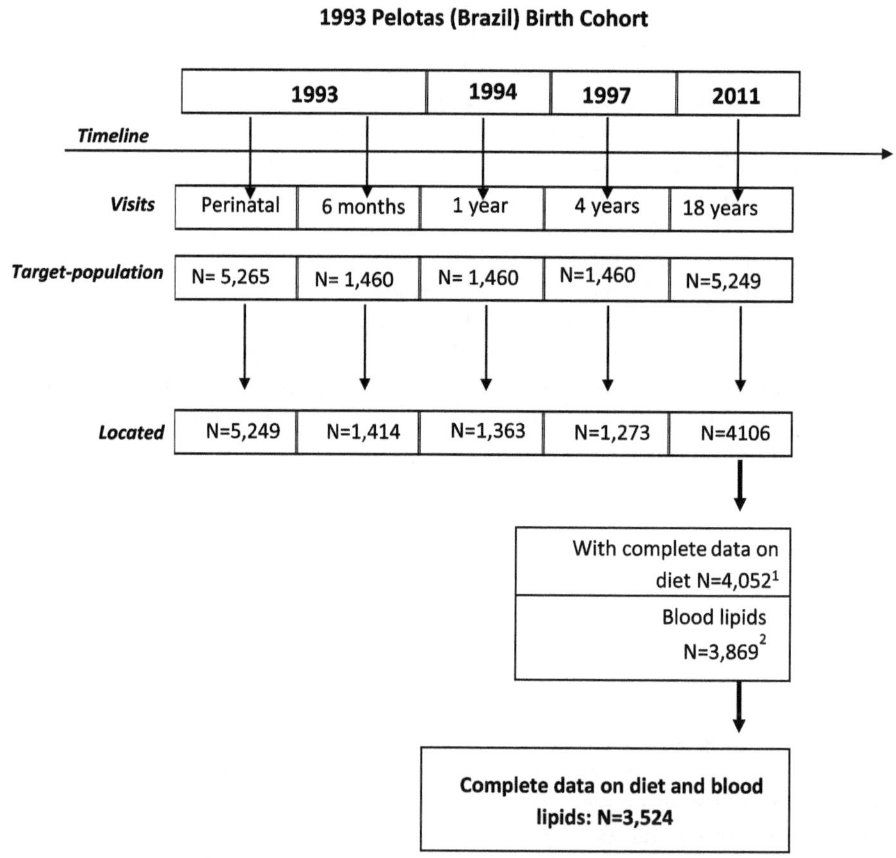

Fig. 1 Description of the 1993 Pelotas (Brazil) Birth Cohort. [1]Subjects excluded of diet data: did not complete the food frequency questionnaire ($n = 22$) and implausible energy report ($n = 205$). [2]Subjects excluded regarding blood lipids: refused to provide blood samples ($n = 180$), pregnancy ($n = 57$) and breastfeeding ($n = 92$), reported use of medication for glucose or lipid control [insulin ($n = 9$), metformin ($n = 2$), statins ($n = 2$)], had haemoglobin A1c ≥6.5% ($n = 12$), one case of hypertriglyceridaemia (triglycerides> 8000)

and for those reported items the platform presents photographed images to identify the usual portion size (small, medium, or large). This electronic platform was developed to be used on the 18th year of follow up of the 1993 Pelotas Birth Cohort, and was based on a recent validation (paper-based FFQ) carried out when subjects from the 1993 Pelotas birth cohort were 15 years [23]. The electronic platform comprises all the food items included in the paper version of the FFQ [22]. The food items listed on the FFQ were based on a validated Brazilian FFQ [24] that was modified considering three 24-h recalls carried out in a sub-sample of the 1993 Pelotas Birth Cohort [23]. The energy intake (EI) ratio calculated based on the FFQ and the energy expenditure (EE) estimated by accelerometer was 1.13 [23]. The validation procedure did not consider macro or micronutrients.

The FFQ comprised 88 items, and eight frequency options were available: (i) five or more times per day; (ii) two to four times per day; (iii) once per day; (iv) five to six times per week; (v) two to four times per week; (vi) once per week; (vii) one to three times per month; and (viii) never or less than one time per month. Daily energy intake in kilocalories and nutrient intake were estimated using the Brazilian Food Composition Table [25], complemented with food items from the United States Department of Agriculture (USDA) National Nutrient Database for Standard Reference [26].

Dietary patterns (main exposure)

FFQ items were combined into 45 food groups based on nutrient composition and frequency of consumption [27]. Those items consumed by 80% or more of the participants or when representative of the Brazilian dietary habits were considered separately (e.g., rice, beans, white bread, sugar, coffee, mate). Three alcoholic items (wine, beer and vodka) were excluded because this food group was consumed by less than 20% of the adolescents at age 18 [28, 29]. The 45 food groups are presented in the Additional file 1.

We applied principal component analysis (PCA) and rotation to derive dietary patterns [30]. A correlation matrix was constructed to assess the correlation between the food groups. The Kaiser-Meyer-Olkin test (≥0.8) and Bartlett's test of sphericity (p-value < 0.05) were applied to verify whether the PCA assumptions were met [27, 29]. Varimax rotation was applied to obtain orthogonal factors. Food groups that showed factor loadings > 0.25 were considered to have strong associations with that factor. A positive factor loading indicated that the food group had a positive association with the pattern, while a negative factor loading indicated an inverse association [30]. Food groups were included in a dietary pattern if their factor loading was shown to be higher for that pattern in comparison to the others, even if these loadings were higher then 0.25 in other dietary patterns.

The number of factors that best represents the data was based on the scree plot and eigenvalues > 1.5 [27]. Dietary patterns were named according to the food items included and the dietary pattern interpretation. Participants received a factor score for each dietary pattern identified [28].

Blood lipids (outcome variable)

A trained nurse was responsible for venous blood sample collection. Samples were kept for 30 min at ambient temperature and then centrifuged for 15 min at 2000 g. It was not possible to obtain fasting blood samples for logistic reasons, and the time of the last meal or snack consumed was registered for statistical adjustment. The average fasting time was 3 h and 20 min (95% CI 1 h – 12 h). Serum aliquots were stored at – 80 °C until analysis. Total cholesterol, HDL-cholesterol, LDL-cholesterol and triglycerides were measured using an automatic enzymatic colorimetric method with a Mindray BS-380 chemistry analyser (Shenzhen Mindray Bio-Medical Electronics Co., Ltd., China). The inter-assay coefficients of variation obtained for total cholesterol, HDL-cholesterol, LDL-cholesterol and triglycerides were 2.0%, 4.5%, 5.0% and 2.4%, respectively.

Covariables

The following independent variables were included in the analyses: sex (girls/boys), skin colour (white, black/ brown), total family income at birth (≤2, 3–5, ≥6 monthly minimum wage), maternal education at birth (< 8, ≥8 years of schooling completed), smoking habits at age 18 (no/yes), age of menarche (≤11; ≥12 years), leisure-time physical activity at age 18, and body mass index (BMI) at age 18.

BMI at age 18 was calculated using the weight measured to the nearest 0.1 kg using an electronic digital scale coupled with the BOD POD system (COSMED, Chicago, IL, USA) divided by the height measured to the nearest 0.1 cm using a portable stadiometer (C.M.S. Weighing Equipment Ltd., London, UK). The z-score of BMI for age and sex was calculated according to the WHO standards [31] and classified using the following cut-offs (BMI for age): underweight (≤ – 1 SD), normal weight (> – 1 SD and < + 1 SD), overweight (≥ + 1 SD and ≤ + 2 SD) and obese (> + 2 SD).

Physical activity was measured using the leisure-time information from the long version of the International Physical Activity Questionnaire (IPAQ) [32], which has been validated for the Brazilian population [33]. The questionnaire was administered to assess habitual physical activity. The number of days a week, and the amount of time spent per day on physical activities (including walking, moderate and vigorous physical activity) were recorded. Individuals who reported spending ≥300 min per week on physical activity were considered active [34].

Statistical analysis

In order to test the association of each dietary patterns and blood lipids fraction, we first assessed the distribution of each lipid fraction to verify normality. We tested the differences in means or medians between categorical variables using Student's *t* tests or Mann-Whitney U tests, ANOVA or Kruskal-Wallis tests, respectively, to evaluate the distribution of blood lipids according to each covariable.

Considering that misreporting of dietary intake may affect the associations between diet and non-communicable disease risk [35], we excluded subjects with implausible energy reports. The plausibility of each energy report was determined by comparing the reported EI with the estimate energy requirements (ER) [36, 37]. An energy report was considered implausible if the EI/ER ratio was outside ± 2 standard deviations range, and those subjects were excluded from the main analysis.

Dietary pattern scores were then categorized into tertiles, and the group with the lowest score was considered the reference category. Blood lipid fractions (total cholesterol, HDL-cholesterol, LDL-cholesterol and triglycerides) were considered as outcomes. The independent association between each dietary pattern and each lipid fraction was tested using crude and adjusted linear regressions. All regressions between dietary patterns and blood lipids were conducted separately for boys and girls. The independent effect of each dietary pattern was tested on each blood lipid fraction, adjusting for all variables with p value < 0.20 in the bivariate model. The adjusted variables were skin colour, maternal education at birth, total family income at birth, smoking habits at age 18, minutes of leisure-time physical activity per week at age 18, BMI at age 18, and age of menarche. Skin colour, maternal education at birth and total family income at birth were complementary socioeconomic measures to adjust for socioeconomic inequalities [20, 21]. The time elapsed since the last meal was included in every regression analysis to control for differences in non-fasting blood collection. In fully adjusted models, total EI was also included to adjust for differences in energy consumption among participants. Triglycerides were log-transformed due to their skewed distribution, and the beta coefficients of the crude and adjusted analyses are shown in their exponential form. The results should be interpreted as the % change (increase or decrease) in triglyceride level associated in relation to the reference group – i.e. a beta coefficient of 1.25 means 25% higher triglycerides in that group in relation to the reference one.

We performed further analyses of participants included and excluded in the current analyses to assess the effects of losses of follow up using chi-square test of proportions for all selected variables aiming to rule out selection bias. All statistical analyses were conducted using Stata 12.1 (Stata Corp., College Station, Texas, USA).

Results

Study participants

The baseline characteristics of the adolescents included in the current study differed from those considered losses to follow up according to sex, skin colour, maternal education at birth and total family income at birth (Additional file 2). At the 18 years follow up, those participants not included in the current study due to losses to follow up or presence of any exclusion criteria comprised a higher proportion of females (64.1%) compared to those that of the included sample (48.8%) (Additional file 3).

Of the 3524 adolescents included in the present analyses, 1718 were girls. Mean BMI of girls and boys were 23.3 ± 4.7 kg/m^2 and 23.3 ± 4.1 kg/m^2, respectively. Sixty-four per cent were white, and the majority lived with total family income ≤2 monthly minimum wages (60.2%). Twenty-six per cent were overweight or obese, and 13.6% declared themselves current smokers. Girls presented significantly higher mean/median lipid concentrations than boys. Differences in blood lipids were observed for all socioeconomic and lifestyle variables, age of menarche and BMI categories (Table 1). Differences in blood lipids according to the referred variables stratified by sex are presented in the Additional file 4.

Dietary patterns

Four dietary patterns were chosen to best describe adolescents' food habits, and these explained 40% of the total variance. The first component had a high loading on all types of meat products, including processed meats (canned tuna/sardines, salt-cured meat, bacon) and fast foods (hamburgers, hot dogs) and was labelled the Meat Products and Fast Foods pattern. The second component loaded highly onto all types of fruits, vegetables and legumes (except black beans) and was labelled the Fruits and Vegetables pattern. The third component, labelled the Candies, Sodas and Dairy Products pattern, was characterized by high loads of chocolate powder, sugar-sweetened sodas, dairy products (milk, yogurt, hard cheese, soft cheese), sweets, chocolates, candies and caramels. The fourth component loaded highly onto black beans, white sugar, margarine/butter, white rice and white bread and was labelled the Common Brazilian Foods pattern (Table 2).

Dietary patterns and blood lipids

In the adjusted analyses, girls at the highest tertile of the Meat Products and Fast Foods pattern presented 1.5 mg/dL lower HDL-cholesterol compared with those at the lowest tertile. Girls at the second and third tertiles of the Candies, Sodas and Dairy Products pattern presented 5% and 10% higher triglycerides than girls in the first tertile, respectively. Girls at the second and third tertiles of the Common Brazilian Foods pattern presented 4 mg/dL lower total cholesterol compared with those classified in the first tertile. Additionally, girls classified in the second and third tertiles of the Common Brazilian Foods pattern had 6% lower triglycerides compared with those in the first tertile. The Fruits and Vegetables pattern was not associated with blood lipids (Table 3).

Boys classified at the third tertile of the Common Brazilian Foods pattern presented 4.6 mg/dL and 3.8 mg/dL lower total and LDL-cholesterol, respectively, compared with those at the first tertile in the adjusted analysis. No associations were found between the Meat Products and Fast Foods; Fruits and Vegetables; or the Candies, Sodas and Dairy Products patterns and the blood lipids in the adjusted models for boys (Table 4).

Discussion

The dietary patterns derived in the present study that characterize the food consumption of 18-year-old adolescents from the 1993 Pelotas Birth Cohort were Meat Products and Fast Foods; Fruits and Vegetables; Candies, Sodas and Dairy Products; and Common Brazilian Foods. These patterns reflect the dietary behaviours of adolescents born in the nineties and are similar to those identified in the 1982 Pelotas Birth Cohort at 22 years, except that the Common Brazilian Foods pattern was the main pattern identified in the previous cohort [38], whereas in the current study, the Meat Products and Fast Foods pattern was dominant. This difference could be due, in part, to different age of the samples when foods were assessed; however differences may also reflect the increasing share of processed foods in the Brazilian diet over the last decades [12].

The dietary patterns identified in the present study are in line with other investigations of children and adolescents [9, 18, 19, 39, 40] including those reported by the Brazilian National School-based Health Survey [41]. The majority of these studies identified a Western or unhealthy pattern, usually characterized by fast foods, meat, sweets and candies, sugar-sweetened beverages, and a healthy or traditional pattern based on traditional foods, fruits and vegetables.

Table 1 Mean/median (SD/IQR) blood lipids of adolescents at age 18 by selected characteristics. The 1993 Pelotas (Brazil) Birth Cohort

Variable	n	%	Lipid profile (mg/dL)			
			Total cholesterol	LDL cholesterol	HDL cholesterol	Triglycerides
			P value* mean (SD)	*P* value* mean (SD)	*P* value* mean (SD)	*P* value* median (IQR)
Sex			< 0.001	< 0.001	< 0.001	0.02
Girls	1718	48.7	170.8 (29.4)	94.5 (20.3)	60.2 (10.9)	71 (58; 91)
Boys	1806	51.3	152.8 (24.5)	84.4 (20.3)	51.7 (8.7)	68 (55; 89)
Skin colour[a]			< 0.001	< 0.001	0.032	< 0.001
White	2199	64.8	163.2 (29.1)	90.2 (23.2)	56.3 (11.1)	71 (58; 95)
Black/brown	1192	35.2	158.8 (27.5)	87.5 (22.1)	55.4 (10.2)	65 (54; 83)
Family income at birth (MMW)			< 0.001	0.007	< 0.001	< 0.001
≤ 2	2120	60.2	159.3 (28.0)	88.1 (22.8)	54.9 (10.3)	67 (56; 86)
3–5	843	23.9	163.8 (27.8)	90.4 (21.6)	56.5 (11.1)	71 (58; 94)
≥ 6	561	15.9	166.9 (30.3)	91.4 (24.2)	58.3 (11.3)	76 (60; 102)
Maternal education at birth (years)[b]			< 0.001	0.034	< 0.001	< 0.001
< 8	2129	60.5	159.6 (28.0)	88.7 (22.7)	54.7 (10.3)	68 (56; 88)
≥ 8	1389	39.5	164.5 (28.9)	90.3 (22.9)	57.5 (11.2)	72 (58; 96)
Smoking habit			< 0.001	0.008	< 0.001	0.530
No	3045	86.4	162.5 (28.4)	89.7 (22.6)	56.7 (10.8)	70 (57; 92)
Yes	479	13.6	155.7 (28.4)	86.8 (23.5)	52.7 (9.8)	69 (57; 89)
Leisure-time physical activity (min/week)			< 0.001	< 0.001	< 0.001	0.008
< 300	1418	40.2	165.3 (28.5)	91.4 (22.9)	57.2 (10.8)	71 (58; 95)
≥ 300	2106	59.8	159.2 (28.2)	87.9 (22.6)	54.9 (10.7)	68 (56; 88)
Age of menarche (years)[c]			0.003	0.028	0.003	0.025
≤ 11	475	27.8	174.2 (30.4)	96.6 (24.4)	61.4 (10.9)	73 (59; 97)
≥ 12	1236	72.2	169.6 (29.0)	93.8 (23.9)	59.7 (10.9)	70 (58; 90)
Body mass index[d]			< 0.001	< 0.001	< 0.001	< 0.001
Under/normal weight	2585	73.3	159.0 (27.8)	86.9 (21.9)	56.5 (10.7)	67 (55; 85)
Overweight/obese	939	26.7	168.7 (29,0)	96.2 (23.8)	54.2 (10.7)	79 (61; 112)
Total N*	3524	100	161.6 (28.5)	89.3 (22.8)	55.8 (10.7)	69 (57; 91)

*P values refer to comparisons of means (SD) or medians (IQR) between groups using Student t tests or Mann-Whitney U tests, ANOVA or Kruskal-Wallis tests, respectively. [a]133 missing values; [b]6 missing values; [c]7 missing values; [d]BMI for age and sex reference in z score: under/normal weight ≤ + 1 SD; overweight/obese: > + 1SD. *Abbreviations: MMW* monthly minimum wages, *SD* Standard deviation, *IQR* Interquartile range

The Common Brazilian Foods pattern that emerged in the present study – albeit not as the main one – does reflect the maintenance of traditional foods in the adolescents diet, as "coffee, sugar, white bread and margarine/butter" and "white rice and black beans" that are part of the basic Brazilian breakfast and lunch [42], respectively. This dietary pattern was significantly associated with lower triglycerides among girls and lower total and LDL-cholesterol concentrations among both girls and boys. We highlighted that this dietary pattern was characterized by foods that may negatively impact blood lipids, as white sugar, margarine/butter, white rice and white bread [9, 10]. The significant association of this pattern with better blood lipids could be explained by the fact that the dietary pattern was constructed based on the frequency of consumption, rather than on the amount of food consumed. This pattern presented a high factor loading of beans, which are rich sources of insoluble fibre, and lower factor loading of foods rich in saturated fat, i.e., meat and dairy products. Although fruits and vegetables also represent foods rich in dietary fibre, black beans are a popular food item in Brazil [42]. It's possible that adolescents that adhered most to this pattern consume a reasonable portion of beans rather than other foods rich in dietary fibre as fruits and vegetables.

The highest factor loading in the Meat Products and Fast Foods pattern was seafood products composed by fish and shrimp. However, the Pelotas market of fish are not those rich in omega-3 and fish is usually consumed fried, as a high frequency of this seafood is probably

Table 2 Factor-loadings[a] of food items for the major factors (dietary patterns) identified at the age of 18 based on a FFQ

Item	Food or food group	Meat Products and Fast Foods	Fruits and Vegetables	Candies, Sodas and Dairy Products	Common Brazilian Foods
1	Seafood	**0.3153**	0.0193	−0.0713	− 0.0962
2	Processed meats	**0.3135**	0.0057	−0.0238	0.0489
3	Pizza	**0.2999**	−0.0739	0.1104	−0.0884
4	Fast foods	**0.2898**	−0.0721	0.1391	−0.0274
5	Giblets	**0.2853**	−0.0189	−0.1368	0.0230
6	Chicken meat	**0.2715**	−0.0014	−0.0152	0.0567
7	Pork meat	**0.2581**	−0.0461	−0.0199	0.0930
8	Canned vegetables	0.2480	0.0077	−0.0661	−0.0318
9	Fried/baked salted pastries	0.2305	−0.0824	0.1460	0.0061
10	Popcorn	0.2097	0.0370	0.0219	0.0243
11	Pasta, polenta, corn	0.1923	0.1208	−0.0870	0.0245
12	French fries	0.1043	0.1107	0.0729	0.0418
13	Light soft drinks	0.1200	0.0675	0.0213	−0.0984
14	Banana	−0.1103	**0.3512**	0.1100	− 0.0207
15	Orange and tangerine	−0.0600	**0.3481**	0.0339	−0.0244
16	Other fruits	0.0272	**0.3591**	0.0420	−0.0959
17	Tomato	−0.1096	**0.3079**	−0.0190	0.1264
18	Other vegetables and legumes	0.1283	**0.3029**	0.1135	0.0056
19	Orange vegetables	0.1251	**0.2704**	−0.1214	−0.0464
20	Whole bread	0.0121	0.2026	−0.0602	−0.0249
21	Tubers	0.1123	0.1931	−0.0776	0.0522
22	Cake	0.0943	0.1775	0.0283	−0.0448
23	Fresh juice	0.0515	0.1530	0.1061	−0.0544
24	Chocolate powder	−0.0787	0.0439	**0.3786**	−0.0442
25	Sugar-sweetened sodas	0.0506	−0.1228	**0.3303**	0.0440
26	Milk and dairy products	−0.1062	0.2339	**0.3174**	−0.0964
27	Sweets and chocolates	0.1159	−0.0037	**0.2906**	−0.0151
28	Candies/caramels	−0.0051	− 0.0634	**0.2784**	−0.1327
29	Ice cream	0.0828	0.0023	**0.2639**	−0.0437
30	Mayonnaise	0.0380	0.0146	0.2222	0.0482
31	Sweet cookies	0.0215	0.0879	0.2016	0.0449
32	Luncheon meats	0.0179	0.0297	0.2008	0.1695
33	Snacks	0.1007	0.1103	0.1607	0.0216
34	Coffee	0.0280	−0.0647	−0.1131	**0.3977**
35	White sugar	−0.0179	− 0.1113	0.0966	**0.3901**
36	Black beans	−0.0150	0.0638	−0.0519	**0.3568**
37	Margarine and butter	0.0047	−0.0007	0.0726	**0.3513**
38	White rice	0.0028	0.0333	−0.0882	**0.2687**
39	White bread	−0.0841	0.0175	0.1077	**0.2516**
40	Vegetable spices	−0.0629	0.1842	−0.1193	0.2317
41	Red meats	0.1168	0.0335	0.0569	0.1696
42	Homemade bread	0.0719	0.0993	−0.1463	0.1553
43	Eggs	0.1231	0.0689	0.0154	0.1350

Table 2 Factor-loadings[a] of food items for the major factors (dietary patterns) identified at the age of 18 based on a FFQ *(Continued)*

Item	Food or food group	Meat Products and Fast Foods	Fruits and Vegetables	Candies, Sodas and Dairy Products	Common Brazilian Foods
44	Artificial juice	0.0034	0.0447	0.0954	0.1340
45	"Mate" drink	−0.0425	0.0996	0.0265	0.1064
	Explained variance (%)	**14.5**	**10.3**	**7.5**	**7.7**

[a]Bold value means those items included in the pattern described in the column

result of fried snack commonly eaten in restaurants and bars. The meat products and fast foods that also composed this pattern are rich sources of saturated fats. As a result, among girls, a high score on the Meat Products and Fast Foods pattern was associated with lower HDL-cholesterol. Our results are in line with other studies that reported a lower HDL-cholesterol among Iranian adolescents associated to red meat consumption [43], and the presence of metabolic syndrome in Brazilian adolescents associated to high consumption of ultra-processed foods [44]. Fast foods consumption among adolescents is commonly reported in studies that reinforce the need of promoting the adoption of healthy food choices [9].

The Candies, Sodas, and Dairy Products pattern was characterized by healthy and unhealthy foods. Milk and dairy products are a rich source of calcium, however milk is usually consumed with chocolate powder, and most dairy products are rich source of saturated fat, as well as yogurts are highly sweetened. This dietary pattern also presented a high factor loading on candies and sodas. The high score on the Candies, Sodas, and Dairy

Table 3 Crude and adjusted linear regressions between dietary patterns and blood lipids among girls at age 18. The 1993 Pelotas (Brazil) Birth Cohort Study ($n = 1718$)

Dietary patterns	Total Cholesterol (mg/dL)		LDL Cholesterol (mg/dL)		HDL Cholesterol (mg/dL)		Triglycerides (mg/dL)[b]	
	Crude β (95% CI)	Adjusted[a] β (95% CI)	Crude β (95% CI)	Adjusted[a] β (95% CI)	Crude β (95% CI)	Adjusted[a] β (95% CI)	Crude β[c] (95% CI)	Adjusted[a] β[c] (95% CI)
Meat Products and Fast Foods								
1st tertile	ref.	ref.	ref.	ref.	ref.	ref.	ref.	ref.
2nd tertile	−0.84 (− 4.25;2.56)	−1.04 (− 4.47;2.38)	−0.25 (− 3.04;2.53)	−0.47 (− 3.29;2.34)	−0.65 (− 1.91;0.61)	−0.75 (− 1.99;0.49)	0.99 (0.95;1.04)	0.99 (0.96;1.04)
3rd tertile	**−6.04 (− 9.46;-2.61)**	−4.74 (− 7.90;0.41)	− 2.69 (− 5.49;0.11)	− 1.70 (− 5.11;1.71)	**−2.54 (− 3.81;-1.27)**	**−1.55 (− 3.05;-0.04)**	**0.95 (0.91;0.99)**	0.97 (0.91;1.02)
Fruits and Vegetables								
1st tertile	ref.	ref.	ref.	ref.	ref.	ref.	ref.	ref.
2nd tertile	0.71 (− 2.70;4.12)	0.85 (− 2.61;4.31)	0.31 (− 2.47;3.11)	0.09 (− 2.75;2.92)	0.05 (− 1.21;1.31)	0.40 (− 0.85;1.65)	1.02 (0.98;1.07)	1.02 (0.98;1.07)
3rd tertile	−2.15 (− 5.58;1.27)	− 0.29 (− 4.21;3.64)	− 0.30 (− 3.10;2.49)	0.19 (− 3.03;341)	**− 1.48 (− 2.76;-0.22)**	−0.24 (− 1.66;1.18)	0.98 (0.93;1.02)	0.98 (0.93;1.03)
Candies, Sodas and Dairy Products								
1st tertile	ref.	ref.	ref.	ref.	ref.	ref.	ref.	ref.
2nd tertile	0.31 (-3.10;3.73)	0.89 (-2.55;4.35)	−0.98 (− 3.77;1.80)	−0.53 (− 3.36;2.31)	0.90 (− 0.37;2.17)	0.92 (− 0.32;2.18)	1.04 (0.99;1.09)	**1.05 (1.01;1.09)**
3rd tertile	− 0.64 (− 4.06;2.78)	0.69 (− 2.77;4.15)	−0.65 (− 3.44;2.14)	2.59 (− 0.99;6.17)	−0.01 (− 1.28;1.26)	1.48 (− 0.10;3.05)	1.03 (0.99;1.08)	**1.10 (1.05;1.16)**
Common Brazilian Foods								
1st tertile	ref.	ref.	ref.	ref.	ref.	ref.	ref.	ref.
2nd tertile	**−5.74 (−9.14;-2.34)**	**−4.30 (−7.75;-0.85)**	**− 4.08 (−6.86;-1.30)**	**− 3.49 (− 6.32;-0.66)**	−0.75 (− 2.01;0.51)	0.29 (− 0.98;1.56)	**0.92 (0.88;0.97)**	**0.94 (0.90;0.99)**
3rd tertile	**−8.98 (− 12.4;-5.58)**	**− 4.95 (− 8.53;-1.36)**	**−5.21 (− 7.99;-2.42)**	**−3.02 (− 5.96;-0.08)**	**− 2.42 (− 3.69;-1.15)**	−0.02 (− 1.49;1.44)	**0.89 (0.85;0.93)**	**0.93 (0.89;0.98)**

[a]Adjusted for hours of fasting, skin colour, maternal education at birth, family income at birth, smoking habit at age 18, age of menarche, body mass index at age 18 and total energy intake at age 18.

[b]Logarithm transformation was used; [c]β's should be interpreted as the % change (increase or decrease) in triglyceride level associated in relation to the reference group

Bold values mean significant at $p < 0.05$.

Table 4 Crude and adjusted linear regressions between dietary pattern and blood lipids among boys at age 18. The 1993 Pelotas (Brazil) Birth Cohort Study ($n = 1806$)

Dietary patterns	Total Cholesterol (mg/dL)		LDL Cholesterol (mg/dL)		HDL Cholesterol (mg/dL)		Triglycerides (mg/dL)[b]	
	Crude β (95% CI)	Adjusted[a] β (95% CI)	Crude β (95% CI)	Adjusted[a] β (95% CI)	Crude β (95% CI)	Adjusted[a] β (95% CI)	Crude β[c] (95% CI)	Adjusted[a] β[c] (95% CI)
Meat Products and Fast Foods								
1st tertile	ref.	ref.	ref.	ref.	ref.	ref.	ref.	ref.
2nd tertile	− 1.07 (− 3.84;1.70)	− 1.10 (− 3.86;1.66)	−0.71 (− 3.01;1.57)	−0.91 (− 3.18;1.37)	0.05 (− 0.94;1.05)	0.13 (− 0.88;1.15)	0.97 (0.93;1.02)	0.98 (0.93;1.02)
3rd tertile	**−3.26 (− 6.04;-0.49)**	− 0.68 (− 4.05;2.69)	**− 2.45 (− 4.74;-0.16)**	−0.54 (− 3.31;2.22)	−0.14 (− 1.14;0.85)	0.21 (− 1.02;1.46)	0.95 (0.91;1.00)	0.98 (0.93;1.04)
Fruits and Vegetables								
1st tertile	ref.	ref.	ref.	ref.	ref.	ref.	ref.	ref.
2nd tertile	0.39 (− 2.39;3.16)	0.22 (− 2.55;3.01)	0.60 (− 1.69;2.89)	0.53 (− 1.75;2.82)	0.47 (− 0.52;1.46)	0.40 (− 0.62;1.43)	0.96 (0.91;1.00)	0.96 (0.92;1.01)
3rd tertile	− 1.99 (− 4.76;0.79)	−1.04 (− 4.38;2.30)	− 1.32 (− 3.62;0.97)	− 0.90 (− 3.64;1.85)	− 0.50 (− 1.50;0.49)	−0.33 (− 1.56;0.90)	0.98 (0.94;1.03)	1.01 (0.95;1.05)
Candies, Sodas and Dairy Products								
1st tertile	ref.	ref.	ref.	ref.	ref.	ref.	ref.	ref.
2nd tertile	0.96 (− 2.35;4.27)	0.65 (− 2.12;3.43)	0.71 (−1.57;3.01)	0.70 (− 1.58;2.98)	0.16 (− 0.83;1.15)	− 0.00 (− 1.03;1.02)	1.00 (0.95;1.04)	1.00 (0.96;1.04)
3rd tertile	−0.74 (− 4.07;2.58)	3.16 (− 0.06;6.39)	− 0.18 (− 2.48;2.10)	1.90 (− 0.75;4.56)	0.81 (− 0.18;1.80)	0.71 (− 0.48;1.90)	1.01 (0.97;1.06)	1.04 (0.99;1.10)
Common Brazilian Foods								
1st tertile	ref.	ref.	ref.	ref.	ref.	ref.	ref.	ref.
2nd tertile	**−3.01 (− 5.76;-0.26)**	−1.48 (−4.28;1.32)	**− 2.38 (− 4.66;-0.11)**	−1.41 (− 3.71;0.89)	0.22 (− 0.77;1.22)	0.25 (− 0.78;1.29)	0.96 (0.91;1.00)	0.99 (0.94;1.03)
3rd tertile	**−7.99 (− 10.74;-5.24)**	**− 4.64 (− 7.91;-1.37)**	**−6.21 (− 8.49;-3.93)**	**−3.82 (− 6.51;-1.13)**	− 0.76 (− 1.75;0.23)	−0.91 (− 2.12;0.30)	**0.94** (0.89;0.98)	1.02 (0.96;1.07)

[a]Adjusted for hours of fasting, skin colour, maternal education at birth, family income at birth, smoking habits at age 18, minutes of leisure-time physical activity per week at age 18, body mass index at age 18, and total energy intake at age 18.
[b]Logarithm transformation was used; [c]β's should be interpreted as the % change (increase or decrease) in triglyceride level associated in relation to the reference group
Bold values mean significant at $P < 0.05$.

Products pattern was associated with higher triglycerides among girls. Sugar-sweetened beverages have been the focus of other studies, most of which show a negative impact on the cardiovascular health of children and adolescents [9]. A prospective study with Australian adolescents revealed a significant association between increased consumption of sugar-sweetened beverages over time and increased triglycerides in both sexes [45].

The Fruits and Vegetables pattern presented a high factor loading for all fruits and vegetables and a very low loading for red meat, indicating a vegetarian-like pattern. Although vegetarian diets are usually associated with better cardiometabolic parameters, such as low LDL-cholesterol and higher HDL-cholesterol [46], in the current study this pattern was not associated with blood lipids. However, adherence to a vegetarian pattern at this age is not indicative of positive health outcomes [47].

Few studies have investigated the associations between dietary patterns on blood lipids in adolescents [18, 19]. Other studies on this topic have included children or adults in the sample [48, 49], and results of these studies are inconsistent. A cluster analysis conducted by Song et al. [19] using data from three consecutive Korean surveys and a sample of 4347 adolescents observed no associations between any of the three dietary patterns identified ('Western', 'traditional' and 'modified') and elevated triglycerides (≥150 mg/dL) or low HDL-cholesterol (≤40 mg/dL), after adjusting for age and the year of the study. In a prospective Finnish cohort [18] composed of 1768 children and adolescents (aged 3 to 18 years), the traditional patterns based on sausages, potatoes, eggs, milk, butter, meats, rye, wheat, margarine and oil, and other cereals, was associated with higher total cholesterol, and LDL-cholesterol in both sexes. The health-conscious pattern based on fish and shellfish, legumes and nuts, root vegetables, fruits and berries, cheese, other dairy products, tea and alcoholic beverages presented no association with blood lipids. All analyses were adjusted for age, smoking status, physical activity and total energy intake [18]. On the other hand, a cross-sectional study conducted among 1214 Inupiat Eskimos (aged 18 to 92 years) observed an association between the traditional dietary pattern characterized by fish and oils, wild greens, stews made up mostly of meat, native meats and fruits and lower triglycerides concentrations. Meanwhile, the beverages and sweets dietary pattern was associated with higher LDL-cholesterol after adjusting for selected confounders [48]. A Canadian study of 635 participants (aged 18 to 55 years) observed that a Western pattern characterized by high consumption of refined grains, French fries and red meat was inversely correlated with LDL-cholesterol particle diameter after adjusting for age [49].

It is also important to discuss the public health implication of our finding. Following the cut-offs proposed by the American Guidelines for Cardiovascular Health and Risk Reduction in Children and Adolescents (10–19 years) [50], the prevalence of boderline/high blood lipids was 32.5% for total cholesterol (≥170 mg/dL), 15.7% for LDL-cholesterol (≥110 mg/dL), 16.2% for low HDL-cholesterol (≤45 mg/dL), and 20% for high triglycerides (≥100 mg/dL). These findings emphasize the need to promote healthy lifestyle and dietary habits early in life. We have previously shown that being active from adolescence to adulthood reduced the risk for high non-fasting triglycerides and current physical active was associated with greater HDL-cholesterol in young adults [51], and it is known that cardiovascular diseases usually manifest in the fourth decade of life, but atherosclerosis begins in the first years [50].

Girls exhibited higher blood lipid concentrations than boys. These findings are in line with the recent school-based Brazilian study of cardiovascular risks in adolescents that observed higher mean concentrations of total cholesterol, LDL-cholesterol and HDL-cholesterol among girls in comparison to boys [5]. Sex differences in blood lipids have also been reported in European studies of adolescents [52, 53]. Girls have more adipose tissue than boys, which may affect blood lipid concentrations [54]. Additionally, an age of menarche younger than 12 years was associated with higher blood lipids, which reflects hormonal conditions that adversely affect blood lipids independently of age and fat free mass [54]. We found that dietary patterns were more closely associated with blood lipids among girls in comparison to boys even after adjustments for socioeconomic and lifestyle factors, BMI and total energy intake.

The present study has some limitations that need to be highlighted. Regarding representativeness, despite of the reasonable sample size, the current study sample differed from targeted population regarding sex, skin colour, maternal education at birth, total family income at birth, smoking habit at age 18, and leisure-time physical activity at age 18. However, the magnitude of such differences is small, minimizing the likelihood of bias. Besides, analyses were stratified by sex and those variables were included in the adjusted models. Blood lipids were collected without fasting for logistical reasons. However, there is no evidence that fasting blood samples are superior to non-fasting blood samples to assay blood lipids for cardiovascular risk assessment in primary prevention [55]. Non-fasting blood better reflects the daily mean plasma lipoprotein concentrations because most individuals consume several meals during the day, and therefore, the postprandial state predominates a 24-h period [55]. In the current study, LDL-cholesterol was directly measured and this lipid fraction does not change with fasting [55, 56]. Triglycerides levels differ on the basis of fasting status, and a systematic difference within subjects according to the time elapsed since the last meal is possible [55, 56]. Thus, hours of fasting were included in all the adjusted models to adjust for this difference. Even though, results should be interpreted with caution. The administered FFQ was developed for the follow-up at age 15 of the 1993 Birth Cohort [23] and was based on a validated FFQ [24], but it was not validated for the follow-up at age 18. We cannot rule out the possibility of misreporting of food consumption. Factor analyses depend on several decisions made by the researcher, such as food group combinations and the number of factors retained. This statistical procedure allows different input of variables to derive dietary patterns (i.e. frequency, grams or portion size) with or without adjustment for total energy intake before the dietary patterns are established. The classification of individuals according to scores in each pattern may allow some individuals comply equally in different patterns. In the current study, we performed the PCA based on frequency of consumption and four meaningful dietary patterns were obtained with factor loading of individual food items very distinct across major patterns. In addition, this is a qualitative analysis rather than a quantitative one, and it cannot be interpreted in the same way as conventional dietary approaches. Another limitation stems from the cross-sectional nature of the analyses and the possibility of reverse causality, as dietary patterns and blood lipids were both measured at age 18. In spite of these limitations, our study has important strengths, such as the large sample size from a population-based study, the high response rate and the application of standard questionnaires.

Conclusion

The present study showed associations between dietary patterns and blood lipids in Brazilian adolescents followed from birth to age 18. Blood lipids were more closely associated with dietary patterns among girls than among boys. However, higher scores for the Common Brazilian Foods pattern were associated with lower total cholesterol for both girls and boys. It is possible that the negative effects of an unhealthy dietary pattern manifest later in life. Our results emphasize the importance of understanding perceptions of dietary patterns among adolescents and of efforts to include traditional foods in their diets.

Additional files

Additional file 1: Forty-five food items of the food frequency questionnaire categorized according to nutrient composition, frequency of consumption or traditional habits. The 1993 Pelotas (Brazil) Birth Cohort.

Additional file 2: Frequency distribution of baseline characteristics of participants included and excluded from the present analyses. The 1993 Pelotas (Brazil) Birth Cohort.

Additional file 3: Frequency distribution of main investigated variables at age 18 between those who were included and excluded from the present analyses. The 1993 Pelotas (Brazil) Birth Cohort.

Additional file 4: Mean/median (SD/IQR) blood lipids of adolescents at age 18 by selected characteristics. The 1993 Pelotas (Brazil) Birth Cohort.

Abbreviations

BMI: Body mass index; CI: Confidence interval; EI: Energy intake; ER: Energy requirements; FFQ: Food frequency lipoprotein; HDL: High density lipoprotein; LDL: Low density lipoprotein; PCA: Principal component analysis

Acknowledgements

We are extremely grateful to all adolescents and their parents who took part in the 1993 Pelotas Birth Cohort.

Funding

The cohort study was supported by the Wellcome Trust (Grant No. 086974/Z/08/Z). Earlier phases of the cohort were funded by the European Union and the Brazilian National Program for Centers of Excellence (PRONEX), the National Research Council (CNPq), and the Ministry of Health. None of theses organizations influenced the study design or collection, analysis, and interpretation of data; the writing of the report; or the decision to submit the manuscript for publication.

Authors' contributions

Formulated the research question: JSV, MCFA, RB. Conceived and design the study: AMBM, MCFA, IO. Analysed the data: JSV, RB, RMB, IO. Wrote and/or reviewed the manuscript: JSV, RMB, GK, RMB, AMBM, MCFA. All authors read and approved the final manuscript.

Competing interests

The authors declare that they have no competing interests.

Author details

[1]Faculty of Nutrition, Federal University of Pelotas, Rua Gomes Carneiro, 1, 2° andar, Pelotas, RS 96010-610, Brazil. [2]Epidemiology, Federal University of Pelotas, Rua Marechal Deodoro, 1160, 3° andar, Pelotas, RS 96020-220, Brazil. [3]Institute of Nutrition, Federal University of Rio de Janeiro, Avenida Carlos Chagas Filho, 367, CCS – Bloco J – 2° andar, sala 29, Cidade Universitária – Ilha do Fundão, Rio de Janeiro, RJ 21941-590, Brazil. [4]Institute of Biology, Federal University of Pelotas, Campus Capão do Leão, s/n, Capão do Leão, RS 96010-900, Brazil.

References

1. De Henauw S, Michels N, Vyncke K, Hebestreit A, Russo P, Intemann T, et al. Blood lipids among young children in Europe: results from the European IDEFICS study. Int J Obes. 2014;38(Suppl 2):S67–75.
2. Khoury M, Manlhiot C, Gibson D, Chahal N, Stearne K, Dobbin S, et al. Universal screening for cardiovascular disease risk factors in adolescents to identify high-risk families: a population-based cross-sectional study. BMC Pediatr. 2016;16:11.
3. Juhola J, Magnussen CG, Viikari JS, Kahonen M, Hutri-Kahonen N, Jula A, et al. Tracking of serum lipid levels, blood pressure, and body mass index from childhood to adulthood: the Cardiovascular Risk in Young Finns Study. J Pediatr. 2011;159:584–90.
4. Nicklas TA, von Duvillard SP, Berenson GS. Tracking of serum lipids and lipoproteins from childhood to dyslipidemia in adults: the Bogalusa Heart Study. Int J Sports Med. 2002;23(Suppl 1):S39–43.
5. Faria Neto JR, Bento VF, Baena CP, Olandoski M, Goncalves LG, Abreu Gde A, et al. ERICA: prevalence of dyslipidemia in Brazilian adolescents. Rev. Saude Publica. 2016;50(Suppl 1):10s.
6. Kelishadi R, Haghdoost AA, Moosazadeh M, Keikha M, Aliramezany M. A systematic review and meta-analysis on screening lipid disorders in the pediatric age group. J Res Med Sci. 2015;20:1191–9.
7. Kim SH, Song YH, Park S, Park MJ. Impact of lifestyle factors on trends in lipid profiles among Korean adolescents: the Korea National Health and Nutrition Examination Surveys study, 1998 and 2010. Korean J Pediatr. 2016; 59:65–73.
8. Ordovas JM. Genetic influences on blood lipids and cardiovascular disease risk: tools for primary prevention. Am J Clin Nutr. 2009;89:1509S–17S.
9. Funtikova AN, Navarro E, Bawaked RA, Fito M, Schroder H. Impact of diet on cardiometabolic health in children and adolescents. Nutr J. 2015;14:118.
10. Siri-Tarino PW, Krauss RM. Diet, lipids, and cardiovascular disease. Curr Opin Lipidol. 2016;27:323–8.
11. Monteiro CA, Cannon G, Moubarac JC, Martins AP, Martins CA, Garzillo J, et al. Dietary guidelines to nourish humanity and the planet in the twenty-first century. A blueprint from Brazil. Public Health Nutr. 2015;18:2311–22.
12. Monteiro CA, Levy RB, Claro RM, de Castro IR, Cannon G. Increasing consumption of ultra-processed foods and likely impact on human health: evidence from Brazil. Public Health Nutr. 2011;14:5–13.
13. Canella DS, Levy RB, Martins AP, Claro RM, Moubarac JC, Baraldi LG, et al. Ultra-processed food products and obesity in Brazilian households (2008–2009). PloS One. 2014;9:e92752.
14. Bel-Serrat S, Mouratidou T, Huybrechts I, Labayen I, Cuenca-Garcia M, Palacios G, et al. Associations between macronutrient intake and serum lipid profile depend on body fat in European adolescents: the Healthy Lifestyle in Europe by Nutrition in Adolescence (HELENA) study. Br J Nutr. 2014;112:2049–59.
15. Bradlee ML, Singer MR, Daniels SR, Moore LL. Eating patterns and lipid levels in older adolescent girls. Nutr Metab Cardiovasc Dis. 2013;23:196–204.
16. Tapsell LC, Neale EP, Satija A, Hu FB. Foods, Nutrients, and Dietary Patterns: Interconnections and Implications for Dietary Guidelines. Adv Nutr. 2016;7:445–54.
17. Joung H, Hong S, Song Y, Ahn BC, Park MJ. Dietary patterns and metabolic syndrome risk factors among adolescents. Korean J Pediatr. 2012;55:128–35.
18. Mikkila V, Rasanen L, Raitakari OT, Marniemi J, Pietinen P, Ronnemaa T, et al. Major dietary patterns and cardiovascular risk factors from childhood to adulthood. The Cardiovascular Risk in Young Finns Study. Br J Nutr. 2007;98:218–25.
19. Song Y, Park MJ, Paik HY, Joung H. Secular trends in dietary patterns and obesity-related risk factors in Korean adolescents aged 10–19 years. Int J Obes. 2010;34:48–56.
20. Victora CG, Araujo CL, Menezes AM, Hallal PC, Vieira Mde F, Neutzling MB, et al. Methodological aspects of the 1993 Pelotas (Brazil) Birth Cohort Study. Rev. Saude Publica. 2006;40:39–46.
21. Goncalves H, Assuncao MC, Wehrmeister FC, Oliveira IO, Barros FC, Victora CG, et al. Cohort profile update: The 1993 Pelotas (Brazil) birth cohort follow-up visits in adolescence. Int J Epidemiol. 2014;43:1082–8.
22. Schneider BC, Motta JVS, Muniz LC, Bielemann RM, Madruga SW, Orlandi SP, et al. Design of a digital and self-reported food frequency questionnaire to estimate food consumption in adolescents and young adults: birth cohorts at Pelotas, Rio Grande do Sul, Brazil. Rev. Bras Epidemiol. 2016;19:419–32.
23. Gigante DP, Reichert FF, Hallal PC, Souza RV, Neutzling MB, Vieira Mde F, et al. Dietary assessment in the 1993 Pelotas (Brazil) birth cohort study: comparing energy intake with energy expenditure. Cad Saude Publica. 2010;26:2080–9.

24. Sichieri R, Everhart JE. Validity of a Brazilian food frequency questionnaire against dietary recalls and estimated energy intake. Nutr Res. 1998;18:1649–59.
25. Tabela Brasileira de Composição de Alimentos. Universidade Estadual de Campinas - NEPA/UNICAMP. 2011. http://www.nepa.unicamp.br/taco/index.php. Accessed 10 Nov 2017.
26. USDA National Nutrient Database for Standard Reference, Release 24. U.S. Department of Agriculture, Agriculture Research Service. 2011. http://ars.usda.gov. Accessed 10 Nov 2017.
27. Newby PK, Tucker KL. Empirically derived eating patterns using factor or cluster analysis: a review. Nutr Rev. 2004;62:177–203.
28. Hu FB. Dietary pattern analysis: a new direction in nutritional epidemiology. Curr Opin Lipidol. 2002;13:3–9.
29. Wirfalt E, Drake I, Wallstrom P. What do review papers conclude about food and dietary patterns? Food Nutr Res. 2013;57. https://doi.org/10.3402/fnr.v57i0.20523.
30. Northstone K, Emmett P, Rogers I. Dietary patterns in pregnancy and associations with socio-demographic and lifestyle factors. Eur J Clin Nutr. 2008;62:471–9.
31. de Onis M, Onyango AW, Borghi E, Siyam A, Nishida C, Siekmann J. Development of a WHO growth reference for school-aged children and adolescents. Bull World Health Organ. 2007;85:660–7.
32. Hagstromer M, Oja P, Sjostrom M. The International Physical Activity Questionnaire (IPAQ): a study of concurrent and construct validity. Public Health Nutr. 2006;9:755–62.
33. Matsudo S, Araujo T, Matsudo V, D. A, E. A, Oliveira L, et al. Questionário Internacional de Atividade Física (IPAQ): Estudo de Validade e Reprodutibilidade no Brasil. Rev. Bras Ativ Saude. 2001;6:5–18.
34. Global Recommendations on Physical Activity for Health. WHO. World Health Organization, Genebra. 2010. http://www.who.int/dietphysicalactivity/publications/9789241599979/en/ Acessed 10 Nov 2017.
35. Jenab M, Slimani N, Bictash M, Ferrari P, Bingham SA. Biomarkers in nutritional epidemiology: applications, needs and new horizons. Hum Genet. 2009;125:507–25.
36. Huang TT, Howarth NC, Lin BH, Roberts SB, McCrory MA. Energy intake and meal portions: associations with BMI percentile in U.S. children. Obes Res. 2004;12:1875–85.
37. McCrory MA, McCrory MA, Hajduk CL, Roberts SB. Procedures for screening out inaccurate reports of dietary energy intake. Public Health Nutr. 2002;5:873–82.
38. Olinto MT, Willett WC, Gigante DP, Victora CG. Sociodemographic and lifestyle characteristics in relation to dietary patterns among young Brazilian adults. Public Health Nutr. 2011;14:150–9.
39. Ambrosini GL, Huang RC, Mori TA, Hands BP, O'Sullivan TA, de Klerk NH, et al. Dietary patterns and markers for the metabolic syndrome in Australian adolescents. Nutr Metab Cardiovasc Dis. 2010;20:274–83.
40. Nobre LN, Lamounier JA, Franceschini SC. Sociodemographic, anthropometric and dietary determinants of dyslipidemia in preschoolers. J Pediatr. 2013;89:462–9.
41. Tavares LF, Castro IR, Levy RB, Cardoso Lde O, Claro RM. Dietary patterns of Brazilian adolescents: results of the Brazilian National School-Based Health Survey (PeNSE). Cad Saude Publica. 2014;30:2679–90.
42. Brasil. Cadernos de atenção básica. Guia alimentar para a população brasileira. Saúde Md, editor. Brasilia: Ministério da Saúde; 2014. p. 156.
43. Kelishadi R, Pour MH, Zadegan NS, Kahbazi M, Sadry G, Amani A, et al. Dietary fat intake and lipid profiles of Iranian adolescents: Isfahan Healthy Heart Program--Heart Health Promotion from Childhood. Prev Med. 2004;39:760–6.
44. Tavares LF, Fonseca SC, Garcia Rosa ML, Yokoo EM. Relationship between ultra-processed foods and metabolic syndrome in adolescents from a Brazilian Family Doctor Program. Public Health Nutr. 2012;15:82–7.
45. Ambrosini GL, Oddy WH, Huang RC, Mori TA, Beilin LJ, Jebb SA. Prospective associations between sugar-sweetened beverage intakes and cardiometabolic risk factors in adolescents. Am J Clin Nutr. 2013;98:327–34.
46. Sabate J, Wien M. Vegetarian diets and childhood obesity prevention. Am J Clin Nutr. 2010;91:1525S–9S.
47. Robinson-O'Brien R, Perry CL, Wall MM, Story M, Neumark-Sztainer D. Adolescent and young adult vegetarianism: better dietary intake and weight outcomes but increased risk of disordered eating behaviors. J Am Diet Assoc. 2009;109:648–55.
48. Eilat-Adar S, Mete M, Nobmann ED, Xu J, Fabsitz RR, Ebbesson SO, et al. Dietary patterns are linked to cardiovascular risk factors but not to inflammatory markers in Alaska Eskimos. J Nutr. 2009;139:2322–8.
49. Bouchard-Mercier A, Paradis AM, Godin G, Lamarche B, Perusse L, Vohl MC. Associations between dietary patterns and LDL peak particle diameter: a cross-sectional study. J Am Coll Nutr. 2010;29:630–7.
50. National Heart Lung and Blood Institute. Expert Panel on Integrated Guidelis for Cardiovascular Health and Risk Reduction in Children and Adolescents Summary Report. NIH Publication No. 12-7486A. 2012.
51. Bielemann RM, Ramires VV, Gigante DP, Hallal PC, Horta BL. Longitudinal and cross-sectional associations of physical activity with triglyceride and HDLc levels in young male adults. J Phys Act Health. 2014;11(4):784–9.
52. Spinneker A, Egert S, Gonzalez-Gross M, Breidenassel C, Albers U, Stoffel-Wagner B, et al. Lipid, lipoprotein and apolipoprotein profiles in European adolescents and its associations with gender, biological maturity and body fat--the HELENA Study. Eur J Clin Nutr. 2012;66:727–35.
53. Ucar B, Kilic Z, Dinleyici EC, Colak O, Gunes E. Serum lipid profiles including non-high density lipoprotein cholesterol levels in Turkish school-children. Anadolu Kardiyol Derg. 2007;7:415–20.
54. Remsberg KE, Demerath EW, Schubert CM, Chumlea WC, Sun SS, Siervogel RM. Early menarche and the development of cardiovascular disease risk factors in adolescent girls: the Fels Longitudinal Study. J Clin Endocrinol Metab. 2005;90:2718–24.
55. Nordestgaard BG, Langsted A, Mora S, Kolovou G, Baum H, Bruckert E, et al. Fasting Is Not Routinely Required for Determination of a Lipid Profile: Clinical and Laboratory Implications Including Flagging at Desirable Concentration Cutpoints-A Joint Consensus Statement from the European Atherosclerosis Society and European Federation of Clinical Chemistry and Laboratory Medicine. Clin Chem. 2016;62:930–46.
56. Steiner MJ, Skinner AC, Perrin EM. Fasting might not be necessary before lipid screening: a nationally representative cross-sectional study. Pediatrics. 2011;128(3):463–70.

11

Dietary fiber intake and reduced risk of ovarian cancer

Bowen Zheng[1†], Hui Shen[2†], Hedong Han[3†], Ting Han[2*] and Yonghong Qin[1*]

Abstract

Background: Epidemiological studies regarding the association between dietary fiber intake and ovarian cancer risk are still inconsistent. We aimed to review the available evidence and conduct a dose-response meta-analysis to investigate the relationship between dietary fiber intake and ovarian cancer risk.

Methods: Relevant studies were identified by searching PubMed, EMBASE, and the Cochrane Library databases before August 2017. Studies that reported relative risk (RR) estimates with 95% confidence intervals (CIs) for the association between dietary fiber intake and risk of ovarian cancer were included. Random-effects models were used to combine the estimated effects extracted from individual study.

Results: Thirteen studies, with a total of 5777 ovarian cancer cases and 142,189 participants, met the inclusion criteria. The pooled multivariable RRs of ovarian cancer for the highest vs. the lowest category of dietary fiber intake was 0.78 (95% CI: 0.70, 0.88) with no evidence of heterogeneity ($I^2 = 4.20\%$, $P = 0.40$). Our dose-response analysis also showed a significant inverse association between dietary fiber intake and ovarian cancer risk (an increment of 10 g/day; combined RR: 0.88; 95% CI: 0.82, 0.93). There was no evidence for a nonlinear association (*P* for nonlinearity = 0.83).

Conclusions: This meta-analysis suggests a significant inverse dose-response association between dietary fiber intake and ovarian cancer risk. Further studies with prospective design that take account of more potential confounders are warranted to confirm this association.

Keywords: Ovarian cancer, Protective factor, Dietary fiber, Meta-analysis

Introduction

Ovarian cancer, the second most common female reproductive malignant tumor (240,000 new cases annually) and the leading cause of death in gynecological malignancy (over 150,000 new deaths annually) worldwide [1], has caused heavy public health burden. In spite of recent advances in surgical treatment, prognosis of ovarian cancer remains poor [2]. Thus, it is of prior importance to identify the significant risks and the protective factors associated with the incidence of ovarian cancer.

Epidemiologic studies have suggested that dietary factors play an important role in the etiology of ovarian cancer, including dietary glycemic load [3], fat [4], dietary phytoestrogen [5], fruit and vegetable [6]. Fiber, mainly consumed through diet with cereal, fruit, and vegetable, was reported to be inversely associated with many types of cancers, such as colorectal cancer [7], breast cancer [8], gastric cancer [9] and endometrial cancer [10]. However, reports regarding the association between dietary fiber intake and risk of ovarian cancer were still conflicting. Six case-control studies suggested that dietary fiber intake was inversely related to risk of ovarian cancer [11–16], while others failed to find similar significant association [5, 17–22]. In addition, the effects of dietary fiber intake on ovarian cancer risk seemed to vary with different types and sources of fiber.

Thus, we conducted this meta-analysis with the following purposes: 1) to comprehensively summarize all the available evidence from case-control and cohort studies on the relationship between dietary fiber and risk

* Correspondence: than927@163.com; yonghongqin@sohu.com; he_dong1102@126.com
†Bowen Zheng, Hui Shen and Hedong Han contributed equally to this work.
[2]Department of Pharmacognosy, School of Pharmacy, Second Military Medical University, 325 Guohe Road, Shanghai 200433, China
[1]Department of Plastic Surgery, Second Hospital of Lanzhou University, Lanzhou 730030, Gansu Province, China

of ovarian cancer; 2) to examine the discrepancy of ovarian cancer risk according to study design, geographic location and types or sources of fiber; 3) to explore the potential dose-response relationship between dietary fiber intake and risk of ovarian cancer.

Materials and methods

Search strategy

The review was registered in PROSPERO-international prospective register of systematic reviews http://www.crd.york.ac.uk/prospero/ (registration number. CRD42016046795).We followed the standard MOOSE [23] and PRISMA criteria [24] to conduct and report this meta-analysis using the databases of PubMed, EMBASE, and the Cochrane library till August 2017. Two investigators (BWZ and HDH) independently identified publications through title and abstract. The eligibility of the publications was further evaluated by full-text assessment. Disagreements between the reviewers were resolved by discussion. We used the following search terms: (diet OR dietary OR fiber OR fibre) AND (ovary OR ovarian) AND (cancer OR neoplasm OR carcinoma OR tumor OR malignancy). Furthermore, the reference lists of retrieved articles were manually scrutinized to identify potential relevant studies.

Study selection

Eligible studies were included in the meta-analysis if they met the following criteria: 1) the study design was observational (case-control, nested case-control or cohort study); 2) the exposure of interest was dietary fiber intake, and the outcome of interest was ovarian cancer risk; 3) the risk estimates, such as relative risks, odds ratios, or hazard ratios with 95% confidence intervals (CIs) were reported; 4) factors were adjusted for ovarian cancer risk.

Data extraction

Two reviewers (BWZ, HHD) independently extracted the data from eligible studies using a predefined data extraction form. The following study characteristics were recorded from each study: the first author's last name, year of publication, study location, study design, No. of participants, No. of cases, dietary assessment, exposure details, contrast (highest vs. lowest), RR (95% CI) (highest vs. lowest), adjustments and New-castle-Ottawa Scale (NOS) score. Validated FFQs meant that FFQs used in the included studies was previously validated. Quality assessment for studies was conducted using the 9-star NOS score [25]. Studies with an NOS score of ≥7 were considered high-quality.

Statistical analysis

Relative risk was used as the common measure of association across the included studies [26]. The DerSimonian and Laird random-effects model [27, 28], which considered both within-study and between-study variation, was used to pool the estimated effects for the highest vs. the lowest categories of dietary fiber intake.

For the dose-response meta-analysis, we used generalized least-squares regression, which considered the correlation between estimates for different exposure levels, to compute study-specific risk estimates [29, 30]. Meanwhile, to examine a potential nonlinear association, we performed a two-stage random-effect dose-response meta-analysis using restricted cubic splines with three knots at fixed percentiles (10, 50, and 90%) of the distribution [31]. A *P*-value for non-linearity was calculated by testing null hypothesis that the coefficient of the second spline was equal to zero. The midpoint or median dietary fiber intake in each category was used as the assigned dose, and half the width of the adjacent category was used to define the corresponding point for the open categories.

Forest plots were used to assess the RR estimates and corresponding 95% CIs. I^2 statistics were used to assess statistical heterogeneity among the studies [32]. The subgroup and meta-regression analyses were conducted according to geographic location, type of control subjects, sample size, study design and adjustments for potential confounders. Publication bias was assessed through the Egger's regression test [33] and funnel plot. We also conducted sensitivity analysis by omitting one study at a time to investigate the influence of a single study on the overall risk estimate.

Stata Version 12.0 software (Stata Corp, College Station, TX) was used for all analyses, and *P*-value < 0.05 was considered to be statistically significant.

Results

Study characteristics

Our literature search identified 4665 articles and 4641 were excluded after review of title or abstract (Fig. 1). Twenty-four full-text articles were further reviewed. We excluded 11 studies due to the following reasons: 7 studies did not reported RRs or 95% CI; 2 were review [34, 35]; 2 reported duplicate population [36, 37]. Thus, 13 studies that contained 5,777 ovarian cancer cases and 142,189 participants, published between 1994 and 2015, were included in this meta-analysis. The characteristics of the included studies were summarized in Table 1. Of the 13 studies, 10 were case-control [11–17, 19–21] and 3 were cohort studies [5, 18, 22]. Among these studies, 6 were conducted in USA [12, 15, 17, 18, 21, 22], 2 in Australia [11, 13], 2 in Canada [16, 19], 1 in Italy [14], 1 in Sweden [5] and 1 in Mexico [20]. All the included studies provided RRs that were adjusted for energy intake and most provided RRs that were adjusted for age, oral contraceptive use, menopausal status and parity. All

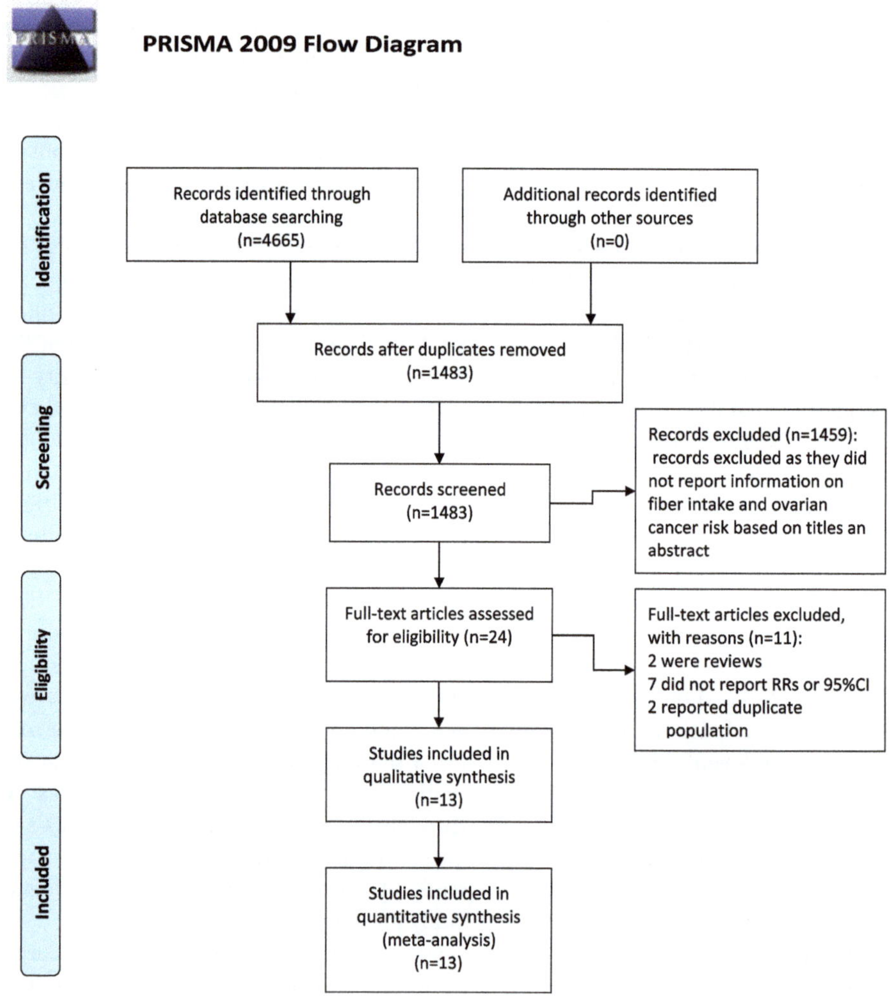

Fig. 1 Selection of studies for inclusion in this meta-analysis

the original studies measured dietary intakes using a food-frequency questionnaire. NOS scores ranged from 6 to 8, and 7 studies were considered high quality.

Dietary fiber intake and ovarian cancer risk

The multivariable-adjusted RR for each study and the combined RR for the highest vs. the lowest categories of dietary fiber intake were shown in Fig. 2. The pooled RR was 0.78 (95% CI: 0.70, 0.88) with no evidence of heterogeneity across the included studies ($I^2 = 4.20\%$, $P = 0.40$).

Dose-response analysis

Nine studies were included in the dose-response analysis (Fig. 3). The summarized RR for ovarian cancer per 10 g/day increase of dietary fiber intake was 0.88 (95% CI: 0.82, 0.93) without heterogeneity ($I^2 = 7.3\%$, $P = 0.38$).There was no evidence for a nonlinear association between dietary fiber intake and ovarian cancer risk (*P* for nonlinearity = 0.83).

Subgroup and meta-regression analyses

The results of subgroup analysis regarding the relationship between dietary fiber intake and risk of ovarian cancer were shown in Table 2. When stratified by study design, the pooled RR was 0.77 (95% CI: 0.66, 0.90) for case-control studies and 0.84 (95% CI: 0.65, 1.10) for cohort studies. In the subgroup analyses by number of cases, the RR was 0.83 (95% CI: 0.65, 1.07) for a sample size < 300 and 0.77 (95% CI: 0.67, 0.87) for a sample size ≥300. In the subgroup analyses by fiber source and fiber type, the RR was 0.80 (95% CI: 0.50, 1.16) for vegetable fiber, 0.90 (0.73, 1.11) for fruit fiber, 1.24 (95% CI: 1.02, 1.51) for cereal fiber, 0.79 (95% CI: 0.51, 1.23) for soluble fiber and 0.60 (95% CI: 0.42, 0.86) for insoluble fiber. The inverse association became insignificant without adjusting for oral contraceptive use (RR: 0.97; 95% CI: 0.76, 1.24) or menopausal status (RR: 0.86; 95% CI: 0.66, 1.11). Meta-regression analysis showed that no variables might account for the heterogeneity across studies (Table 2).

Table 1 Baseline characteristics of all the studies included in the meta-analysis

First Author, Year, Country	Study design	Age (years)	No. of Cases /Participants	Dietary assessment	Exposure details	Contrast (Highest vs. lowest)	RR (95% CI) (Highest vs. lowest)	Adjustments	NOS
Qin,2015, USA	PB-CC	Cases:57.5 Control:54.5	406/1015	Validated 110-item FFQ	Total fiber	≥10.9 vs. ≤6.5 g/d	0.79 (0.53,1.17)	Age, education, region, total energy intake, parity, oral contraceptive use, menopause status, tubal ligation and family history of breast/ovarian cancer, alcohol.	7
Hedelin,2011, Sweden	Cohort	30–49 at entry	163/47140	Validated 80-item FFQ	Total fiber Cereal fiber Vegetable fiber	2.5–10 vs. ≤1.82 g/d 1.5–5.7 vs. ≤0.90 g/d 2.5–10 vs. ≤1.82 g/d	0.82 (0.50,1.35) 1.17 (0.74,1.87) 1.02 (0.63,1.64)	Age, oral contraceptives, age at menarche, parity, hormone replacement therapy, and intake of total energy intake, alcohol, saturated fat, meat, and fish.	8
Nagle,2011, Australia	PB-CC	Cases:57.6 Control:56.3	1366/2780	136-item FFQ	Total fiber	38–77 vs. 10–27 g/d	0.78 (0.62,0.98)	Age, oral contraceptive use, level of post school education, parity, BMI, menopausal status, energy intake.	8
Silvera,2007, USA	Cohort	59.4 ± 7.2	264/49613	Validated 86-item FFQ	Total fiber Soluble fiber Insoluble fiber Cereal fiber Vegetable fiber Fruit fiber	> 24.0 vs. < 15.6 g/d > 7.4 vs. < 4.4 g/d > 5.1 vs. < 2.8 g/d > 5.2 vs. < 2.6 g/d > 10.1 vs. < 5.5 g/d > 5.8 vs. < 2.2 g/d	0.77 (0.52,1.14) 0.79 (0.51,1.23) 0.72 (0.47,1.10) 1.09 (0.71,1.70) 0.94 (0.63,1.40) 0.76 (0.51,1.12)	Age, BMI, alcohol, hormone replacement therapy, use of oral contraceptives, parity, age at Menarche, menopausal status, total energy intake, physical activity, study center, treatment allocation.	8
Pan,2004, Canada	PB-CC	Cases:55.1 Control:55.2	442/2577	Validated 69-item FFQ	Total fiber	Q4 vs. Q1	0.91 (0.66,1.25)	10-year age group, province of residence, education, alcohol consumption, cigarette pack-years, BMI, total caloric intake, recreational Physical activity, number of live births, menstruation years, menopause status.	7
McCann,2003, USA	PB-CC	40–85	124/820	FFQ	Total fiber	> 34 vs. < 19 g/d	0.43 (0.20,0.94)	Age, education, total months menstruating, difficulty becoming pregnant, oral contraceptive use, menopausal status, total energy	6
Zhang,2004, Australia	HB-CC	< 75	254/906	Validated 120-item FFQ	Insoluble fiber	≥15.3 vs. ≤9.7 g/d	0.36 (0.21,0.62)	Age, education, family income, BMI, total energy intake, smoking, alcohol, ovarian cancer in first degree relatives, parity, menopausal status, oral contraceptive use.	6
Salazar-Martinez, 2002, Mexico	HB-CC	20–79	84/713	Validated 116-item FFQ	Total fiber	≥24 vs. ≤ 13 g/d	1.15(0.65,2.05)	Age, total energy intake, number of live births, recent changes in weight, physical activity, diabetes.	6

Table 1 Baseline characteristics of all the studies included in the meta-analysis *(Continued)*

First Author, Year, Country	Study design	Age (years)	No. of Cases /Participants	Dietary assessment	Exposure details	Contrast (Highest vs. lowest)	RR (95% CI) (Highest vs. lowest)	Adjustments	NOS
Goodman, 2002, USA	PB-CC	54.8	558/1165	256-item FFQ	Total fiber	≥29.4 vs. ≤ 15.3 g/d	1.01 (0.63,1.63)	Age, ethnicity, study center, education, use of oral contraceptives, parity, tubal ligation, energy intake.	7
Pelucchi,2001, Italy	HB-CC	18–79	1031/3442	Validated 78-item FFQ	Total fiber Insoluble fiber Vegetable fiber Fruit fiber Grain fiber	Q5 vs. Q1 Q5 vs. Q1 Q5 vs. Q1 Q5 vs. Q1 Q5 vs. Q1	0.68 (0.53,0.88) 0.70 (0.54,0.89) 0.59 (0.46,0.77) 0.96 (0.75,1.22) 1.32 (1.03,1.71)	Age, center, education, occupational physical activity, parity, oral contraceptive use, family history of ovarian and/or breast cancer in first-degree relatives, menopausal status, total energy intake	6
McCann,2001, USA,	HB-CC	20–87	496/1921	44-item FFQ	Total fiber	≥30 vs. ≤16 g/d	0.57 (0.38,0.87)	Age, education, region of residence, regularity of menstruation, family history of ovarian cancer, parity, age at menarche, oral contraceptive use, total energy intake	6
Kushi,1999, USA	Cohort	55–69	139/29083	Validated 126-item FFQ	Total fiber	> 23.6 vs. < 16.3 g/d	1.01 (0.61,1.68)	Age, total energy intake, number of live births, age at menopause, family history of ovarian cancer in a first-degree relative, hysterectomy/unilateral oophorectomy status, waist-to-hip ratio, level of physical activity, cigarette smoking, and educational level.	7
Risch,1994, Canada	PB-CC	35–79	450/1014	200-item FFQ	Total fiber Vegetable fiber Fruit fiber Cereal fiber	For 10 g/d increase	0.82 (0.71,0.94) 0.63 (0.49,0.80) 1.03 (1.75,1.43) 0.88 (0.70,1.10)	Age, number of full-term pregnancies, oral contraceptive use, total dally calories, saturated tat/total fat.	6

Abbreviations: *RR* relative risk, *CI* confidence interval, *PB-CC* population-based case-control, *HB-CC* hospital-based case-control, *NOS* Newcastle–Ottawa Quality Assessment Scale, *FFQ* food frequency questionnaire, *BMI* body mass index

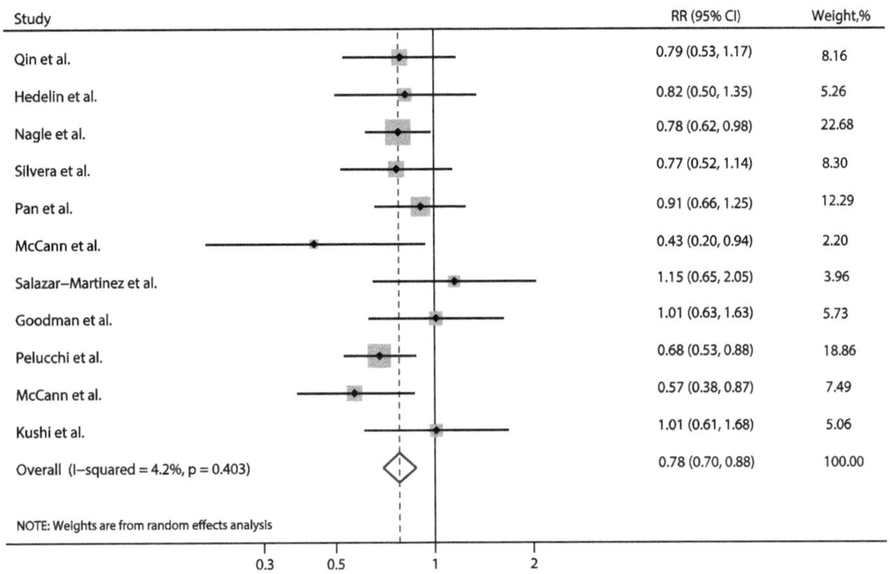

Fig. 2 Forest plot of dietary fiber intake and risk of ovarian cancer for highest vs. lowest categories

Publication bias and sensitivity analysis

Funnel plot shapes demonstrated a symmetrical distribution (Fig. 4) and no evidence of publication bias was detected by the Egger's regression test ($p = 0.73$). Sensitivity analysis shown that none of the studies influenced the combined results substantially, with a range from 0.77 (95% CI: 0.68, 0.87) to 0.81 (95% CI: 0.71, 0.91).

Discussion

To the best of our knowledge, this is the first meta-analysis to summarize evidence between total dietary fiber intake and different types or sources of dietary fiber intake and risk of ovarian cancer. The meta-analysis of 13 observational studies involving 5,777 ovarian cancer cases supports the hypothesis that a significant inverse association between dietary fiber intake and risk of ovarian cancer. The risk of ovarian cancer was reduced by 22% in the group of highest dietary fiber intake compared with the lowest. Furthermore, a 12% reduction in risk of ovarian cancer was found for per 10 g increase per day. No evidence for a nonlinear association between dietary fiber intake and ovarian cancer was found.

Although no evidence of heterogeneity was found across the included studies, we conducted subgroup analyses to test whether the effect of dietary fiber intake on ovarian cancer risk differed in subpopulations. In the

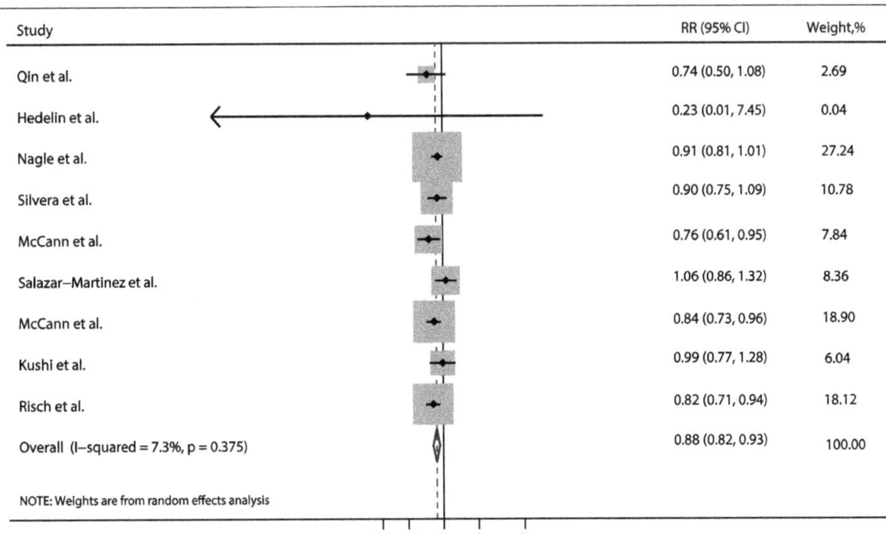

Fig. 3 Frost plot of relative risk of ovarian cancer for an increment of 10 g/day dietary fiber intake

Table 2 Subgroup analysis of dietary fiber intake and ovarian cancer risk

Subgroup	Studies, n	RR (95% CI)	I^2 (%)	P^a	P^b
Total	11	0.78 (0.70,0.88)	4.20	0.40	
Study design					
Case-control	8	0.77 (0.66,0.90)	25	0.23	0.17
Cohort	3	0.84 (0.65,1.10)	0	0.70	
Type of control subjects					
Population-based	8	0.82 (0.72,0.94)	0	0.69	0.16
Hospital-based	3	0.72 (0.52,0.99)	48.20	0.15	
Geographic location					
North America	7	0.79 (0.66,0.95)	19.40	0.28	0.87
Others	4	0.77 (0.66,0.89)	0	0.41	
No. of cases					
< 300	5	0.83 (0.65,1.07)	15.40	0.32	0.16
≥ 300	6	0.77 (0.67,0.87)	5.10	0.38	
Study quality					
NOS < 7	4	0.68 (0.50,0.91)	42.90	0.15	0.09
NOS ≥7	7	0.84 (0.73,0.96)	0	0.92	
Validation FFQ					
Yes	7	0.81 (0.70,0.93)	0	0.60	0.59
No	4	0.72 (0.54,0.94)	43.00	0.15	
Fiber type					
Vegetable fiber	3	0.80 (0.55,1.16)	66.90	0.05	
Fruit fiber	2	0.90 (0.73,1.11)	0	0.32	
Cereal fiber	3	1.24 (1.02,1.51)	0	0.73	
Fiber source					
Soluble fiber	1	0.79 (0.51,1.23)	–	–	
Insoluble fiber	3	0.60 (0.42,0.86)	61.00	0.08	
Adjustments					
BMI					
Yes	3	0.81 (0.69,0.96)	0	0.71	
No	8	0.77 (0.64,0.92)	25.40	0.23	
Parity					
Yes	10	0.79 (0.70,0.89)	0	0.52	
No	1	0.43 (0.20,0.93)	–	–	
Oral contraceptive use					
Yes	8	0.74 (0.65,0.84)	0	0.54	
No	3	0.97 (0.76,1.24)	0	0.77	
physical activity					
Yes	6	0.80 (0.70,0.91)	0	0.46	
No	5	0.73 (0.57,0.94)	24.80	0.26	
Menopausal status					
Yes	6	0.76 (0.67,0.86)	0	0.53	
No	5	0.86 (0.66,1.11)	28.70	0.23	

Abbreviations: *RR* relative risk, *CI* confidence interval, *NOS* Newcastle–Ottawa Quality Assessment Scale, *BMI* body mass index, *P*-value[a], *p* for heterogeneity within each subgroup, *P*-value[b], p for heterogeneity between subgroups

analysis stratified by study design, protective effect of dietary fiber intake was significant in case-control studies but not in cohort studies. There were only three cohort studies with 566 cancer cases, which might not have sufficient power to detect a statistically significant effect. In addition, null association in studies with a relatively small sample size (No. of cases < 300) may also be explained by insufficient statistical power. Additionally, we observed a significant positive association with cereal fiber intake, which probably caused by a high ratio between starch and fiber intake in the Italian population in the study conducted by Pelucchi et al. [14], as the potential promotional action of starch may overwhelm possible protective action of fiber. However, this result should be interpreted carefully and confirmed by further studies because of limited information. The present meta-analysis also indicated that the association was significantly modified by oral contraceptive use and menopausal status, which was corresponding to the previous studies that ovarian cancer risk differed by menopausal status [38] and oral contraceptive use [39].

Several plausible mechanisms have been proposed to explain the hypothesis that dietary fiber intake protects against ovarian cancer. Dietary fiber may decrease circulating estrogen concentrations by changing bacterial macroflora, increasing excretion and consequently lowering serum levels and availability of oestrogens, which reduces the bioavailability of steroid hormones, which in turn is related to the progression of ovarian cancer [8, 40–42]. In addition to the estrogen-related pathway, dietary fiber is believed to reduce glycemic load and improve insulin sensitivity, thus influence insulin-like growth factors which are suggested to be risk factor for ovarian cancer [43, 44].

Our study had several important strengths. This meta-analysis involving 5,777 ovarian cancer cases comprehensively assessed the association between dietary fiber intake and ovarian cancer risk without heterogeneity across studies, enhancing the statistical power to detect a significant association and providing more precise risk estimates. Moreover, most of the included studies were adjusted for important confounders, such as age, energy intake, parity and oral contraceptive use. The sensitivity analysis showed stable and robust results after removal of one study at a time. In addition, outcomes assessment with regards to diagnosis of ovarian cancer in the included studies were histologically confirmed. Finally, the significant inverse dose-response relationship found in this meta-analysis strengthened the association between dietary fiber intake and risk of ovarian cancer.

Potential limitations should be considered in this study. First, we had no access to the individual patient-level data, which would provide a more reliable assessment of relationship between dietary fiber intake

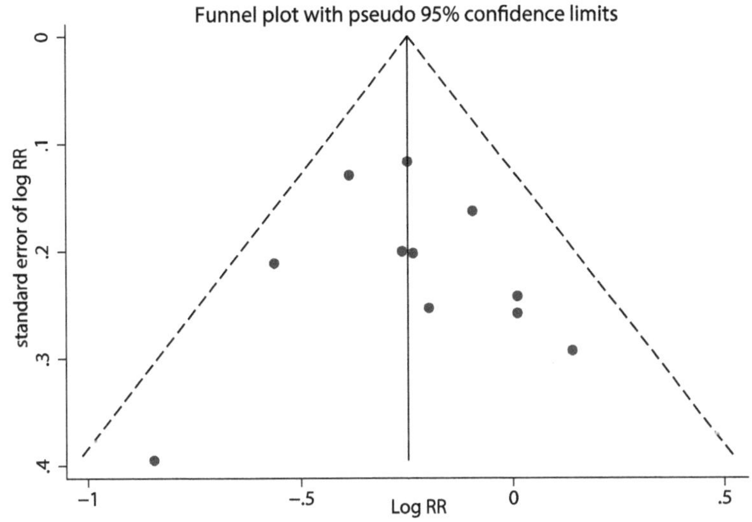

Fig. 4 Funnel plot of studies reporting dietary fiber intake and ovarian cancer risk

and risk of ovarian cancer. Second, the results in our study were mainly based on case-control studies, which may introduce selection bias or recall bias that were inherited in retrospective studies. Third, in observational studies, other factors potentially accounted for the observed association cannot be ruled out. However, potential confounders including energy intake, parity and oral contraceptive use were adjusted in the included studies and the inverse association persisted when analyses were restricted to studies that adjusted for these confounders. Fourth, assessing dietary fiber intake with an FFQ at baseline could have led to overestimation of the range of fiber intake and thus may underestimate the pooled relative risk [45, 46]. Information on the "validated FFQs" was extracted from studies included in this meta-analysis, which meant that the tools used for quantitative dietary measurements were reported with some sort of evaluation in these studies. The evaluation may be tested only in a specific population/setting of interest and for the dietary components of interest but was probably related to smaller bias comparing with the untested FFQs. Moreover, result of subgroup analysis suggested that the inverse association remained significant without application of a validated FFQ. Fifth, the estimates of fiber intakes from different dietary assessment methods and different compositional databases could account for discrepancy among the included studies, so results from this meta-analysis should be interpreted cautiously. Sixth, data in this meta-analysis was mainly from western population, further studies concerning other populations were warranted to generalize this inverse association.

Fiber is mainly consumed through daily diet with cereal, fruit, and vegetable. The mean dietary fiber intake in United States and most European countries is 15 g/day, which is considerably less than the recommended amount (approximately 25–38 g/day) [47, 48]. Considering the public health burden of ovarian cancer, increasing dietary fiber intake in the general population is of importance for ovarian cancer prevention.

Conclusion

This meta-analysis provides evidence for the hypothesis that a higher intake of dietary fiber is inversely associated with ovarian cancer risk, consistent with a dose-response relationship. This evidence is largely limited to case-control studies. Further studies with prospective design that are adequately adjusted for potential confounders and clarified types or sources of fiber are needed to confirm our findings.

Abbreviations

BMI: body mass index; CI: confidence interval; FFQ: food frequency questionnaire; HB-CC: hospital-based case-control; NOS: Newcastle–Ottawa Quality Assessment Scale; PB-CC: population-based case-control; RR: relative risk

Acknowledgements

The authors thank the staff of the Department of Health Statistics, Second Military Medical University, China and Department of Pharmacognosy, School of Pharmacy, Second Military Medical University, China for their dedicated assistance in literature searching and screening.

Funding

None.

Authors' contributions

BWZ, HS and HDH made study protocol, designed the research and performed the literature search. BWZ and HDH had full access to the study data and carried out all analysis. BWZ and HDH wrote the draft of this paper. HS and TH revised the article critically; and all authors contributed to the manuscript writing, made critical revision, read and approved the final manuscript.

Competing interests
All of the authors declare that they have no competing interest.

Author details
[1]Department of Plastic Surgery, Second Hospital of Lanzhou University, Lanzhou 730030, Gansu Province, China. [2]Department of Pharmacognosy, School of Pharmacy, Second Military Medical University, 325 Guohe Road, Shanghai 200433, China. [3]Department of Health Statistics, Second Military Medical University, Shanghai 200433, China.

References

1. Torre LA, Bray F, Siegel RL, Ferlay J, Lortet-Tieulent J, Jemal A. Global cancer statistics, 2012. CA Cancer J Clin. 2015;65:87–108.
2. Falconer H, Yin L, Gronberg H, Altman D. Ovarian cancer risk after salpingectomy: a nationwide population-based study. J Natl Cancer Inst. 2015;107:dju410.
3. Turati F, Galeone C, Gandini S, Augustin LS, Jenkins DJ, Pelucchi C, La Vecchia C. High glycemic index and glycemic load are associated with moderately increased cancer risk. Mol Nutr Food Res. 2015;59:1384–94.
4. Qiu W, Lu H, Qi Y, Wang X. Dietary fat intake and ovarian cancer risk: a meta-analysis of epidemiological studies. Oncotarget. 2016;7:37390–406.
5. Hedelin M, Lof M, Andersson TML, Adlercreutz H, Weiderpass E. Dietary phytoestrogens and the risk of ovarian Cancer in the Women's lifestyle and health cohort study. Cancer Epidemiol Biomark Prev. 2011;20:308–17.
6. Tang L, Lee AH, Su D, Binns CW. Fruit and vegetable consumption associated with reduced risk of epithelial ovarian cancer in southern Chinese women. Gynecol Oncol. 2014;132:241–7.
7. Kunzmann AT, Coleman HG, Huang WY, Kitahara CM, Cantwell MM, Berndt SI. Dietary fiber intake and risk of colorectal cancer and incident and recurrent adenoma in the prostate, lung, colorectal, and ovarian Cancer screening trial. Am J Clin Nutr. 2015;102:881–90.
8. Aune D, Chan DS, Greenwood DC, Vieira AR, Rosenblatt DA, Vieira R, Norat T. Dietary fiber and breast cancer risk: a systematic review and meta-analysis of prospective studies. Ann Oncol. 2012;23:1394–402.
9. Zhang Z, Xu G, Ma M, Yang J, Liu X. Dietary Fiber intake reduces risk for gastric Cancer: a meta-analysis. Gastroenterology. 2013;145:113–20.
10. Bidoli E, Pelucchi C, Zucchetto A, Negri E, Dal Maso L, Polesel J, Montella M, Franceschi S, Serraino D, La Vecchia C, Talamini R. Fiber intake and endometrial cancer risk. Acta Oncol. 2010;49:441–6.
11. Nagle CM, Kolahdooz F, Ibiebele TI, Olsen CM, Lahmann PH, Green AC, Webb PM. Carbohydrate intake, glycemic load, glycemic index, and risk of ovarian cancer. Ann Oncol. 2011;22:1332–8.
12. McCann SE, Freudenheim JL, Marshall JR, Graham S. Risk of human ovarian cancer is related to dietary intake of selected nutrients, phytochemicals and food groups. J Nutr. 2003;133:1937–42.
13. Zhang M. Reproductive and dietary risk factors for epithelial ovarian cancer in China. Gynecol Oncol. 2004;92:320–6.
14. Pelucchi C, La Vecchia C, Chatenoud L, Negri E, Conti E, Montella M, Calza S, Dal Maso L, Franceschi S. Dietary fibres and ovarian cancer risk. Eur J Cancer. 2001;37:2235–9.
15. McCann SE, Moysich KB, Mettlin C. Intakes of selected nutrients and food groups and risk of ovarian cancer. Nutr Cancer. 2001;39:19–28.
16. Risch HA, Jain M, Marrett LD, Howe GR. Dietary fat intake and risk of epithelial ovarian cancer. J Natl Cancer Inst. 1994;86:1409–15.
17. Qin B, Moorman PG, Alberg AJ, Barnholtz-Sloan JS, Bondy M, Cote ML, Funkhouser E, Peters ES, Schwartz AG, Terry P, Schildkraut JM, Bandera EV. Dietary carbohydrate intake, glycaemic load, glycaemic index and ovarian cancer risk in African-American women. Br J Nutr. 2016;115:694–702.
18. Silvera SAN, Jain M, Howe GR, Miller AB, Rohan TE. Dietary fiber intake and ovarian cancer risk: a prospective cohort study. Cancer Causes Control. 2007; 18:335–41.
19. Pan SY, Ugnat AM, Mao Y, Wen SW, Johnson KC. A case-control study of diet and the risk of ovarian cancer. Cancer Epidemiol Biomark Prev. 2004;13:1521–7.
20. Salazar-Martinez E, Lazcano-Ponce EC. Gonzalez lira-lira G, Escudero-De Los Rios P, Hernandez-Avila M: nutritional determinants of epithelial ovarian cancer risk: a case-control study in Mexico. Oncology. 2002;63:151–7.
21. Goodman MT. Association of Dairy Products, lactose, and calcium with the risk of ovarian Cancer. Am J Epidemiol. 2002;156:148–57.
22. Kushi LH, Mink PJ, Folsom AR, Anderson KE, Zheng W, Lazovich D, Sellers TA. Prospective study of diet and ovarian cancer. Am J Epidemiol. 1999;149: 21–31.
23. Stroup DF, Berlin JA, Morton SC, Olkin I, Williamson GD, Rennie D, Moher D, Becker BJ, Sipe TA, Thacker SB. Meta-analysis of observational studies in epidemiology: a proposal for reporting. Meta-analysis of observational studies in epidemiology (MOOSE) group. Jama. 2000;283:2008–12.
24. Liberati A, Altman DG, Tetzlaff J, Mulrow C, Gotzsche PC, Ioannidis JP, Clarke M, Devereaux PJ, Kleijnen J, Moher D. The PRISMA statement for reporting systematic reviews and meta-analyses of studies that evaluate health care interventions: explanation and elaboration. PLoS Med. 2009;6:e1–e34.
25. Wells GA, Shea B, O'Connell D, Peterson J, Welch V, et al. (2011) The Newcastle-Ottawa Scale (NOS) for assessing the quality of nonrandomized studies in meta-analysis. Available: www.ohri.ca/programs/clinical_epidemiology/oxford.asp. Accessed 25 November 2012.
26. Zhang J, Yu KF. What's the relative risk? A method of correcting the odds ratio in cohort studies of common outcomes. Jama. 1998;280:1690–1.
27. Jackson D, White IR, Thompson SG. Extending DerSimonian and Laird's methodology to perform multivariate random effects meta-analyses. Stat Med. 2010;29:1282–97.
28. Borenstein M, Higgins JP. Meta-analysis and subgroups. Prev Sci. 2013;14: 134–43.
29. Orsini NBCRG. Generalized least squares for trend estimation of summarized dose-response. Stata J. 2006;6:40–57.
30. Greenland S, Longnecker MP. Methods for trend estimation from summarized dose-response data, with applications to meta-analysis. Am J Epidemiol. 1992;135:1301–9.
31. Larsson SC, Orsini N, Wolk A. Vitamin B6 and risk of colorectal cancer: a meta-analysis of prospective studies. JAMA. 2010;303:1077–83.
32. Higgins JP, Thompson SG, Deeks JJ, Altman DG. Measuring inconsistency in meta-analyses. Bmj. 2003;327:557–60.
33. Egger M, Davey Smith G, Schneider M, Minder C. Bias in meta-analysis detected by a simple, graphical test. Bmj. 1997;315:629–34.
34. Crane TE, Khulpateea BR, Alberts DS, Basen-Engquist K, Thomson CA. Dietary intake and ovarian cancer risk: a systematic review. Cancer Epidemiology Biomarkers and Prevention. 2014;23:255–73.
35. Brekelmans CT. Risk factors and risk reduction of breast and ovarian cancer. Curr Opin Obstet Gynecol. 2003;15:63–8.
36. Qin B, Moorman PG, Kelemen LE, Alberg AJ, Barnholtz-Sloan JS, Bondy M, Cote ML, Funkhouser E, Peters ES, Schwartz AG, Terry P, Schildkraut JM, Bandera EV. Dietary quality and ovarian Cancer risk in African-American women. Am J Epidemiol. 2017;185:1281–9.
37. Qin B, Moorman PG, Alberg AJ, Barnholtz-Sloan JS, Bondy M, Cote ML, Funkhouser E, Peters ES, Schwartz AG, Terry P, Schildkraut JM, Bandera EV. Dairy, calcium, vitamin D and ovarian cancer risk in African-American women. Br J Cancer. 2016;115:1122–30.
38. Moorman PG, Calingaert B, Palmieri RT, Iversen ES, Bentley RC, Halabi S, Berchuck A, Schildkraut JM. Hormonal risk factors for ovarian cancer in premenopausal and postmenopausal women. Am J Epidemiol. 2008;167: 1059–69.
39. Beral V, Doll R, Hermon C, Peto R, Reeves G. Ovarian cancer and oral contraceptives: collaborative reanalysis of data from 45 epidemiological studies including 23,257 women with ovarian cancer and 87,303 controls. Lancet. 2008;371:303–14.
40. Pillow PC, Duphorne CM, Chang S, Contois JH, Strom SS, Spitz MR, Hursting SD. Development of a database for assessing dietary phytoestrogen intake. Nutr Cancer. 1999;33:3–19.
41. Rose DP, Goldman M, Connolly JM, Strong LE. High-fiber diet reduces serum estrogen concentrations in premenopausal women. Am J Clin Nutr. 1991;54:520–5.
42. Cunat S, Hoffmann P, Pujol P. Estrogens and epithelial ovarian cancer. Gynecol Oncol. 2004;94:25–32.
43. Franceschi S, Dal Maso L, Augustin L, Negri E, Parpinel M, Boyle P, Jenkins DJ, La Vecchia C. Dietary glycemic load and colorectal cancer risk. Ann Oncol. 2001;12:173–8.
44. Yu H, Rohan T. Role of the insulin-like growth factor family in cancer development and progression. J Natl Cancer Inst. 2000;92:1472–89.
45. Prentice RL. Dietary assessment and the reliability of nutritional epidemiology reports. Lancet. 2003;362:182–3.
46. Willett WC, Sampson L, Stampfer MJ, Rosner B, Bain C, Witschi J, Hennekens CH, Speizer FE. Reproducibility and validity of a semiquantitative food frequency questionnaire. Am J Epidemiol. 1985;122:51–65.

12

Dietary patterns during pregnancy and risk of gestational diabetes: a prospective cohort study in Western China

Jonathan K. L. Mak[1], Ngoc Minh Pham[1,2], Andy H. Lee[1], Li Tang[3], Xiong-Fei Pan[4], Colin W. Binns[1] and Xin Sun[3*]

Abstract

Background: Previous research has demonstrated the association between maternal dietary patterns and gestational diabetes (GDM), but evidence in Asian populations remains limited and inconsistent. This study investigated the association between dietary patterns during early pregnancy and the risk of GDM among pregnant women in Western China.

Methods: A prospective cohort study was conducted among 1337 pregnant women in Western China. Dietary intakes were assessed at 15–20 weeks of gestation using a validated food frequency questionnaire. GDM was diagnosed by oral glucose tolerance tests at 24–28 weeks of gestation. Exploratory factor analysis was performed to derive dietary patterns, and logistic regression models were used to examine the association between dietary patterns and GDM.

Results: A total of 199 women (14.9%) developed GDM. Three dietary patterns were identified, namely, a plant-based pattern, a meat-based pattern and a high protein-low starch pattern. Notwithstanding a lack of association between dietary patterns and GDM risk in the whole cohort, there was a significant reduction in GDM risk among overweight women (BMI ≥24 kg/m^2); the odds ratio being 0.29 (95% confidence interval 0.09 to 0.94) when comparing the highest versus the lowest score of the high protein-low starch pattern.

Conclusions: There was no significant association between early pregnancy dietary patterns and GDM risk later in pregnancy for women in Western China, but high protein-low starch diet was associated with lower risk for GDM among women who were overweight at pre-pregnancy.

Keywords: China, Dietary patterns, Pregnancy, Body mass index, Gestational diabetes

Background

Gestational diabetes mellitus (GDM) is a common pregnancy complication in which women without diabetes develop glucose intolerance during pregnancy [1]. Global estimates of its prevalence vary from < 1 to 28% contingent on diagnostic criteria and screening approaches used [2], but have risen by over 30% during the past two decades [3]. In Asia, the GDM prevalence is between 12% [3] and 14% [4], while in China, a recent meta-analysis has shown the total incidence of GDM was approximately 15% [5]. GDM has been recognized as an underlying cause of maternal complications (e.g., pre-eclampsia, pregnancy-induced hypertension and caesarean section) and adverse infant outcomes such as macrosomia and preterm birth [6, 7]. It also increases the risk of long-term metabolic conditions for both mother and offspring [3, 8].

Accumulating evidence has suggested that dietary intake before and during pregnancy is associated with the risk of GDM [9, 10]. On one hand, high consumption of macronutrients (e.g., red meat, processed meat and eggs) and micronutrients (such as dietary heme iron, animal protein, total fat and cholesterol) can increase the GDM risk [11–17]. On the other hand, increasing the intakes of fiber [18], nuts [14], and vegetable-derived protein [14, 15] may lower the GDM risk. Foods or nutrients are commonly consumed in combination rather than separately. As such, studying single food items may be unable to discern the relationship due to the interaction between macro- and

* Correspondence: sunx79@hotmail.com
[3]Chinese Evidence-based Medicine Center, West China Hospital, Sichuan University, Chengdu 610041, China

micronutrients. Dietary pattern analysis, which represents a large and complex set of interrelated dietary factors, is a useful approach to evaluating the diet-GDM relationship. Prudent dietary patterns, such as vegetarian or Mediterranean-style diet, have been shown to reduce the risk of GDM [19]. Meanwhile, a Westernized or less healthy diet, characterized by high intakes of red and processed meat, refined grains and fried foods, is associated with increased risk of GDM [20–22]. Since dietary habits are different between racial and ethnic populations [23], it is of interest to examine the role of dietary patterns in the etiology of GDM, especially in Asia where there has been a rapid nutrition transition to a more Westernized diet [24], with increasing prevalence of GDM [3, 4].

Currently, studies of dietary patterns and GDM in Asia remain scarce with conflicting results. For instance, a study in Southern China showed a positive association between a seafood and sweets pattern and risk of GDM [25], whereas an inverse association was found for a seafood and noodle pattern and risk of GDM in a multi-ethnic Asian cohort [26]. It is unclear whether diet may impact the GDM burden, and whether there are regional differences in the association between dietary patterns and GDM risk. Given that GDM is strongly associated with pre-pregnancy body mass index (BMI) [27], its relationship with maternal dietary patterns may be modified by pregravid BMI levels [28]. The aim of this study was to investigate the association between dietary patterns during early pregnancy and the risk of GDM in Western China, taking into consideration the potential effect modification of pre-pregnancy BMI and other confounding factors.

Methods

Study design and participants

A prospective cohort study was conducted among pregnant women in Western China to identify modifiable risk factors (maternal lifestyle and nutritional status) of adverse pregnancy and infant health outcomes. Full details of the study protocol and recruitment procedures were described elsewhere [29]. Briefly, participants were recruited from four maternity hospitals in Chengdu, Sichuan Province. From May 2015 to August 2015, all pregnant women at 15 to 20 weeks of gestation who attended antenatal care at these hospitals were approached and assessed for eligibility. Eligible women were those aged 18–40 years, with singleton pregnancy, without severe chronic or infectious disease (e.g. HIV), and without any infertility treatment such as in vitro fertilization and intrauterine insemination. Only women who returned their signed consent form were included. In total, 1901 pregnant women were followed up from 15 to 20 weeks of gestation until 12 months postpartum. The study protocol was approved by the Ethics Committee of West China School of Public Health, Sichuan University, and the Human Research Ethics Committee of Curtin University.

Exposure assessment

Dietary intake was assessed at baseline during 15–20 weeks of gestation via face-to-face interviews conducted by trained nurses, using a semi-quantitative Food Frequency Questionnaire (FFQ) originally developed for residents in Chongqing city (a municipality geographically adjacent to Sichuan province), Western China, with the exception of 10 items (four for oil and six for condiments) which are uncommon or deemed difficult to estimate [30]. The FFQ is based on a previous semi-quantitative FFQ validated among women in Chengdu, Sichuan province [31], with reported mean correlation coefficient of 22 nutrients and intra-class correlation coefficients being 0.66 and 0.65, respectively. It contained 109 food and beverage items in 17 predefined groups, with quantities and frequencies recorded in detail. A standard portion (in grams) was defined for each food item listed. A photo booklet was available to show participants about the standard portion sizes, and they were asked to estimate their intake portion for each food, with the options of 0, 0.5, 0.8, 1.0, 1.5, 2.0 and 3.0 or above. They also chose their intake frequencies: 1–3 times per month, 1–2 times per week, 3–4 times per week, 5–6 times per week, once per day, twice per day, three times per day, and four times or more per day. A daily food frequency intake was then computed. Total food intakes in grams per day were calculated using the product of daily frequency intake and amount of food intake per meal in standard portions. In addition, we adjusted food intakes for energy consumption using a density method by calculating the amount of food intake per 1000 kcal of energy [32].

For the analysis of dietary patterns, 109 food and beverage items originally included in the FFQ were combined into 32 food and beverage groups based on their similarities in nutrient profile (see Appendix 1). Exploratory factor analysis with the principle component method [33] was applied to derive dietary patterns, based on the energy-adjusted intakes of food. Number of factors retained was determined by identifying a break point in the scree plot [34] and interpretability of patterns. Factors were rotated by orthogonal/varimax transformation to improve interpretability and utility. Dietary patterns were named according to the food items that contributed most to the pattern. We chose factor loadings ≥0.3 to represent a high correlation between the food group and the dietary pattern. Accordingly, factor scores for each dietary pattern were calculated by the sum of food intake weighted by the corresponding factor loadings.

Outcome assessment

GDM status was determined using oral glucose tolerance tests (OGTT). Between 24 and 28 weeks of gestation, participants who were not previously diagnosed as diabetic were routinely scheduled for a 75 g, 2-h OGTT. Blood samples were collected at fasting, at 1 and 2 h after they received the 75 g oral glucose. GDM cases were confirmed using the IADPSG diagnostic criteria [35], including at least one of the following values being met: fasting serum glucose ≥5.1 mmol/L, 1-h serum glucose ≥10.0 mmol/L, or 2-h post prandial serum glucose ≥8.5 mmol/L.

Assessment of covariates

Information on socio-demographic and health characteristics, including maternal age, education, parity, family history of diabetes and cigarette smoking, was collected during the baseline survey. Maternal age was categorized into four groups (< 25, 25–29, 30–34, ≥35 years) for statistical analysis. Educational status was classified by three levels (junior secondary school or below, senior/technical secondary school, university or above). Physical activity during pregnancy was assessed using a validated Pregnancy Physical Activity Questionnaire [36] and expressed in terms of metabolic equivalent tasks (MET) [37]. Height was measured by a stadiometer, and self-reported pre-pregnancy weight was obtained from medical records. Pre-pregnancy body mass index (BMI) was then calculated as pre-pregnancy weight (kg) divided by height squared (m^2). Participants with BMI < 18.5, 18.5–23.9 and ≥ 24 kg/m^2 were classified as underweight, normal and overweight, respectively [38].

Statistical analysis

Baseline characteristics were compared between groups using t-tests or analysis of variance (ANOVA) for continuous variables, and χ^2 tests for categorical variables. Logistic regression models were used to ascertain the associations between different dietary patterns and risk of GDM, with the lowest tertile taken as the reference level. Crude and adjusted odds ratios (OR) together with 95% confidence intervals (CI) were presented (see Appendix 2). Linear trend analysis was also performed for the logistic regressions. Potential covariates included age, pre-pregnancy BMI, family history of diabetes, parity, education and total physical activity. We examined potential effect modification by age groups, pre-pregnancy BMI (< 24 kg/m^2, or ≥ 24 kg/m^2) and family history of diabetes (yes, no, or don't know) on the association between dietary patterns and GDM risk. We tested the significance of interaction by adding multiplicative interaction terms in the models. All statistical analyses were performed using Stata (version 14.2, Stata Corp, Texas, USA). A two-tailed *p*-value less than 0.05 was considered as statistically significant.

Results

Characteristics of participants

After excluding participants with a history of diabetes before pregnancy ($n = 2$), incomplete information on OGTT ($n = 450$) and those with missing data on diet ($n = 112$), 1337 women were available for analysis. No significant difference was observed between the included and excluded women in terms of age, pre-pregnancy BMI, education, parity, smoking habit and family history of diabetes.

Table 1 summarizes participant characteristics according to the GDM status. Overall, the mean age of participants was 25.8 years (SD = 4.1), and women aged below 25 years accounted for 39.4% of the cohort. The mean pre-pregnancy BMI was 20.7 kg/m^2 (SD = 2.8), while the prevalence of overweight or obese (BMI ≥24 kg/m^2) was 12.6%. In total, 199 women (14.9%) were diagnosed with GDM, who tended to be older, had a higher pre-pregnancy BMI and a greater likelihood of family history of diabetes when compared to their non-GDM counterparts ($p < 0.05$).

Dietary pattern analysis

We identified three major dietary patterns that accounted for 21.2% of the total variation, with their rotated factor loadings presented in Table 2. The first pattern, named the 'plant-based pattern,' was characterized by high intakes of green leafy vegetables, cruciferous vegetables, gourd/melon family vegetables, red or orange vegetables, potatoes, root vegetables, bean vegetables, bean products, mushrooms, fruits, and low intake of lean pork meat. It accounted for 9.0% of the total variance. The second pattern, called the 'meat-based pattern,' was represented by high intakes of pork, pig blood curd, ox tripe, organ meat, processed meat, squid and mushrooms. It explained 7.1% of the total variance. The third pattern was typified by high intakes of foods rich in protein, including eggs, milk, fish and lean pork meat, and low intakes of noodles and bread. We named it the 'high protein-low starch pattern,' which explained 5.0% of the total variance.

Table 3 describes participants' characteristics and their dietary intakes according to tertiles of dietary pattern scores. For the plant-based pattern, women with a higher score were older, more highly educated and physically active than those with a lower score. They had higher intakes of total energy and lower intake of total fat. Also, they consumed more vegetables, fruit, nuts/seeds, fish, eggs, protein and carbohydrate, but less red meat. Regarding the meat-based pattern, women with a higher score were older and had more children than those with a lower score. They had higher intakes of total energy, vegetables, red meat, protein and total fat, but had lower intakes of fruit, nuts/seeds, milk, eggs, grains and carbohydrate. For the high protein-low starch pattern, women with a higher score were more educated and had a

Table 1 Baseline characteristics of participants by prospective development of GDM [a]

Characteristics	Overall (n = 1337)	GDM (n = 199)	Non-GDM (n = 1138)	p^b
Age (year)	25.8 ± 4.1	26.8 ± 4.2	25.7 ± 4.0	< 0.001
By category				0.002
< 25	527 (39.4)	63 (31.7)	464 (40.8)	
25–29	589 (44.1)	86 (43.2)	503 (44.2)	
30–34	184 (13.8)	40 (20.1)	144 (12.7)	
≥ 35	37 (2.8)	10 (5.0)	27 (2.4)	
Pre-pregnancy BMI (kg/m^2)	20.7 ± 2.8	21.8 ± 3.2	20.5 ± 2.7	< 0.001
By category				< 0.001
< 18.5	304 (22.7)	28 (14.1)	276 (24.3)	
18.5–23.9	865 (64.7)	130 (65.3)	735 (64.6)	
≥ 24	168 (12.6)	41 (20.6)	127 (11.2)	
Family history of diabetes				0.006
Yes	72 (6.2)	19 (11.2)	53 (5.4)	
No	1013 (87.5)	136 (80.5)	877 (88.7)	
Don't know	73 (6.3)	14 (8.3)	59 (6.0)	
Education				0.513
Junior secondary school or below	321 (24.0)	51 (25.6)	270 (23.7)	
Senior/technical secondary school	524 (39.2)	82 (41.2)	442 (38.8)	
University or above	492 (36.8)	66 (33.2)	426 (37.4)	
Parity				0.747
0	932 (69.8)	137 (68.8)	795 (70.0)	
≥ 1	403 (30.2)	62 (31.2)	341 (30.0)	
Active smoking before pregnancy				0.289
Yes	73 (5.5)	14 (7.0)	59 (5.2)	
No	1264 (94.5)	185 (93.0)	1079 (94.8)	
Total physical activity (MET-hour/week)	149.7 ± 84.2	145.4 ± 82.6	150.5 ± 84.5	0.439

BMI body mass index, *GDM* gestational diabetes mellitus, *MET* Metabolic equivalent task
[a]Numbers are presented as n (%) or mean ± SD
[b]Based on t-tests or χ^2 tests

lower pregravid BMI when compared to women with a lower score. Those with a higher versus lower score had higher total energy intake and higher consumption of fruit, nuts/seeds, red meat, lean pork, fish, milk, eggs, protein and total fat, while their intake of vegetables, grains, and carbohydrate was lower.

Dietary patterns and risk of gestational diabetes

There was no significant association between any dietary pattern and the risk of GDM. Compared with the lowest tertile of dietary pattern scores, multivariable-adjusted ORs for the corresponding highest tertile for the plant-based, meat-based and high protein-low starch patterns were 0.97 (95% CI 0.64 to 1.47, $p > 0.05$), 0.89 (95% CI 0.58 to 1.36, $p > 0.05$) and 0.73 (95% CI 0.48 to 1.10, $p > 0.05$), respectively (Appendix 2).

In subgroup analyses, a significant reduction in GDM risk was observed among overweight women, when comparing the highest tertile of high protein-low starch pattern scores to the lowest tertile (OR 0.29; 95% CI 0.09 to 0.94; p for trend = 0.049, Figure 1), despite the lack of significance for the interaction between pre-pregnancy BMI and high protein-low starch pattern score (p for interaction = 0.134). There was no effect modification by pregravid BMI on the association between the plant-based pattern and meat-based pattern and GDM risk. Neither age nor family history of diabetes modified the risk of GDM in relation to the identified dietary patterns (data not shown for brevity).

Discussion

In the present prospective cohort study of 1337 pregnant women in Western China, three dietary patterns called the plant-based pattern, meat-based pattern and high protein-low starch pattern were identified. Despite the lack of association between the three dietary patterns and the risk of GDM in the whole cohort, we observed a significant inverse association between the high protein-low starch pattern and risk of GDM only among overweight women. Our finding suggested that increasing the intake of high protein-low starch foods during early pregnancy may be beneficial towards the prevention of GDM for overweight or obese women at pre-pregnancy.

Unlike prior research [11], the present study found no significant association between the identified dietary patterns and the risk of GDM in all participants. One possible reason may be due to the different dietary patterns derived in different studies. Dietary pattern analysis is a holistic approach to determining the role of combinations of foods and nutrients consumed in cardiometabolic health including GDM [39]. However, results remain inconsistent due to the heterogeneity of diet composition across the world regions [23]. Similarly, within-country differences in dietary patterns exist. In China, for example, Southern Chinese eat rice as the staple food, unlike their northern counterparts who eat bread and buns regularly [40], which may contribute to the inconsistency regarding the association between dietary patterns and GDM risk in Chinese mothers [25, 41].

An alternative explanation is our study participants had fewer risk factor clusters in addition to GDM than those in previous studies. According to a population-based study

Table 2 Rotated factor loadings of the three major dietary patterns [a]

Food groups	Plant-based pattern	Meat-based pattern	High protein-low starch pattern
Green leafy vegetables	**0.65**	0.26	0.06
Root vegetables	**0.56**	0.15	0.04
Gourd/melon family vegetables	**0.55**	−0.05	− 0.07
Red/orange vegetables	**0.51**	−0.15	− 0.01
Cruciferous vegetables	**0.48**	0.11	0.08
Bean vegetables	**0.41**	0.00	−0.20
Potatoes	**0.40**	−0.02	−0.21
Mushrooms	**0.39**	**0.39**	0.11
Bean products	**0.35**	−0.01	−0.06
Fruits	**0.31**	−0.12	0.18
Organ meat	0.13	**0.67**	−0.01
Ox tripe	−0.05	**0.59**	−0.06
Pig blood curd	0.10	**0.50**	0.00
Squid	0.03	**0.45**	−0.04
Pork	0.16	**0.39**	0.24
Processed meat	0.01	**0.37**	−0.19
Eggs	0.02	−0.12	**0.48**
Milk	0.03	−0.24	**0.40**
Lean pork meat	**−0.34**	0.10	**0.40**
Fish	0.27	0.22	**0.40**
Noodles	−0.01	0.04	**−0.44**
Bread	0.11	−0.01	**−0.43**
Sea vegetables	0.26	0.27	0.11
Pickled vegetables	0.11	0.07	−0.13
Nuts and seeds	0.28	−0.12	0.28
Beef	0.23	0.27	0.03
Poultry	0.26	0.26	0.26
Processed eggs	−0.09	0.23	0.15
Rice	−0.28	−0.18	− 0.24
Maize	0.21	−0.08	−0.07
Alcohol	−0.03	0.04	−0.10
Coffee/Tea	−0.02	0.01	−0.05
Variance explained (%)	9.04	7.10	5.01

[a]Factor loadings ≥ ± 0.30 are bolded

of 98,271 adults in Western China [42], the prevalence of overweight or obese (BMI ≥24 kg/m^2) was much higher than our cohort (28.0% versus 12.6%). Moreover, our participants were younger (mean age 25.8 years) than those (28.9 and 28.0 years) of two previous studies in China [25, 41]. The effect of dietary patterns, if any, on the risk of GDM may not be discernible among women with an apparently low risk profile of developing GDM in the present study.

An inverse association was found between the consumption of high protein-low starch foods and the risk of GDM among overweight Chinese women. This dietary pattern was characterized by a high intake of eggs, milk, fish and lean pork, as well as a low intake of starchy carbohydrates. The apparent reduction in GDM risk may be partly due to the antidiabetic effects of milk [43] and fish [44]. Overweight/obesity is associated with insulin resistance [45], impaired insulin section [46] and elevated inflammation levels [47]. A major protein in milk, whey proteins [48, 49], has been demonstrated to increase insulin sensitivity [50], regulate blood glucose levels and decrease low-grade inflammation, oxidative stress as well as body weight [51]. In

Table 3 Baseline characteristics and dietary intakes of participants by tertiles of dietary pattern scores[a]

Variable	Plant-based pattern			Meat-based pattern			High protein-low starch pattern		
	Tertile 1	Tertile 3	p [b]	Tertile 1	Tertile 3	p [b]	Tertile 1	Tertile 3	p [b]
Age (year), mean ± SD	25.5 ± 3.9	26.1 ± 4.1	0.053	25.4 ± 4.0	26.1 ± 4.2	0.034	25.8 ± 4.1	25.9 ± 4.3	0.830
Pre-pregnancy BMI (kg/m^2)			0.701			0.518			0.047
< 18.5	109 (24.4)	97 (21.8)		104 (23.3)	95 (21.4)		96 (21.5)	97 (21.8)	
18.5–23.9	278 (62.3)	290 (65.2)		279 (62.6)	301 (67.6)		284 (63.7)	307 (69.0)	
≥ 24	59 (13.2)	58 (13.0)		63 (14.1)	49 (11.0)		66 (14.8)	41 (9.2)	
Family history of diabetes	24 (6.1)	28 (7.4)	0.677	24 (6.4)	18 (4.7)	0.360	23 (5.9)	27 (7.1)	0.454
Education			0.011			0.184			0.024
Junior secondary school or below	132 (29.6)	93 (20.9)		105 (23.5)	117 (26.3)		121 (27.1)	103 (23.2)	
Senior/technical secondary school	163 (36.6)	173 (38.9)		189 (42.4)	156 (35.1)		186 (41.7)	175 (39.3)	
University or above	151 (33.9)	179 (40.2)		152 (34.1)	172 (38.7)		139 (31.2)	167 (37.5)	
Parity			0.293			< 0.001			0.037
0	299 (67.0)	316 (71.0)		338 (75.8)	285 (64.0)		292 (65.5)	325 (73.2)	
≥ 1	147 (33.0)	129 (29.0)		108 (24.2)	160 (36.0)		154 (34.5)	119 (26.8)	
Active smoking before pregnancy									
Yes	26 (5.8)	18 (4.0)	0.249	23 (5.2)	30 (6.7)	0.314	29 (6.5)	25 (5.6)	0.332
No	420 (94.2)	427 (96.0)		423 (94.8)	415 (93.3)		417 (93.5)	420 (94.4)	
Total physical activity (MET-hour/week)	141.1 ± 81.1	157.7 ± 87.7	0.013	144.3 ± 83.9	156.7 ± 85.2	0.082	146.2 ± 80.3	149.9 ± 86.1	0.468
Total energy consumption (kcal/day)	1757.2 ± 775.7	2026.3 ± 855.5	< 0.001	1709.0 ± 569.8	2045.1 ± 956.7	< 0.001	1736.7 ± 770.0	2017.1 ± 814.7	< 0.001
Energy-adjusted food intake (g/1000 kcal/day)									
Vegetables[c]	85.9 ± 34.1	256.1 ± 104.7	< 0.001	165.6 ± 110.4	171.7 ± 99.8	< 0.001	164.3 ± 96.7	160.9 ± 98.9	0.787
Fruits	65.4 ± 61.0	131.5 ± 97.6	< 0.001	120.3 ± 102.8	81.9 ± 66.9	< 0.001	80.6 ± 69.8	115.4 ± 101.0	< 0.001
Nuts and seeds	7.6 ± 7.4	15.1 ± 13.3	< 0.001	14.0 ± 13.6	10.2 ± 9.2	< 0.001	8.2 ± 7.7	15.4 ± 13.8	< 0.001
Red meat[d]	51.2 ± 31.2	37.1 ± 24.2	< 0.001	28.3 ± 22.0	56.1 ± 28.4	< 0.001	31.4 ± 23.0	52.6 ± 30.5	< 0.001
Lean pork meat	34.5 ± 26.6	23.4 ± 18.5	< 0.001	24.5 ± 22.2	33.2 ± 25.1	< 0.001	19.9 ± 18.2	38.1 ± 26.3	< 0.001
Fish	10.3 ± 9.9	19.3 ± 20.2	< 0.001	11.0 ± 15.1	19.4 ± 20.0	< 0.001	9.1 ± 8.7	21.2 ± 23.5	< 0.001
Milk	89.2 ± 85.9	96.1 ± 77.4	0.002	127.8 ± 101.2	76.0 ± 66.4	< 0.001	60.7 ± 60.2	136.0 ± 98.7	< 0.001
Eggs	18.4 ± 18.8	19.9 ± 13.9	0.015	23.7 ± 19.8	18.1 ± 16.5	< 0.001	11.5 ± 11.5	29.1 ± 20.7	< 0.001
Grains[e]	203.3 ± 70.5	173.1 ± 54.7	< 0.001	199.6 ± 61.9	171.1 ± 61.2	< 0.001	224.3 ± 61.1	147.1 ± 46.9	< 0.001
Nutrient intake (% energy)									
Protein	13.4 ± 2.8	14.6 ± 2.4	< 0.001	13.3 ± 2.5	14.9 ± 2.7	< 0.001	12.3 ± 2.2	15.7 ± 2.4	< 0.001
Total fat	50.4 ± 7.6	43.8 ± 6.8	< 0.001	45.7 ± 7.5	48.4 ± 8.5	< 0.001	42.5 ± 7.4	51.3 ± 6.8	< 0.001
Carbohydrate	37.1 ± 8.8	43.6 ± 7.3	< 0.001	42.6 ± 8.2	38.0 ± 9.0	< 0.001	46.7 ± 7.3	34.3 ± 7.2	< 0.001

BMI body mass index, *MET* Metabolic equivalent task

[a]Numbers are presented as n (%) or mean ± SD. Tertile 2 are not presented for brevity

[b]Based on ANOVA or χ^2 tests

[c]Included green leafy vegetables, cruciferous vegetables, gourd/melon family vegetables, red/orange vegetables, root vegetables, bean vegetables and mushrooms

[d]Included pork, beef, ox tripe, pig blood curd, processed meat and organ meat

[e]Included rice, noodles, bread and maize

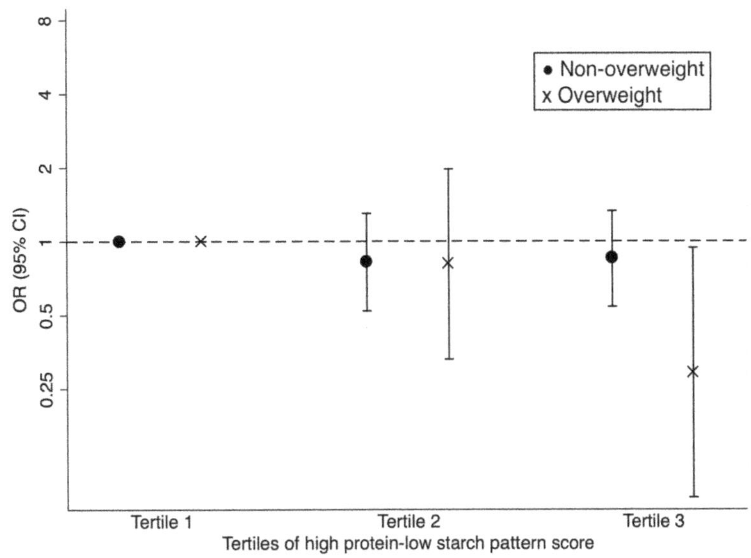

Fig. 1 Association between the high protein-low starch pattern and gestational diabetes according to pre-pregnancy body mass index levels. The model is adjusted for age, family history of diabetes, education, parity and total physical activity. Circle (•) represents women with BMI < 24 kg/m^2; cross (x) denotes women with BMI ≥24 kg/m^2

addition, fatty acids in fish possess anti-inflammatory properties [52], while egg-derived phospholipids [53] can elevate high-density lipoproteins [54], which have been suggested to control glucose homeostasis [55]. Besides the potent anti-oxidative and anti-inflammatory properties of egg lutein and zeaxanthin [56], egg whites may have insulin-sensitizing effects [57]. Another possibility is that adherence to the high protein-low starch pattern can lead to greater weight loss in overweight individuals [58], while a high body weight is an established risk factor for GDM. Finally, a lower intake of starchy carbohydrates (e.g., noodles and bread) may reduce the risk of GDM through improved insulin resistance and insulin sensitivity as well as regulation of blood glucose levels [59, 60].

A major strength of this study is our cohort design, in which information on dietary intake was obtained during early pregnancy before the diagnosis of GDM. This allows assessment of the temporal relationship between dietary patterns and risk of developing GDM. In addition, dietary data were collected via direct interviews using a validated and reliable FFQ, and GDM was determined through OGTT to minimize potential exposure measurement errors and misclassification of the outcome, respectively. The analysis of dietary patterns, instead of separate food items or nutrients, enables the description of overall diet of pregnant women by accounting for interactions between food groups and/or nutrients. Indeed, a dietary pattern is amenable to interpretation by the general public and provides a base for development of dietary guidelines [61].

Several limitations should be considered. Firstly, the use of exploratory factor analysis with the principal component method requires some arbitrary decisions to include variables, the number of retained factors, the method of rotation and labelling of the factors [33]. This approach may limit the generalizability of our results. Secondly, habitual dietary intakes may not be fully captured by the FFQ which is limited by its pre-coded food items [62]. The level of accuracy in individual portion size estimation is another issue because Chinese adults normally eat communally and share their dishes with others [40]. Thirdly, dietary intake was assessed at a single time point, even though the habitual diet of pregnant women may change over time [63]. Finally, despite the adjustment for plausible factors associated with diet and GDM in the logistic regression models, residual confounding cannot be ruled out.

Conclusion

This is the first study in Western China to investigate the prospective association between dietary patterns during early pregnancy and the risk of GDM. Three major dietary patterns were identified among Western Chinese women: plant-based, meat-based and high protein-low starch pattern. Overall, our study indicated a lack of association between dietary patterns and the GDM risk. However, there was a significant inverse association between the high protein-low starch pattern characterized by high intake of milk, eggs, fish and lean meat and low intake of starch, and the incidence of GDM for Chinese women who were overweight at pre-pregnancy. Further research is needed to elucidate the role of diet in the prevention of GDM in China.

Appendix 1

Table 4 Food groups used in dietary pattern analysis

#	Food group	Food items
1	Green leafy vegetables	Lettuce leaves, lettuce head, Chinese mallow, Swiss chard, young garlic shoot, celery, pak choi, *Houttuynia cordata*, flower Chinese cabbage, pea seedlings, spinach, garlic bolt, water spinach, bamboo shoots, green Chinese onion, Chinese toon, Chinese chives, caraway
2	Cruciferous vegetables	Cabbage, cauliflower
3	Gourd/melon family vegetables	Cucumber, eggplant, bitter gourd, green chilies, towel gourd
4	Red/orange vegetables	Carrot, pumpkin, tomato
5	Potatoes	Potato
6	Root vegetables	Lotus root, sweet potato, white radish, garlic
7	Bean vegetables	Broad bean, soybean, soybean sprouts, green bean, mung bean sprouts, string bean, pea
8	Bean products	Tofu, dried tofu, soybean milk, bean curd jelly, Chinese vermicelli, Chinese jelly noodles
9	Mushrooms	Mushroom, black fungus, oyster mushroom, needle mushroom, white fungus
10	Sea vegetables	Seaweed, sea lettuce
11	Pickled vegetables	Pickled Chinese cabbage, pickled garlic, pickled radish, preserved Szechuan pickle
12	Fruits	Apple, orange, banana, pear
13	Nuts and seeds	Peanut, walnut, sesame, sunflower seed
14	Pork	Pork, pork ribs, pork fat, trotters
15	Pig blood curd	Pig blood curd
16	Lean pork meat	Lean pork
17	Beef	Beef
18	Ox tripe	Ox tripe
19	Organ meat	Pork liver, pig kidney, pork intestine, duck gizzard, duck intestine
20	Poultry	Chicken, duck, goose
21	Processed meat	Sausage, preserved meat
22	Fish	Silver carp, crucian, grass carp, eel, hair tail
23	Squid	Squid
24	Milk	Milk
25	Eggs	Egg, duck egg
26	Processed eggs	Preserved egg, salted duck egg
27	Rice	Polished round-grained rice, glutinous rice, rice noodles
28	Noodles	Noodles, instant noodles
29	Bread	Bread, steamed bun, steamed twisted roll, flour
30	Maize	Corn, maize flour
31	Alcohol	Beer, Chinese liquor
32	Coffee/Tea	Coffee, tea

Appendix 2

Table 5 Odds ratios (95% confidence interval) for gestational diabetes mellitus (GDM) according to dietary pattern scores

Dietary patterns	Tertile 1	Tertile 2	Tertile 3	*p*-trend
Plant-based pattern				
GDM cases /pregnancies	63/446	64/446	72/445	
Model 1[a]	1.00	1.02 (0.70, 1.48)	1.17 (0.81, 1.69)	0.367
Model 2[b]	1.00	0.95 (0.63, 1.43)	0.97 (0.65, 1.46)	0.919
Model 3[c]	1.00	0.94 (0.62, 1.42)	0.97 (0.64, 1.47)	0.915
Meat-based pattern				
GDM case/pregnancies	65/446	73/446	61/445	
Model 1[a]	1.00	1.15 (0.80, 1.65)	0.93 (0.64, 1.36)	0.628
Model 2[b]	1.00	1.05 (0.70, 1.57)	0.82 (0.54, 1.25)	0.318
Model 3[c]	1.00	1.08 (0.72, 1.62)	0.89 (0.58, 1.36)	0.534
High protein-low starch pattern				
GDM case/pregnancies	77/446	60/446	62/445	
Model 1[a]	1.00	0.74 (0.52, 1.07)	0.78 (0.54, 1.12)	0.148
Model 2[b]	1.00	0.83 (0.56, 1.23)	0.73 (0.49, 1.11)	0.137
Model 3[c]	1.00	0.84 (0.56, 1.26)	0.73 (0.48, 1.10)	0.132

[a]Crude model
[b]Adjusted for age, pre-pregnancy body mass index and family history of diabetes
[c]Additionally adjusted for parity, education and total physical activity

Abbreviations

ANOVA: Analysis of variance; BMI: Body mass index; CI: Confidence interval; FFQ: Food frequency questionnaire; GDM: Gestational diabetes mellitus; IADPSG: International Association of Diabetes and Pregnancy Study Groups; MET: Metabolic equivalent task; OGTT: Oral glucose tolerance test; OR: Odds ratio; SD: Standard deviation

Acknowledgements

The authors would like to thank all the participants, health professionals and researchers who contributed to this cohort study.

Funding

This study was supported by the China Medical Board (Grant No. 14–199).

Authors' contributions

AHL, CWB and XS designed the research protocol; LT and XFP conducted the study; JKLM and NMP analyzed the data; JKLM drafted the manuscript; AHL, NMP and CWB critically revised the manuscript, and XS was responsible for the final contents. All authors read and approved the final manuscript.

Competing interests

The authors declare that they have no competing interests.

Author details

[1]School of Public Health, Curtin University, Perth, WA, Australia. [2]Thai Nguyen University of Medicine and Pharmacy, Thai Nguyen, Vietnam. [3]Chinese Evidence-based Medicine Center, West China Hospital, Sichuan University, Chengdu 610041, China. [4]Department of Epidemiology and Biostatistics, School of Public Health, Tongji Medical College, Huazhong University of Science and Technology, Wuhan, China.

References

1. American Diabetes Association. Gestational diabetes mellitus. Diabetes Care. 2004;27(Suppl 1):S88–90.
2. Jiwani A, Marseille E, Lohse N, Damm P, Hod M, Kahn JG. Gestational diabetes mellitus: results from a survey of country prevalence and practices. J Matern Neonatal Med. 2012;25:600–10.
3. Zhu Y, Zhang C. Prevalence of gestational diabetes and risk of progression to type 2 diabetes: a global perspective. Curr Diab Rep. 2016;16:7.
4. Nguyen CL, Pham NM, Binns CW, Duong DV, Lee AH. Prevalence of gestational diabetes mellitus in eastern and southeastern Asia: a systematic review and meta-analysis. J Diabetes Res. 2018;2018:1–10.
5. Gao C, Sun X, Lu L, Liu F, Yuan J. Prevalence of gestational diabetes mellitus in mainland China: a systematic review and meta-analysis. J Diabetes Investig. 2018. https://doi.org/10.1111/jdi.12854.
6. Wendland EM, Torloni MR, Falavigna M, Trujillo J, Dode MA, Campos MA, et al. Gestational diabetes and pregnancy outcomes - a systematic review of the World Health Organization (WHO) and the International Association of Diabetes in Pregnancy Study Groups (IADPSG) diagnostic criteria. BMC Pregnancy Childbirth. 2012;12:23.
7. Billionnet C, Mitanchez D, Weill A, Nizard J, Alla F, Hartemann A, et al. Gestational diabetes and adverse perinatal outcomes from 716,152 births in France in 2012. Diabetologia. 2017;60:636–44.
8. Damm P, Houshmand-Oeregaard A, Kelstrup L, Lauenborg J, Mathiesen ER, Clausen TD. Gestational diabetes mellitus and long-term consequences for mother and offspring: a view from Denmark. Diabetologia. 2016;59:1396–9.

9. Zhang C, Ning Y. Effect of dietary and lifestyle factors on the risk of gestational diabetes: review of epidemiologic evidence. Am J Clin Nutr. 2011;94:1975S–9S.
10. Schoenaker DAJM, Mishra GD, Callaway LK, Soedamah-Muthu SS. The role of energy, nutrients, foods, and dietary patterns in the development of gestational diabetes mellitus: a systematic review of observational studies. Diabetes Care. 2016;39:16–23.
11. Zhang C, Schulze MB, Solomon CG, Hu FB. A prospective study of dietary patterns, meat intake and the risk of gestational diabetes mellitus. Diabetologia. 2006;49:2604–13.
12. Qiu C, Frederick IO, Zhang C, Sorensen TK, Enquobahrie DA, Williams MA. Risk of gestational diabetes mellitus in relation to maternal egg and cholesterol intake. Am J Epidemiol. 2011;173:649–58.
13. Bowers K, Yeung E, Williams MA, Qi L, Tobias DK, Hu FB, et al. A prospective study of prepregnancy dietary iron intake and risk for gestational diabetes mellitus. Diabetes Care. 2011;34:1557–63.
14. Bao W, Bowers K, Tobias DK, Hu FB, Zhang C. Prepregnancy dietary protein intake, major dietary protein sources, and the risk of gestational diabetes mellitus: a prospective cohort study. Diabetes Care. 2013;36:2001–8.
15. Bao W, Bowers K, Tobias DK, Olsen SF, Chavarro J, Vaag A, et al. Prepregnancy low-carbohydrate dietary pattern and risk of gestational diabetes mellitus: a prospective cohort study. Am J Clin Nutr. 2014;99:1378–84.
16. Bo S, Menato G, Lezo A, Signorile A, Bardelli C, DeMichieli F, et al. Dietary fat and gestational hyperglycaemia. Diabetologia. 2001;44:972–8.
17. Bowers K, Tobias DK, Yeung E, Hu FB, Zhang C. A prospective study of prepregnancy dietary fat intake and risk of gestational diabetes. Am J Clin Nutr. 2012;95:446–53.
18. Zhang C, Liu S, Solomon CG, Hu FB. Dietary fiber intake, dietary glycemic load, and the risk for gestational diabetes mellitus. Diabetes Care. 2006;29:2223–30.
19. Pham NM, Do V. Van, lee AH. Polyphenol-rich foods and risk of gestational diabetes: a systematic review and meta-analysis. Eur J Clin Nutr. https://doi.org/10.1038/s41430-018-0218-7.
20. Shin D, Lee K, Song W. Dietary patterns during pregnancy are associated with risk of gestational diabetes mellitus. Nutrients. 2015;7:9369–82.
21. Schoenaker DAJM, Soedamah-Muthu SS, Callaway LK, Mishra GD. Pre-pregnancy dietary patterns and risk of gestational diabetes mellitus: results from an Australian population-based prospective cohort study. Diabetologia. 2015;58:2726–35.
22. Donazar-Ezcurra M, Lopez-Del Burgo C, Martinez-Gonzalez MA, Basterra-Gortari FJ, de Irala J, Bes-Rastrollo M. Pre-pregnancy adherences to empirically derived dietary patterns and gestational diabetes risk in a Mediterranean cohort: the Seguimiento Universidad de Navarra (SUN) project. Br J Nutr. 2017;118:715–21.
23. Imamura F, Micha R, Khatibzadeh S, Fahimi S, Shi P, Powles J, et al. Dietary quality among men and women in 187 countries in 1990 and 2010: a systematic assessment. Lancet Glob Health. 2015;3:e132–42.
24. Kelly M. The nutrition transition in developing asia: dietary change, drivers and health impacts. In: Jackson P, Spiess WEL, Sultana F, editors. Eating, Drinking: Surviving. Cham: Springer; 2016. p. 83–90.
25. He J-R, Yuan M-Y, Chen N-N, Lu J-H, Hu C-Y, Mai W-B, et al. Maternal dietary patterns and gestational diabetes mellitus: a large prospective cohort study in China. Br J Nutr. 2015;113:1292–300.
26. de Seymour J, Chia A, Colega M, Jones B, McKenzie E, Shirong C, et al. Maternal dietary patterns and gestational diabetes mellitus in a multi-ethnic asian cohort: the GUSTO study. Nutrients. 2016;8:574.
27. Ogonowski J, Miazgowski T, Kuczynska M, Krzyzanowska-Swiniarska B, Celewicz Z. Pregravid body mass index as a predictor of gestational diabetes mellitus. Diabet Med. 2009;26:334–8.
28. Tryggvadottir EA, Medek H, Birgisdottir BE, Geirsson RT, Gunnarsdottir I. Association between healthy maternal dietary pattern and risk for gestational diabetes mellitus. Eur J Clin Nutr. 2016;70:237–42.
29. Tang L, Pan X-F, Lee AH, Binns CW, Yang C-X, Sun X. Maternal lifestyle and nutritional status in relation to pregnancy and infant health outcomes in Western China: protocol for a prospective cohort study. BMJ Open. 2017;7:e014874.
30. Zhou Z-Y, Takezaki T, Mo B-Q, Sun H-M, Wang W-C, Sun L-P, et al. Development of a semi-quantitative food frequency questionnaire to determine variation in nutrient intakes between urban and rural areas of Chongqing, China. Asia Pac J Clin Nutr. 2004;13:273–83.
31. Tang Y, Liu Y, Xu L, Jia Y, Shan D, Li W, et al. Validity and reproducibility of a revised semi-quantitative food frequency questionnaire (SQFFQ) for women of age-group 12-44 years in Chengdu. J Health Popul Nutr. 2015;33:50–9.
32. Willett WC, Howe GR, Kushi LH. Adjustment for total energy intake in epidemiologic studies. Am J Clin Nutr. 1997;65:1220S–8S discussion 1229S–1231S.
33. Rencher AC, Christensen WF. Exploratory factor analysis. In: Methods of multivariate analysis. Hoboken: John Wiley & Sons, Inc.; 2012. p. 435–77.
34. Cattell RB. The scree test for the number of factors. Multivariate Behav Res. 1966;1:245–76.
35. Metzger BE, Gabbe SG, Persson B, Buchanan TA, Catalano PA, Damm P, et al. International association of diabetes and pregnancy study groups recommendations on the diagnosis and classification of hyperglycemia in pregnancy. Diabetes Care. 2010;33:676–82.
36. Xiang M, Konishi M, Hu H, Takahashi M, Fan W, Nishimaki M, et al. Reliability and validity of a Chinese-translated version of a pregnancy physical activity questionnaire. Matern Child Health J. 2016;20:1940–7.
37. Ainsworth BE, Haskell WL, Herrmann SD, Meckes N, Bassett DR Jr, Tudor-Locke C, et al. 2011 compendium of physical activities: a second update of codes and MET values. Med Sci Sport Exerc. 2011;43:1575–81.
38. Zhou B-F, Cooperative Meta-Analysis Group of the Working Group on Obesity in China. Predictive values of body mass index and waist circumference for risk factors of certain related diseases in Chinese adults–study on optimal cut-off points of body mass index and waist circumference in Chinese adults. Biomed Environ Sci. 2002;15:83–96.
39. Hu FB. Dietary pattern analysis: a new direction in nutritional epidemiology. Curr Opin Lipidol. 2002;13:3–9.
40. Ma G. Food, eating behavior, and culture in Chinese society. J Ethn Foods. 2015;2:195–9.
41. Du HY, Jiang H, O K, Chen B, Xu LJ, Liu SP, et al. Association of dietary pattern during pregnancy and gestational diabetes mellitus: a prospective cohort study in Northern China. Biomed Environ Sci 2017;30:887–897.
42. Li X, Jiang Y, Hu N, Li Y, Zhang M, Huang Z, et al. Prevalence and characteristic of overweight and obesity among adults in China, 2010. Chinese J Prev Med. 2012;46:683–6.
43. Gijsbers L, Ding EL, Malik VS, de Goede J, Geleijnse JM, Soedamah-Muthu SS. Consumption of dairy foods and diabetes incidence: a dose-response meta-analysis of observational studies. Am J Clin Nutr. 2016;103:1111–24.
44. Villegas R, Xiang YB, Elasy T, Li HL, Yang G, Cai H, et al. Fish, shellfish, and long-chain n-3 fatty acid consumption and risk of incident type 2 diabetes in middle-aged Chinese men and women. Am J Clin Nutr. 2011;94:543–51.
45. Kahn BB, Flier JS. Obesity and insulin resistance. J Clin Invest. 2000;106:473–81.
46. Polonsky KS, Given BD, Hirsch L, Shapiro ET, Tillil H, Beebe C, et al. Quantitative study of insulin secretion and clearance in normal and obese subjects. J Clin Invest. 1988;81:435–41.
47. Balistreri CR, Caruso C, Candore G. The role of adipose tissue and adipokines in obesity-related inflammatory diseases. Mediat Inflamm. 2010;2010:802078.
48. Walstra P, Jenness R. Dairy chemistry and physics. New York: John Wiley & Sons; 1984.
49. Fox PF. Milk proteins: general and historical aspects. In: Fox PF, McSweeney PLH, editors. Advanced dairy chemistry, volume 1: proteins. New York: Kluwer Academic/Plenum Publishers; 2003. p. 1–48.
50. Belobrajdic DP, McIntosh GH, Owens JA. A high-whey-protein diet reduces body weight gain and alters insulin sensitivity relative to red meat in wistar rats. J Nutr. 2004;134:1454–8.
51. Sousa GT, Lira FS, Rosa JC, de Oliveira EP, Oyama LM, Santos RV, et al. Dietary whey protein lessens several risk factors for metabolic diseases: a review. Lipids Heal Dis. 2012;11:67.
52. Wall R, Ross RP, Fitzgerald GF, Stanton C. Fatty acids from fish: the anti-inflammatory potential of long-chain omega-3 fatty acids. Nutr Rev. 2010;68:280–9.
53. Sunwoo HH, Gujral N. Chemical composition of eggs and egg products. In: Cheung PCK, Mehta BM, editors. Handbook of food chemistry. Heidelberg: Springer; 2015. p. 331–63.
54. Blesso CN. Egg phospholipids and cardiovascular health. Nutrients. 2015;7:2731–47.
55. Drew BG, Rye KA, Duffy SJ, Barter P, Kingwell BA. The emerging role of HDL in glucose metabolism. Nat Rev Endocrinol. 2012;8:237–45.
56. Ciccone MM, Cortese F, Gesualdo M, Carbonara S, Zito A, Ricci G, et al. Dietary intake of carotenoids and their antioxidant and anti-inflammatory effects in cardiovascular care. Mediat Inflamm. 2013;2013:782137.
57. Jahandideh F, Chakrabarti S, Davidge ST, Wu J. Egg white hydrolysate shows insulin mimetic and sensitizing effects in 3T3-F442A pre-adipocytes. PLoS One. 2017;12:e0185653.
58. Foster GD, Wyatt HR, Hill JO, McGuckin BG, Brill C, Mohammed BS, et al. A randomized trial of a low-carbohydrate diet for obesity. N Engl J Med. 2003;

348:2082–90.

59. de Luis DA, Izaola O, Aller R, de la Fuente B, Bachiller R, Romero E. Effects of a high-protein/low carbohydrate versus a standard hypocaloric diet on adipocytokine levels and insulin resistance in obese patients along 9 months. J Diabetes Complicat. 2015;29:950–4.
60. Zuniga YL, Rebello SA, Oi PL, Zheng H, Lee J, Tai ES, et al. Rice and noodle consumption is associated with insulin resistance and hyperglycaemia in an Asian population. Br J Nutr. 2014;111:1118–28.
61. Tapsell LC, Neale EP, Satija A, Hu FB. Foods, nutrients, and dietary patterns: interconnections and implications for dietary guidelines. Adv Nutr. 2016;7:445–54.
62. Sempos CT. Some limitations of semiquantitative food frequency questionnaires. Am J Epidemiol. 1992;135:1127–32.
63. Chen LW, Low YL, Fok D, Han WM, Chong YS, Gluckman P, et al. Dietary changes during pregnancy and the postpartum period in Singaporean Chinese, Malay and Indian women: the GUSTO birth cohort study. Public Health Nutr. 2014;17:1930–8.

13

Comparison of the NHANES dietary screener questionnaire to the Automated Self-Administered 24-Hour Recall for Children in the Healthy Communities Study

Sridharshi Chintha Hewawitharana[1*], Frances Elizabeth Thompson[2], Catherine M. Loria[3], Warren Strauss[4], Jyothi Nagaraja[4], Lorrene Ritchie[1] and Karen Lucy Webb[1]

Abstract

Background: A dietary screener questionnaire (DSQ) was used to assess dietary outcomes among children in the Healthy Communities Study (HCS), a study of the relationships between programs and policies to prevent child obesity and child diet, physical activity and weight outcomes.

Methods: To compare dietary intake estimates derived from the DSQ against those from the Automated Self-Administered 24-Hour Recalls for Children (ASA24-Kids) among children, a measurement error model, using structural equation modelling, was utilized to estimate slopes, deattenuated correlation coefficients, and attenuation factors by age and sex, ethnicity, and BMI status.

Participants/setting: A randomly selected sub-sample of HCS participants aged 4–15 years in 130 communities throughout the U.S. who completed the DSQ and up to two ASA24-Kids recalls ($n = 656$;13% of HCS participants).

Results: For most nutrient/foods examined, the DSQ yielded larger mean intake estimates than the ASA24-Kids, and agreement between the two measures varied by food/nutrient, age and sex, ethnicity, and BMI category. Deattenuated correlation coefficients of 0.4 or greater were observed for added sugars from SSBs (0.54), fruits and vegetables (0.40), and dairy foods (0.50). Lower deattenuated correlation coefficients were seen for total added sugars (0.37), whole grains (0.34), and fiber (0.34). Attenuation factors were most severe for total added sugars intake among overweight children, and for several other dietary outcomes among children aged 9–11 years.

Conclusions: The DSQ was found to be a tool with acceptable agreement with the ASA24-Kids for measuring multiple dietary outcomes of interest in the HCS, although there may be potential due to measurement error to underestimate results (bias towards the null). In future studies, measurement error modelling and regression calibration may be possible solutions to correct for bias due to measurement error in most food/nutrient intake estimates from the DSQ when used among children.

Keywords: ASA24-kids, FFQ, Dietary screener, DSQ, Concurrent validity

* Correspondence: shewawitharana@ucanr.edu
[1]Nutrition Policy Institute, University of California, Agriculture and Natural Resources Division, 2115 Milvia Street, Third floor, Berkeley, CA 94704, USA

Background

Assessing dietary intakes can be done in multiple ways, but each method has advantages and disadvantages [1]. For example, the use of recovery biomarkers allows intakes to be measured without relying on self-report but limits outcomes to those for which there are known recovery biomarkers. In contrast, assessing diet through methods reliant on self-report such as 24-hour recalls, food frequency questionnaires, and dietary screeners allow for the examination of a greater number of food groups and nutrients of interest, but also contain varying degrees of measurement error due to factors such as recall error and social desirability bias. Measurement error not only varies by dietary assessment tool, but also by dietary intake and study population.

In addition to the expected amount of measurement error, other concerns such as feasibility, cost, and participant burden play a role in determining the most appropriate tool to use in a study. Researchers must make tradeoffs to obtain the most accurate measures for the study population and resources available, and accept the type and magnitude of measurement error associated with the method of choice. For example, 24-hour recalls tend to have less measurement error than food frequency questionnaires and dietary screeners, but are more resource-intensive and require more from participants to complete. Regardless of the dietary assessment method used, it is crucial for researchers to be aware of the nature, direction and magnitude of measurement error so as to interpret results appropriately.

This paper aims to describe the measurement error present in intake estimates of added sugars, added sugars from sugar-sweetened beverages (SSBs), fruits and vegetables, whole grains, fiber, and dairy derived from the NHANES dietary screener questionnaire (DSQ) among children 4–15 years of age. In this study, we have evaluated agreement with intake estimates derived from the Automated Self-Administered 24-Hour Recall for Children (ASA24-Kids), using data from the Healthy Communities Study (HCS) (see Additional file 1).

The HCS aimed to assess associations between community programs and policies to prevent childhood obesity and outcomes including nutrition and physical activity behaviors and BMI, in a large, diverse sample of children from 130 communities across the United States. To accomplish this, a measure of dietary intake that could easily be administered by a large number of field data collectors for a large sample of children across the country was required. Dietary assessments were made on the entire HCS sample of over 5000 children, using a modified version of the DSQ [2] that was developed by the National Cancer Institute (NCI) and used with children and adults in the National Health and Nutrition Examination Survey (NHANES) [3].

This short food frequency questionnaire-based method was selected for use in the HCS because it assessed dietary factors related to obesity risk and because it was feasible to administer to a large study population in a short time by field interviewers who had no special nutrition training [2, 4]. It also allowed for comparison to national data using the same method and enabled the calculation of quantitative intake estimates from reported frequencies [2]. Previously, DSQ intake estimates for foods such as fruits and vegetables have been shown to correlate well with estimates from interviewer-administered 24-hour recalls among adults [5]. However, as a brief dietary screener, the DSQ relies on complex cognitive tasks to calculate usual frequency of intake of various foods and is thus more challenging and potentially less accurate when used with children [1].

While the DSQ was the most feasible dietary assessment tool to be used in the HCS, information was lacking on the measurement error associated with intake estimates in relation to a more accurate dietary assessment method, especially among children. Dietary assessments on a subset of the HCS sample were therefore made using a 24-hour dietary recall to describe and quantify the measurement error present in DSQ intake estimates. The ASA24-Kids recall was selected as the reference method with which to compare the DSQ in the HCS. The ASA24-Kids was the most feasible, affordable comparison method because it is a standardized, automated online interview and does not require specialist trained nutrition researchers for data collection. While past studies have shown that some children at younger ages find it difficult to accurately report their own intakes using the ASA24-Kids, other studies have shown that among adults, the ASA24 yields results comparable to that of interviewer-administered 24-hour recalls [6–8]. Two recalls were collected from each of the sub sample respondents to adjust for in-person variation [2].

Methods

Study population

Sampling, measures, and methods used in the HCS have been described in detail elsewhere [2, 9–14]. In brief, HCS study participants ($n = 5138$) were recruited from a large, stratified sample of 130 high school catchments areas, or "communities", across the U.S. [9]. By design, the HCS oversampled lower income and minority communities and was not a representative sample of US children. Within each community, up to two elementary and two middle schools, were selected as the recruitment base for household/child participants [9]. Up to 81 children in grades K-8 were selected per community to complete the standard set of assessments, including the DSQ [9]. Letters requesting participation and study interest forms were sent home and those households returning an interest form were scheduled for home visits [9]. A random subsample of about 14% of the households consenting to participate in the HCS were selected for the enhanced protocol which included more detailed measures of dietary intake, such as the ASA24-Kids recall, in addition to the standard set of assessments. The study population for this paper comprises the sub-sample of the HCS participants with a completed DSQ who completed at least one ASA24-Kids recall.

The research protocol was approved by OMB and the Battelle Memorial Institute IRB. Parents provided written informed consent for child participation [2].

Dietary assessment measures

The 27-item DSQ was adapted from the version administered to those aged 2–69 years of age in NHANES 2009–2010 [2]. An expert committee was convened by the lead investigators to advise on dietary assessment methods. Modifications of the DSQ for the HCS were minimal. In an attempt to reduce time required for home visits, DSQ items were prioritized and variables selected that have shown moderate to strong evidence of a relationship to obesity, including sugar sweetened beverages, fruits and vegetables among others. Questions about meat intake were excluded and a question about the frequency of chip and cracker consumption was added, although the latter was used only to assess the frequency of intake of discretionary foods, and, as such, was not used for quantitative intake estimates analyzed in this paper. [2]. While fast food intake was not assessed by the DSQ, a question about frequency of intake was included. Participants or their proxy reported the frequency of consuming selected foods and food groups over the past 30 days in number of times per day, week, or month. Quantitative estimates for intakes of each of the food groups and nutrients were calculated from the DSQ using publically available scoring algorithms derived from NHANES 2009–2010 data. To calculate scores, the reported frequencies of consumption were standardized to daily frequencies, to which age and sex specific median quantities of selected food groups were applied, and calibration equations were computed, derived from regressing DSQ with 24-hour recalls [15].

The ASA24-Kids is a 24-hour recall web-based program which was developed by the NCI for use with children and is available in English and Spanish [16, 17]. It is based on the Automated Multiple Pass Method used in interviewer administered recalls for NHANES, and adapted for online administration [18–20]. The ASA24-Kids consists of an 'interview' conducted by an animated character that queries the respondent in stages about all foods and beverages consumed in the previous 24 hours. During each stage or "pass", the respondent is probed for forgotten foods and beverages; time and eating occasion; and amounts consumed using photographs of graduated serving sizes [21]. The ASA24-Kids (2012 and 2014 versions) utilized the Food and Nutrient Database for Dietary Studies 4.1 as the basis for calculating intakes of nutrients, and food groups. "MyPyramid" serving equivalents were calculated within the ASA24-Kids program using the MyPyramid Equivalents Database 2.0 [16].

Data collection

Dietary data was collected during home visits, with the parent/guardian and child present. The DSQ and ASA24-Kids recalls were collected in English or Spanish, according to participant preference [2]. For both dietary assessments, the primary respondent was selected based on the child's age as follows: the parent/adult proxy with child assistance for children 4–8 years; the child with parent/adult proxy assistance for children 9–11 years; the child with parent/adult proxy assistance only if needed for children 12–15 years [2].

Trained field data collectors (FDCs) administered the DSQ, giving a neutral, scripted introduction and directions to the parent or adult caregiver and child concerning who should respond and how to obtain clarification from parents when the child was the primary respondent [2]. The FDC entered respondents' answers into a pre-programmed electronic tablet [2]. Out of range responses prompted a neutral scripted probe by the interviewer to verify or correct responses [2].

Respondents in the enhanced protocol sub-sample completed the ASA24-Kids on an HCS tablet computer supplied by FDCs during home visits [2]. Study participants were asked to complete two recalls. The first was collected on the same day as the interviewer administration of the DSQ, and the second recall occurred at a follow up home visit approximately 7–10 days later. The FDCs' role in administering the ASA24-Kids was restricted to logging onto the program, troubleshooting, and providing minimal assistance [2]. To avoid potential reactivity, respondents were unaware that they would be completing 24-hour recalls prior to the home visit [2].

Participant sex, age, race, and ethnicity were determined by survey responses and BMI was calculated from measured height and weight recorded by trained FDCs.

Training and quality assurance

FDCs were trained to administer the DSQ and oversee completion of the ASA24-Kids [2]. To assure adherence to the protocol, field supervisors and senior research staff conducted quality assurance checks of FDCs on selected home visits [2].

Data quality was monitored monthly for missing data, irregularities in administration time, extreme values at the low and high ends of the distribution, and percentage of 'don't know' and 'refusal' responses for the DSQ [2]. Data obtained from the ASA24-Kids was also reviewed monthly, for response rates, incompletes, documentation about reasons for missing or incomplete recalls, comparison with age and sex specific values from NHANES 2010, and review of outliers [2]. FDCs with incomplete or other data issues participated in refresher training and were monitored subsequently [2].

Statistical analyses

Box-Cox transformations were used to find the best transformation to achieve normal distributions for each food group or nutrient intake on the completed recalls ($n = 656$). Transformed data were reviewed, and extreme outliers were excluded from analysis for those particular nutrients or food groups. Extreme outliers were defined as those with nutrients or food groups at least two times the interquartile range lower or higher than the lower and upper bounds of the interquartile range (25th and 75th percentiles). For each intake of interest, full records were excluded if intake estimates from both recalls were missing or identified as extreme outliers, or if the DSQ intake estimate was missing ($n = 7$ for total added sugars; $n = 4$ for added sugars from SSBs; $n = 9$ for fruits and vegetables; n = 4 for whole grains; $n = 18$ for fiber; and $n = 3$ for dairy). All statistical analyses were conducted using SAS (version 9.4, 2013, SAS Institute Inc.).

Mean differences between the DSQ and ASA24-Kids intake estimates (mean of two recall days if available) were assessed by paired t-tests. A measurement error model using structural equation modelling, similar to that described by Freedman et al. [22], was applied to estimate relationships between estimated usual intake, as derived from the recalls, and the DSQ intake estimates. ASA24-Kids intake estimates were modelled as true usual intake plus random error. The modelling removed intra-individual variation to estimate true usual intake, with the assumption that the recalls were unbiased at the individual level and only contained intra-individual random error [23]. DSQ intakes were then modelled as a function of the estimated true usual intake plus error, both random and systematic. This model was fit by age group and sex, ethnicity, and BMI category to the DSQ and ASA24-Kids recall data and yielded estimates of measurement error characteristics of the DSQ. Models were not adjusted for covariates because we sought to assess the direct relationship between these two measurement methods and how these measures relate to a theoretical estimate of true intake using a structural equation modelling approach; the addition of covariates to the model would have distorted these relationships. The slope (β_1) in the regression of reported intake from the DSQ on estimated true usual intake, using the recalls, as well as the deattenuated correlation coefficient between reported and estimated usual intakes (R), and the attenuation factor ($\lambda = R^2/\ \beta_1$) were then estimated using full information maximum likelihood estimation.

If the DSQ were unbiased, the regression of reported intake on true usual intake would have a slope of one and an intercept of zero [23]. Deattenuated correlations assess the agreement between reported intake and estimated usual intake, adjusted for intra-individual variation. The attenuation factor indicates the degree to which the observed log relative risk between the observed exposure of a dietary intake derived from the DSQ and an outcome of interest is biased due to measurement error [23]. Attenuation factors typically range from 0 to 1, indicating bias towards the null (underestimation of true association), with values closer to zero indicating more severe attenuation [23]. Attenuation factors greater than one indicate bias away from the null (overestimation of true association) [23].

Results

Of the 5138 participants in the HCS, 5123 completed a DSQ, and 712 (14%) were randomly selected for the enhanced protocol. Of those, 656 participants (92.1%) completed one recall and 551 participants (77.4%) completed both recalls. The sample size for the analysis of each intake variable ranged from 638 to 653. The sample comprised approximately 50% females (Table 1). A higher proportion of participants were 4–8 years old, than 9–11 year olds, or 12–15 year olds. Over half of the participants were white, non-Hispanic, were of normal weight, and had a family income of less than $35,000 per year. Approximately 40% had parents who had attained a high school education or less. Overall there were no statistically significant differences in sociodemographic characteristics between the enhanced protocol subsample and the entire HCS sample.

Relative to the ASA24-Kids recalls, the mean intake estimates from the DSQ for all nutrients/foods were significantly higher for the total sample and for nearly all subgroups (Table 2). Differences in means between the two measures were not significantly different for girls aged 9–11 years on added sugars from SSBs, for girls aged 9–15 years on fruits and vegetables, and for girls aged 4–8 years for whole grains.

Deattenuated correlation coefficients of 0.4 or above were observed for the overall sample on three of the six nutrient/food intakes measured by DSQ and ASA24-Kids; the highest deattenuated correlation was observed for sugars from SSBs (0.54), followed by dairy (0.50), and fruits and vegetables (0.40) (Table 3). Values for the other three intake variables ranged from 0.34 for whole grains and fiber to 0.37 for total added sugar. Deattenuated correlations varied among the 14 sub-groups as defined by children's age and sex (6 groups), race (3 groups) ethnicity

Table 1 Comparison of sociodemographics of Enhanced Protocol sub-sample and Total sample, Healthy Communities Study, USA, 2013–2015

	Number of Participants (*n* (%))		*P*-value[a]
	Enhanced Protocol Sub-Sample (*n* = 656)	Total HCS Sample (*n* = 5138)	
1. Demographics			
Sex/Age Category			0.83
Male	323 (49.2)	2524 (49.1)	
4-8y	136 (20.7)	1099 (21.4)	
9-11y	100 (15.2)	815 (15.9)	
12-15y	87 (13.3)	610 (11.9)	
Female	333 (50.8)	2614 (50.9)	
4-8y	132 (20.1)	1097 (21.4)	
9-11y	113 (17.2)	824 (16.0)	
12-15y	88 (13.4)	693 (13.5)	
BMI Category			0.26
Normal weight	366 (55.8)	3022 (58.8)	
Overweight	105 (16.0)	789 (15.4)	
Obese	180 (27.4)	1264 (24.6)	
Missing	5 (0.8)	63 (1.2)	
Race			0.35
White	360 (54.9)	2924 (56.9)	
African American	136 (20.7)	960 (18.7)	
American Indian/ Alaskan Native	7 (1.1)	59 (1.2)	
Native Hawaiian/ Pacific Islander	1 (0.2)	8 (0.2)	
Asian	14 (2.1)	167 (3.3)	
Multiracial	45 (6.9)	227 (4.4)	
Missing	93 (14.2)	793 (15.4)	
Ethnicity			0.26
Hispanic	265 (40.4)	2225 (43.3)	
Non-Hispanic	375 (57.2)	2767 (53.9)	
Missing	16 (2.4)	146 (2.9)	
2. By socioeconomic status			
Income per year			0.57
Less than $20,000	168 (25.6)	1261 (24.5)	
$20,000–$35,000	144 (22.0)	1109 (21.6)	
$35,000–$50,000	88 (13.4)	602 (11.7)	
$50,000–$75,000	59 (9.0)	517 (10.1)	
$75,000–$100,000	54 (8.2)	383 (7.5)	
Greater than or equal to $100,000	96 (14.6)	840 (16.4)	
Missing	47 (7.2)	426 (8.3)	
Maximum parent educational attainment[b]			0.39
Did not attend high school	41 (6.3)	434 (8.5)	
Some high school, no diploma	95 (14.5)	713 (13.9)	
High school diploma, GED or equivalent	136 (20.7)	979 (19.1)	
Some college, no degree	91 (13.9)	646 (12.6)	
Associate or bachelor degree	175 (26.7)	1347 (26.2)	
Masters, doctoral, or professional degree	98 (14.9)	844 (16.4)	
Missing	20 (3.1)	175 (3.4)	

[a]Differences in categorical variables assessed via Chi-squared test
[b]Highest level of education attained by parent

(2 groups), or BMI (3 groups). The greatest number of deattenuated correlation coefficients at or above 0.4 among sub-groups were seen for added sugars from SSBs (11), dairy (11), and fruits and vegetables (9). Lowest deattenuated correlations (0.15 or below) were seen among children aged 9–11 years for several dietary intakes including total added sugars (both sexes), whole grains (girls), and dairy (boys). African American children tended to have lower deattenuated correlations as compared to White children or children of other races. Hispanic children had notably higher deattenuated correlations than non-Hispanic children for intakes of total added sugars and sugars from SSBs, but substantially lower deattenuated correlations for intakes of fruits and vegetables, and whole grains. Compared to normal weight children, deattenuated correlations were higher among overweight or obese children for intakes of dairy, added sugars from SSBs, and whole grains; and lower for intake of fruits and vegetables.

Attenuation was greater than 0.2 for more than 90% of the age and sex-, race-, ethnicity-, and BMI category-specific food group/nutrient intakes (Table 3). Attenuation factors for intake of sugars from SSBs were higher, while those for fruit and vegetable intake were lower, among children with higher BMI. For all intake estimates, there was a greater degree of attenuation among African American children compared to White children and children of other races. For all intake estimates other than those for total added sugars and fiber, there was a greater degree of attenuation for Hispanics than for non-Hispanics. Attenuation was most severe ($\lambda = 0.01–0.18$) for added sugars among boys and girls 9–11 years and among overweight children; whole grain intake among females 9–11 years; and dairy intake among boys 9–11 years.

Table 2 Differences between children's dietary intakes measured via DSQ and ASA24-Kids, Healthy Communities Study, USA, 2013–2015

Food Group/ Nutrient	DSQ		ASA24-Kids		Mean difference between dietary intakes as measured by DSQ and ASA24-Kids			
	Mean ± SD	Median	Mean ± SD	Median	Mean Difference[a]	Percent Change[b]	Paired t-test test statistic	*P*-value
1. Total added sugars (tsp/day)								
All (*n* = 649)	19.0 ± 7.4	17.2	12.2 ± 8.3	10.7	− 6.8	− 55.7%	− 17.8	< 0.01
Sex and age								
Male (*n* = 321)	20.1 ± 7.8	18.2	13.0 ± 8.7	11.3	− 7.1	− 54.6%	− 12.3	< 0.01
4-8y (*n* = 136)	18.3 ± 5.0	17.1	11.0 ± 6.7	9.4	− 7.2	− 66.4%	− 11.0	< 0.01
9-11y (*n* = 98)	19.6 ± 8.3	17.6	13.8 ± 8.1	13.3	− 5.7	− 42.0%	− 5.0	< 0.01
12-15y (*n* = 87)	23.5 ± 9.7	20.8	15.2 ± 11.3	12.8	− 8.3	− 54.6%	− 6.3	< 0.01
Female (*n* = 328)	17.9 ± 6.8	16.3	11.3 ± 7.8	10.3	− 6.6	− 53.4%	− 12.8	< 0.01
4-8y (*n* = 131)	16.0 ± 3.9	15.1	10.6 ± 6.3	10.0	− 5.5	− 50.9%	− 9.2	< 0.01
9-11y (*n* = 112)	18.2 ± 5.2	17.2	12.8 ± 9.1	10.9	− 5.5	− 42.2%	− 5.6	< 0.01
12-15y (*n* = 85)	20.3 ± 10.4	17.5	10.6 ± 7.9	9.8	−9.7	− 91.5%	−8.6	< 0.01
BMI category[c]								
Normal weight (*n* = 363)	18.9 ± 7.6	17.1	12.0 ± 8.1	10.6	− 6.9	− 57.5%	− 13.5	< 0.01
Overweight (*n* = 104)	18.5 ± 5.9	17.2	12.0 ± 8.8	10.9	− 6.5	− 54.2%	− 6.8	< 0.01
Obese (*n* = 177)	19.4 ± 7.8	17.5	12.7 ± 8.7	10.9	− 6.7	− 52.8%	− 9.0	< 0.01
Race								
White (*n* = 357)	18.3 ± 6.1	17.0	12.8 ± 8.3	11.1	−5.5	− 43.0%	− 11.8	< 0.01
African American (*n* = 135)	22.9 ± 11.1	19.8	12.8 ± 9.2	11.0	−10.1	−78.9%	− 8.7	< 0.01
Other (*n* = 66)	17.1 ± 4.2	16.3	11.5 ± 6.7	10.7	−5.6	− 48.7%	− 6.3	< 0.01
Ethnicity								
Hispanic (*n* = 262)	18.4 ± 5.8	17.2	11.1 ± 7.5	10.2	−7.4	− 65.8%	−15.1	< 0.01
Non-Hispanic (*n* = 371)	19.2 ± 7.9	17.1	13.0 ± 8.8	11.1	−6.2	− 47.7%	−11.3	< 0.01
2. Added sugars from sugar sweetened beverages (tsp/day)								
All (*n* = 652)	7.1 ± 4.8	5.6	4.9 ± 5.4	3.6	− 2.1	− 44.9%	− 9.7	< 0.01
Sex and age								
Male (*n* = 321)	7.4 ± 3.8	6.3	5.4 ± 5.9	4.0	−1.9	− 37.0%	−6.9	< 0.01
4-8y (*n* = 136)	6.1 ± 2.7	5.2	4.0 ± 3.6	3.4	− 2.1	−52.5%	−6.5	< 0.01
9-11y (*n* = 98)	6.6 ± 3.2	5.6	5.6 ± 5.6	3.8	−1.0	− 17.9%	− 2.1	0.04
12-15y (*n* = 87)	10.3 ± 4.4	8.8	7.5 ± 8.2	5.6	− 2.8	− 37.3%	− 3.9	< 0.01
Female (*n* = 331)	6.8 ± 5.5	4.9	4.4 ± 4.9	3.2	−2.3	−54.5%	−6.9	< 0.01

Table 2 Differences between children's dietary intakes measured via DSQ and ASA24-Kids, Healthy Communities Study, USA, 2013–2015 *(Continued)*

Food Group/ Nutrient	DSQ		ASA24-Kids		Mean difference between dietary intakes as measured by DSQ and ASA24-Kids			
	Mean ± SD	Median	Mean ± SD	Median	Mean Difference[a]	Percent Change[b]	Paired t-test test statistic	*P*-value
4-8y (*n* = 132)	5.3 ± 2.7	4.3	3.8 ± 3.7	2.8	−1.5	− 39.5%	−4.5	< 0.01
9-11y (*n* = 112)	6.0 ± 2.9	4.7	5.1 ± 5.3	4.0	− 0.8	−17.6%	− 1.6	0.11
12-15y (*n* = 87)	10.0 ± 8.9	6.8	4.5 ± 5.8	3.2	−5.5	− 122.2%	−6.2	< 0.01
BMI category[c]								
Normal weight (*n* = 365)	6.8 ± 4.4	5.4	4.8 ± 5.6	3.3	− 2.1	−41.7%	−6.7	< 0.01
Overweight (*n* = 104)	7.0 ± 3.7	5.8	4.4 ± 4.5	3.6	− 2.5	− 59.1%	− 5.5	< 0.01
Obese (*n* = 178)	7.7 ± 5.9	5.8	5.7 ± 5.6	4.5	− 2.1	− 35.1%	− 4.8	< 0.01
Race								
White (*n* = 358)	6.6 ± 4.2	5.4	5.0 ± 5.6	3.5	− 1.6	− 32.0%	− 5.7	< 0.01
African American (*n* = 136)	9.3 ± 6.6	7.4	5.4 ± 5.3	4.3	− 3.9	− 72.2%	− 6.2	< 0.01
Other (*n* = 67)	6.5 ± 3.8	5.3	4.7 ± 4.3	4.7	− 1.8	− 38.3%	− 2.9	< 0.01
Ethnicity								
Hispanic (*n* = 262)	6.7 ± 4.2	5.7	4.7 ± 5.1	3.6	−2.0	− 42.6%	− 6.4	< 0.01
Non-Hispanic (*n* = 374)	7.2 ± 4.6	5.5	5.2 ± 5.7	3.7	− 2.1	− 38.5%	− 7.2	< 0.01
3. Fruits and vegetables (cup equivalents/day)								
All (*n* = 647)	2.5 ± 0.9	2.3	2.1 ± 1.4	1.9	− 0.4	− 19.0%	− 7.2	< 0.01
Sex and age								
Male (*n* = 321)	2.7 ± 1.0	2.4	2.1 ± 1.4	1.8	− 0.6	−28.6%	− 7.6	< 0.01
4-8y (*n* = 136)	2.5 ± 0.8	2.4	2.0 ± 1.3	1.9	− 0.5	−25.0%	−4.0	< 0.01
9-11y (*n* = 98)	2.7 ± 1.0	2.4	2.2 ± 1.6	1.7	− 0.5	− 22.7%	− 3.2	< 0.01
12-15y (*n* = 87)	3.0 ± 1.1	2.7	2.0 ± 1.4	1.8	− 1.0	− 50.0%	−6.4	< 0.01
Female (*n* = 326)	2.3 ± 0.7	2.2	2.1 ± 1.3	1.9	− 0.2	− 9.5%	− 2.4	0.02
4-8y (*n* = 130)	2.4 ± 0.7	2.3	2.1 ± 1.3	1.8	− 0.3	− 14.3%	−2.6	0.01
9-11y (*n* = 111)	2.3 ± 0.6	2.2	2.2 ± 1.2	2.2	− 0.1	−4.5%	− 0.9	0.36
12-15y (*n* = 85)	2.2 ± 0.7	2.0	2.1 ± 1.6	1.8	− 0.1	−4.8%	− 0.6	0.55
BMI category[c]								
Normal weight (*n* = 363)	2.6 ± 0.9	2.3	2.1 ± 1.4	1.9	− 0.4	− 23.8%	− 5.8	< 0.01
Overweight (*n* = 104)	2.5 ± 0.8	2.3	2.0 ± 1.3	1.8	− 0.5	− 25.0%	− 3.5	< 0.01
Obese (*n* = 175)	2.4 ± 0.8	2.2	2.0 ± 1.3	1.8	− 0.3	− 20.0%	− 3.1	< 0.01

Table 2 Differences between children's dietary intakes measured via DSQ and ASA24-Kids, Healthy Communities Study, USA, 2013–2015 *(Continued)*

	DSQ		ASA24-Kids		Mean difference between dietary intakes as measured by DSQ and ASA24-Kids			
Food Group/ Nutrient	Mean ± SD	Median	Mean ± SD	Median	Mean Difference[a]	Percent Change[b]	Paired t-test test statistic	*P*-value
Race								
White ($n = 355$)	2.6 ± 0.9	2.4	2.1 ± 1.3	1.9	−0.5	−23.8%	−6.5	< 0.01
African American ($n = 134$)	2.3 ± 0.7	2.1	1.9 ± 1.2	1.7	−0.4	−21.1%	−3.0	< 0.01
Other ($n = 67$)	2.6 ± 0.9	2.3	2.1 ± 1.4	1.9	−0.6	−23.8%	−3.3	< 0.01
Ethnicity								
Hispanic ($n = 279$)	2.5 ± 0.8	2.3	2.1 ± 1.4	1.9	−0.3	−19.0%	−3.5	< 0.01
Non-Hispanic ($n = 373$)	2.5 ± 0.9	2.3	2.1 ± 1.3	1.8	−0.5	−19.0%	−6.5	< 0.01
4. Whole grains (oz equivalents/day)								
All ($n = 652$)	0.7 ± 0.4	0.6	0.5 ± 0.7	0.3	−0.2	−40.0%	−7.1	< 0.01
Sex and age								
Male ($n = 322$)	0.8 ± 0.5	0.7	0.5 ± 0.8	0.3	−0.2	−60.0%	−5.2	< 0.01
4-8y ($n = 136$)	0.8 ± 0.4	0.7	0.5 ± 0.6	0.3	−0.2	−60.0%	−4.3	< 0.01
9-11y ($n = 99$)	0.8 ± 0.6	0.7	0.6 ± 1.0	0.3	−0.2	−33.3%	−2.0	0.05
12-15y ($n = 87$)	0.7 ± 0.3	0.6	0.5 ± 0.7	0.2	−0.2	−40.0%	−3.3	< 0.01
Female ($n = 330$)	0.6 ± 0.4	0.5	0.4 ± 0.6	0.2	−0.2	−50.0%	−4.9	< 0.01
4-8y ($n = 132$)	0.6 ± 0.3	0.6	0.5 ± 0.7	0.3	−0.1	−20.0%	−1.2	0.22
9-11y ($n = 111$)	0.7 ± 0.4	0.6	0.4 ± 0.4	0.2	−0.3	−75.0%	−5.5	< 0.01
12-15y ($n = 87$)	0.6 ± 0.5	0.5	0.4 ± 0.6	0.1	−0.2	−50.0%	−2.8	0.01
BMI category[c]								
Normal weight ($n = 364$)	0.7 ± 0.4	0.6	0.5 ± 0.7	0.3	−0.2	−40.0%	−5.4	< 0.01
Overweight ($n = 105$)	0.7 ± 0.4	0.6	0.5 ± 0.6	0.3	−0.2	−40.0%	−3.2	< 0.01
Obese ($n = 178$)	0.7 ± 0.4	0.5	0.5 ± 0.7	0.2	−0.2	−40.0%	−3.1	< 0.01
Race								
White ($n = 358$)	0.7 ± 0.4	0.6	0.5 ± 0.7	0.3	−0.2	−40.0%	−4.5	< 0.01
African American ($n = 135$)	0.7 ± 0.5	0.6	0.4 ± 0.5	0.2	−0.4	−75.0%	−6.5	< 0.01
Other ($n = 67$)	0.7 ± 0.4	0.6	0.6 ± 0.6	0.3	−0.1	−16.7%	−1.6	0.12
Ethnicity								
Hispanic ($n = 264$)	0.7 ± 0.4	0.6	0.5 ± 0.7	0.2	−0.2	−40.0%	−4.5	< 0.01
Non-Hispanic ($n = 372$)	0.7 ± 0.4	0.6	0.5 ± 0.6	0.3	−0.2	−40.0%	−5.2	< 0.01

Table 2 Differences between children's dietary intakes measured via DSQ and ASA24-Kids, Healthy Communities Study, USA, 2013–2015 *(Continued)*

Food Group/ Nutrient	DSQ		ASA24-Kids		Mean difference between dietary intakes as measured by DSQ and ASA24-Kids			
	Mean ± SD	Median	Mean ± SD	Median	Mean Difference[a]	Percent Change[b]	Paired t-test test statistic	*P*-value
5. Fiber (g/day)								
All ($n = 638$)	15.4 ± 3.9	14.7	12.5 ± 6.5	11.4	−2.9	− 23.2%	− 10.6	< 0.01
Sex and age								
Male ($n = 318$)	16.5 ± 4.4	16.0	12.8 ± 7.2	11.7	− 3.7	−28.9%	−8.6	< 0.01
4-8y ($n = 136$)	15.4 ± 3.8	15.1	12.5 ± 6.5	12.0	−2.9	−23.2%	−4.8	< 0.01
9-11y ($n = 99$)	16.2 ± 4.7	15.6	13.7 ± 7.5	11.7	−2.5	−18.2%	−3.1	< 0.01
12-15y ($n = 87$)	18.7 ± 4.4	17.7	12.3 ± 7.8	10.7	−6.4	− 52.0%	−7.3	< 0.01
Female ($n = 320$)	14.2 ± 2.9	13.7	12.2 ± 5.8	11.3	−2.0	−16.4%	−6.4	< 0.01
4-8y ($n = 129$)	14.4 ± 2.7	14.0	11.8 ± 5.2	11.3	−2.6	− 22.0%	− 5.7	< 0.01
9-11y ($n = 109$)	14.0 ± 2.7	13.7	12.7 ± 5.8	11.3	−1.3	−10.2%	−2.5	0.02
12-15y ($n = 82$)	14.1 ± 3.3	13.3	12.1 ± 6.7	11.3	−2.0	−16.5%	−2.9	0.01
BMI category[c]								
Normal weight ($n = 359$)	15.7 ± 4.2	15.0	12.8 ± 6.8	11.7	−2.9	− 22.7%	− 7.6	< 0.01
Overweight ($n = 103$)	15.3 ± 3.8	14.8	11.8 ± 6.6	10.7	−3.6	− 29.7%	− 5.4	< 0.01
Obese ($n = 171$)	14.6 ± 3.3	14.2	12.0 ± 5.8	11.2	− 2.6	− 21.7%	−5.4	< 0.01
Race								
White ($n = 352$)	15.7 ± 4.0	15.1	12.8 ± 6.6	11.5	− 2.8	− 22.7%	− 7.9	< 0.01
African American ($n = 131$)	14.4 ± 3.9	13.4	11.3 ± 5.1	11.0	− 3.1	− 27.4%	− 5.7	< 0.01
Other ($n = 66$)	15.4 ± 3.7	14.9	12.2 ± 6.9	11.6	− 3.2	− 26.2%	− 3.7	< 0.01
Ethnicity								
Hispanic ($n = 255$)	15.5 ± 4.0	15.0	12.6 ± 7.0	11.0	−2.8	− 23.0%	− 6.2	< 0.01
Non-Hispanic ($n = 368$)	15.2 ± 3.9	14.5	12.4 ± 6.1	11.7	−2.9	− 22.6%	− 8.6	< 0.01
6. Dairy (cup equivalents/day)								
All ($n = 653$)	2.5 ± 0.7	2.4	1.8 ± 1.2	1.6	−0.7	− 38.9%	− 14.6	< 0.01
Sex and age								
Male ($n = 323$)	2.7 ± 0.7	2.7	2.0 ± 1.3	1.9	−0.7	− 35.0%	− 9.6	< 0.01
4-8y ($n = 136$)	2.8 ± 0.6	2.7	2.0 ± 1.1	1.9	−0.8	−40.0%	− 8.6	< 0.01
9-11y ($n = 100$)	2.8 ± 0.8	2.6	2.1 ± 1.3	2.1	−0.7	−33.3%	−4.6	< 0.01
12-15y ($n = 87$)	2.5 ± 0.7	2.5	2.0 ± 1.4	1.7	−0.6	− 25.0%	−3.8	< 0.01
Female ($n = 330$)	2.2 ± 0.6	2.2	1.6 ± 1.1	1.4	−0.7	− 37.5%	−11.2	< 0.01

Table 2 Differences between children's dietary intakes measured via DSQ and ASA24-Kids, Healthy Communities Study, USA, 2013–2015 *(Continued)*

	DSQ		ASA24-Kids		Mean difference between dietary intakes as measured by DSQ and ASA24-Kids			
Food Group/ Nutrient	Mean ± SD	Median	Mean ± SD	Median	Mean Difference[a]	Percent Change[b]	Paired t-test test statistic	*P*-value
4-8y ($n = 131$)	2.3 ± 0.5	2.2	1.7 ± 1.1	1.6	−0.6	− 35.3%	− 6.0	< 0.01
9-11y ($n = 113$)	2.5 ± 0.7	2.3	1.7 ± 1.2	1.6	−0.8	− 47.1%	− 6.6	< 0.01
12-15y ($n = 86$)	1.9 ± 0.5	1.8	1.2 ± 0.9	1.1	− 0.7	− 58.3%	− 7.2	< 0.01
BMI category[c]								
Normal weight ($n = 364$)	2.5 ± 0.7	2.4	1.8 ± 1.2	1.7	−0.7	−38.9%	− 11.3	< 0.01
Overweight ($n = 105$)	2.4 ± 0.7	2.3	1.8 ± 1.2	1.6	−0.6	− 33.3%	−5.7	< 0.01
Obese ($n = 179$)	2.5 ± 0.8	2.3	1.8 ± 1.2	1.6	−0.7	−38.9%	−7.9	< 0.01
Race								
White ($n = 359$)	2.5 ± 0.7	2.4	2.0 ± 1.2	1.9	−0.6	− 25.0%	− 8.7	< 0.01
African American ($n = 134$)	2.4 ± 0.7	2.3	1.4 ± 1.1	1.3	−0.9	−71.4%	−8.9	< 0.01
Other ($n = 67$)	2.5 ± 0.8	2.3	1.9 ± 1.3	1.8	−0.6	−31.6%	−4.5	< 0.01
Ethnicity								
Hispanic ($n = 265$)	2.5 ± 0.7	2.4	1.7 ± 1.2	1.6	−0.8	− 47.1%	− 10.2	< 0.01
Non-Hispanic ($n = 372$)	2.5 ± 0.7	2.4	1.8 ± 1.2	1.7	−0.6	−38.3%	− 10.0	< 0.01

[a](ASA24-Kids – DSQ)
[b](ASA24-Kids – DSQ)/ASA24-Kids
[c]BMI categories defined as follows: 'normal weight' was defined as having a BMI under the 85th percentile BMI for age and sex; 85th up to 95th percentile for 'overweight'; and at or above 95th percentile for 'obese'

Table 3 Slopes[a], deattenuated correlations[b], and attenuation factors[c] of DSQ dietary intakes, Healthy Communities Study, USA, 2013–2015

Food group/nutrient	Slope (SEE)	Deattenuated Correlation (SEE)	Attenuation Factor (SEE)
1. Total added sugars (tsp/day)			
All (*n* = 649)	0.55 (0.11)	0.37 (0.06)	0.25 (0.04)
Sex and age			
Male (*n* = 321)	0.49 (0.14)	0.35 (0.08)	0.25 (0.06)
4-8y (*n* = 136)	0.47 (0.27)	0.36 (0.16)	0.27 (0.12)
9-11y (*n* = 98)	0.10 (0.23)	0.06 (0.15)	0.04 (0.10)[d]
12-15y (*n* = 87)	0.65 (0.29)	0.47 (0.15)	0.34 (0.11)
Female (*n* = 328)	0.57 (0.19)	0.37 (0.10)	0.24 (0.06)
4-8y (*n* = 131)	0.78 (0.97)	0.46 (0.33)	0.27 (0.14)
9-11y (*n* = 112)	0.05 (0.12)	0.06 (0.13)	0.07 (0.16)[d]
12-15y (*n* = 85)	1.60 (0.88)	0.68 (0.21)	0.29 (0.08)
BMI category[e]			
Normal weight (*n* = 363)	0.55 (0.15)	0.36 (0.08)	0.23 (0.05)
Overweight (*n* = 104)	0.39 (0.37)	0.26 (0.20)	0.18 (0.13)[d]
Obese (*n* = 177)	0.61 (0.19)	0.45 (0.10)	0.33 (0.08)
Race			
White (*n* = 357)	0.56 (0.15)	0.45 (0.09)	0.36 (0.07)
African American (*n* = 135)	0.36 (0.22)	0.20 (0.12)	0.12 (0.07)[d]
Other (*n* = 66)	0.28 (0.23)	0.27 (0.20)	0.26 (0.19)
Ethnicity			
Hispanic (*n* = 262)	1.01 (0.46)	0.60 (0.15)	0.36 (0.07)
Non-Hispanic (*n* = 371)	0.43 (0.11)	0.32 (0.07)	0.24 (0.05)
2. Added sugars from sugar sweetened beverages (tsp/day)			
All (*n* = 652)	0.66 (0.07)	0.54 (0.04)	0.44 (0.04)
Sex and age			
Male (*n* = 321)	0.71 (0.10)	0.76 (0.06)	0.81 (0.07)
4-8y (*n* = 136)	0.75 (0.29)	0.59 (0.15)	0.46 (0.11)
9-11y (*n* = 98)	0.72 (0.26)	0.77 (0.15)	0.83 (0.15)
12-15y (*n* = 87)	0.57 (0.13)	0.76 (0.10)	1.02 (0.16)
Female (*n* = 331)	0.60 (0.11)	0.40 (0.06)	0.27 (0.05)
4-8y (*n* = 132)	0.88 (0.56)	0.56 (0.21)	0.36 (0.11)
9-11y (*n* = 112)	0.19 (0.08)	0.27 (0.11)	0.39 (0.17)
12-15y (*n* = 87)	0.93 (0.23)	0.50 (0.10)	0.27 (0.06)

Table 3 Slopes[a], deattenuated correlations[b], and attenuation factors[c] of DSQ dietary intakes, Healthy Communities Study, USA, 2013–2015 *(Continued)*

Food group/nutrient	Slope (SEE)	Deattenuated Correlation (SEE)	Attenuation Factor (SEE)
BMI category[e]			
Normal weight ($n = 365$)	0.50 (0.09)	0.45 (0.06)	0.40 (0.06)
Overweight ($n = 104$)	1.00 (0.54)	0.65 (0.20)	0.43 (0.11)
Obese ($n = 178$)	0.82 (0.13)	0.63 (0.07)	0.48 (0.06)
Race			
White ($n = 358$)	0.63 (0.08)	0.62 (0.05)	0.62 (0.06)
African American ($n = 136$)	0.69 (0.24)	0.39 (0.11)	0.22 (0.07)
Other ($n = 67$)	0.38 (0.22)	0.31 (0.16)	0.25 (0.14)
Ethnicity			
Hispanic ($n = 262$)	1.19 (0.40)	0.73 (0.13)	0.45 (0.06)
Non-Hispanic ($n = 374$)	0.57 (0.07)	0.56 (0.05)	0.55 (0.06)
3. Fruits and vegetables (cup equivalents/day)			
All ($n = 647$)	0.36 (0.06)	0.40 (0.05)	0.44 (0.06)
Sex and age			
Male ($n = 321$)	0.42 (0.10)	0.41 (0.08)	0.40 (0.08)
4-8y ($n = 136$)	0.31 (0.12)	0.36 (0.11)	0.42 (0.13)
9-11y ($n = 98$)	0.44 (0.17)	0.46 (0.13)	0.48 (0.15)
12-15y ($n = 87$)	0.59 (0.26)	0.46 (0.15)	0.36 (0.12)
Female ($n = 326$)	0.32 (0.07)	0.44 (0.07)	0.61 (0.10)
4-8y ($n = 130$)	0.39 (0.09)	0.54 (0.10)	0.75 (0.15)
9-11y ($n = 111$)	0.40 (0.18)	0.50 (0.15)	0.62 (0.18)
12-15y ($n = 85$)	0.19 (0.11)	0.28 (0.14)	0.42 (0.22)
BMI category[e]			
Normal weight ($n = 363$)	0.42 (0.07)	0.46 (0.06)	0.50 (0.07)
Overweight ($n = 104$)	0.49 (0.30)	0.42 (0.18)	0.36 (0.15)
Obese ($n = 175$)	0.20 (0.11)	0.23 (0.11)	0.26 (0.13)
Race			
White ($n = 355$)	0.46 (0.09)	0.47 (0.07)	0.49 (0.07)
African American ($n = 134$)	0.08 (0.13)	0.09 (0.14)	0.10 (0.15)[d]
Other ($n = 67$)	0.53 (0.21)	0.56 (0.16)	0.60 (0.18)

Table 3 Slopes[a], deattenuated correlations[b], and attenuation factors[c] of DSQ dietary intakes, Healthy Communities Study, USA, 2013–2015 *(Continued)*

Food group/nutrient	Slope (SEE)	Deattenuated Correlation (SEE)	Attenuation Factor (SEE)
Ethnicity			
Hispanic (*n* = 279)	0.29 (0.10)	0.32 (0.09)	0.35 (0.10)
Non-Hispanic (*n* = 373)	0.44 (0.08)	0.47 (0.07)	0.51 (0.07)
4. Whole grains (oz equivalents/day)			
All (*n* = 652)	0.33 (0.07)	0.34 (0.06)	0.35 (0.06)
Sex and age			
Male (*n* = 322)	0.34 (0.10)	0.36 (0.08)	0.37 (0.09)
4-8y (*n* = 136)	0.38 (0.12)	0.42 (0.11)	0.47 (0.13)
9-11y (*n* = 99)	0.28 (0.19)	0.26 (0.15)	0.24 (0.14)
12-15y (*n* = 87)	0.40 (0.26)	0.47 (0.21)	0.56 (0.23)
Female (*n* = 330)	0.29 (0.09)	0.29 (0.08)	0.30 (0.08)
4-8y (*n* = 132)	0.14 (0.07)	0.26 (0.11)	0.47 (0.20)
9-11y (*n* = 111)	1.08 (38.71)	0.09 (1.87)	0.01 (0.10)[d]
12-15y (*n* = 87)	0.50 (0.17)	0.47 (0.13)	0.44 (0.13)
BMI category[e]			
Normal weight (*n* = 364)	0.27 (0.07)	0.30 (0.07)	0.32 (0.08)
Overweight (*n* = 105)	0.59 (0.39)	0.44 (0.20)	0.33 (0.13)
Obese (*n* = 178)	0.51 (0.19)	0.54 (0.13)	0.56 (0.12)
Race			
White (*n* = 358)	0.36 (0.10)	0.37 (0.08)	0.39 (0.08)
African American (*n* = 135)	0.55 (0.25)	0.35 (0.13)	0.22 (0.08)
Other (*n* = 67)	0.97 (0.84)	0.70 (0.33)	0.51 (0.17)
Ethnicity			
Hispanic (*n* = 264)	0.17 (0.06)	0.22 (0.07)	0.27 (0.09)
Non-Hispanic (*n* = 372)	0.53 (0.17)	0.45 (0.10)	0.38 (0.08)
5. Fiber (g/day)			
All (*n* = 638)	0.31 (0.06)	0.34 (0.06)	0.37 (0.06)
Sex and age			
Male (*n* = 318)	0.21 (0.07)	0.24 (0.08)	0.26 (0.09)
4-8y (*n* = 136)	0.22 (0.12)	0.26 (0.12)	0.29 (0.14)
9-11y (*n* = 99)	0.28 (0.15)	0.30 (0.14)	0.31 (0.15)
12-15y (*n* = 87)	0.18 (0.11)	0.24 (0.14)	0.31 (0.18)

Table 3 Slopes[a], deattenuated correlations[b], and attenuation factors[c] of DSQ dietary intakes, Healthy Communities Study, USA, 2013–2015 *(Continued)*

Food group/nutrient	Slope (SEE)	Deattenuated Correlation (SEE)	Attenuation Factor (SEE)
Female (*n* = 320)	0.44 (0.11)	0.54 (0.09)	0.64 (0.11)
4-8y (*n* = 129)	0.56 (0.29)	0.56 (0.18)	0.57 (0.16)
9-11y (*n* = 109)	0.53 (0.26)	0.63 (0.18)	0.74 (0.19)
12-15y (*n* = 82)	0.35 (0.14)	0.48 (0.14)	0.67 (0.21)
BMI category[e]			
Normal weight (*n* = 359)	0.27 (0.07)	0.32 (0.07)	0.37 (0.08)
Overweight (*n* = 103)	0.42 (0.23)	0.40 (0.16)	0.39 (0.16)
Obese (*n* = 171)	0.35 (0.22)	0.32 (0.15)	0.29 (0.13)
Race			
White (*n* = 352)	0.32 (0.07)	0.36 (0.07)	0.41 (0.08)
African American (*n* = 131)	0.19 (0.24)	0.14 (0.16)	0.10 (0.11)[d]
Other (*n* = 66)	0.28 (0.17)	0.36 (0.18)	0.46 (0.23)
Ethnicity			
Hispanic (*n* = 255)	0.31 (0.10)	0.34 (0.09)	0.38 (0.10)
Non-Hispanic (*n* = 368)	0.35 (0.09)	0.36 (0.07)	0.37 (0.08)
6. Dairy (cup equivalents/day)			
All (*n* = 653)	0.47 (0.08)	0.50 (0.06)	0.54 (0.06)
Sex and age			
Male (*n* = 323)	0.36 (0.10)	0.39 (0.09)	0.43 (0.09)
4-8y (*n* = 136)	0.60 (0.22)	0.65 (0.14)	0.69 (0.14)
9-11y (*n* = 100)	0.19 (0.28)	0.15 (0.21)	0.12 (0.16)[d]
12-15y (*n* = 87)	0.26 (0.10)	0.38 (0.13)	0.54 (0.20)
Female (*n* = 330)	0.47 (0.12)	0.50 (0.09)	0.54 (0.09)
4-8y (*n* = 131)	0.34 (0.10)	0.49 (0.11)	0.71 (0.17)
9-11y (*n* = 113)	0.42 (0.25)	0.40 (0.18)	0.39 (0.16)
12-15y (*n* = 86)	0.77 (0.92)	0.51 (0.37)	0.34 (0.18)
BMI Category[e]			
Normal weight (*n* = 364)	0.42 (0.09)	0.48 (0.07)	0.54 (0.08)
Overweight (*n* = 105)	0.55 (0.31)	0.51 (0.19)	0.48 (0.17)
Obese (*n* = 179)	0.91 (0.42)	0.71 (0.18)	0.56 (0.11)

Table 3 Slopes[a], deattenuated correlations[b], and attenuation factors[c] of DSQ dietary intakes, Healthy Communities Study, USA, 2013–2015 *(Continued)*

Food group/nutrient	Slope (SEE)	Deattenuated Correlation (SEE)	Attenuation Factor (SEE)
Race			
White ($n = 359$)	0.52 (0.13)	0.54 (0.09)	0.55 (0.09)
African American ($n = 134$)	0.22 (0.12)	0.25 (0.12)	0.27 (0.14)
Other ($n = 67$)	0.86 (0.34)	0.84 (0.17)	0.81 (0.15)
Ethnicity			
Hispanic ($n = 265$)	0.56 (0.17)	0.52 (0.11)	0.49 (0.09)
Non-Hispanic ($n = 372$)	0.42 (0.08)	0.49 (0.07)	0.57 (0.09)

[a]Slopes in the regression of dietary intake reported from Dietary Screener Questionnaire on true usual intake, as estimated from multiple ASA24-Kids recalls in a measurement error model. If the DSQ were unbiased, slopes would equal 1 [23]

[b]Deattenuated correlations between reported and true usual intakes

[c]Attenuation factors resulting from measurement error in reported intake for each dietary factor. The attenuation factor indicates the degree to which the observed log relative risk between the observed exposure of a dietary intake derived from the DSQ and an outcome of interest is biased due to measurement error [23]. Values between 0 and 1 indicate bias towards the null (underestimation of true association) and values greater than 1 indicate bias away from the null (overestimation of true association) [23]

[d]Attenuation factor is very close to 0; careful consideration is needed when determining whether to adjust these intake estimates for measurement error

[e]BMI categories defined as follows: 'normal weight' was defined as having a BMI under the 85th percentile BMI for age and sex; 85th up to 95th percentile for 'overweight'; and at or above 95th percentile for 'obese'

Intake patterns

Although most of the intake estimates derived from the DSQ were significantly different from those from ASA24-Kids recalls, some patterns of intake among subgroups were similar using both methods. For total added sugars, fiber, and dairy foods, males consumed more than females on both measures (Table 2). While older males consumed more added sugars than younger males in both the DSQ and ASA24-Kids, this pattern was not seen among females. For added sugars from SSBs, males consumed more than females, and older children consumed more than younger ones on both measures. Intake patterns by sex and age group for fruits and vegetables, and for whole grains were inconsistent between the two methods. In addition, both instruments showed that, on average, obese children had greater intakes of total added sugars and added sugars from SSBs than overweight or normal weight children, and, that non-Hispanic children had higher consumption of these than Hispanic children. Normal weight children had greater intake of fruits and vegetables than overweight or obese children as measured by both instruments.

Discussion

This is the first study we are aware of which evaluates the performance of the DSQ among children. Unlike other dietary screeners which only yield consumption frequency, the DSQ yields quantified intake estimates based on reported frequencies of consumption. For three dietary outcomes examined in the HCS, added sugars from SSBs; fruits and vegetables; and dairy foods, deattenuated correlations were 0.4 or greater. This is an important finding for two reasons: i) many community policies and programs for obesity prevention target these foods, and ii) the level of agreement between the two dietary assessment methods suggests that the DSQ appears to be an acceptable tool for measuring these dietary outcomes for purposes of the analysis of the association between community programs and policies and dietary outcomes in studies such as the HCS and potentially for similar study populations and research questions.

The lower deattenuated correlations observed for total added sugars, compared with those for added sugars from SSBs may reflect the greater ease with which respondents can report beverage frequency than they can in reporting a wider range of foods they consume containing added sugars. Some research also suggests that foods consumed very frequently and foods consumed rarely, characteristic of many beverages, are more consistently reported than are foods that are consumed moderately frequently [24].

The variable levels of agreement seen between the two assessment methods for different age groups, in part, may be a function of the accuracy with which the selected primary respondents in the study are able to report dietary intakes. The higher correlations, suggestive of less measurement error, observed among children aged 12–15 years on several dietary outcomes may indicate that these youth were cognitively mature enough to serve as their own primary respondents. Reasonable agreement between both methods was also seen among children aged 4–8 years for several dietary outcomes, suggesting that caregiver adults were an adequate proxy reporter for this group. The higher degree of measurement error among children aged 9–11 years, especially males, as indicated by lower attenuation factors and deattenuated correlations for several dietary outcomes, suggests that they may have had difficulty in reporting their food and beverage intakes accurately, even with the assistance of a parent, findings which are consistent with those of numerous other studies [6, 25, 26].

There is substantial evidence that higher BMI is associated with higher measurement error in reporting diet, particularly underreporting of total energy intake [26–30]. Thus, it might be expected that overweight or obese children would underreport sugars from SSBs and other foods high in energy. However, relatively little is known about differential bias in reporting particular food groups among adults or children by BMI status, or the tendency for more biased reporting by overweight or obese respondents using different dietary assessment methods. Surprisingly, our study found that intake estimates of sugars from SSBs were less attenuated and had greater deattenuated correlation coefficients among overweight and obese children, indicating closer agreement between the two methods for overweight or obese children than for other children. By contrast, the degree of attenuation/measurement error in estimates of fruit and vegetable intake was higher in successively higher BMI categories. Further research is needed to identify the effect of BMI status, and hence misreporting bias on estimated intakes of selected *food groups* (beyond its effect on the accuracy of reporting energy intake).

We found that race and ethnicity were associated with the level of agreement between the two dietary assessment methods. Hispanic and African American children showed a higher degree of measurement error than children of other races and ethnicities. Previous validity studies have shown mixed results regarding performance of various dietary assessment methods among Hispanics compared with non-Hispanics; some studies found no significant differences in measures of agreement [23, 31–33], while others have found differences [1, 25, 34]. While efforts were made to design the DSQ to accommodate various Hispanic and Asian subgroups, it may not have included sufficient number or variety of important ethnic-specific foods. Alternatively, the scoring algorithms did not take into account the relative portion sizes of food items within a food group typical of Hispanic groups. Tucker et al. found that among Hispanic (Puerto Rican) adults, there was a tendency to consume larger portions of particular fruits and smaller portions of particular vegetables than the general U.S. population, comparing estimates from the 1982–1984 Hispanic Health and Nutrition Examination Survey with NHANES [34]. It is also possible that Hispanic respondents may have had more difficulty navigating the online ASA24-Kids recall due to language difficulty, or less familiarity with computers than adult and child respondents of other ethnicities. Although the Spanish language version of ASA24-Kids was offered, it was not often selected by respondents. Similar to previous studies comparing methods between African Americans and other races, we found that there was more measurement error in intake estimates among African Americans [35–37]. This may be due to similar factors to those we suggested for Hispanics (differences in foods consumed, and in portions of particular types of foods).

A limitation of our study was the uncertain validity of our reference method. For practical reasons, the ASA24-Kids was the best available method for collecting detailed dietary intake data in the HCS against which to compare data from the DSQ. The assumptions that 24-hour recalls provide unbiased estimates of usual food intake, and, further, that the ASA24-Kids, as a self-administered method, provides no additional bias over a standard interviewer-administered 24-hour recall are relatively unexplored assumptions. The use of an imperfect reference method, the ASA24-Kids recalls, may have led to inflated estimates of deattenuated correlation coefficients if the error within recall intake estimates was correlated with the error present in DSQ intake estimates.

With regards to the first assumption, it is possible that the ASA24-Kids recall method underestimated dietary intakes. We found that almost all of the intake estimates from the HCS recalls were significantly lower than those from the DSQ. In addition, the majority of mean nutrient/food intakes from the ASA24-Kids were lower than the NHANES 2009–2010 age and sex specific means, but most means were within 20% (see Additional file 2). It is widely known that 24-hour recalls underestimate energy intake [27, 38–41], but the presence and amount of reporting bias for food groups and many nutrients are currently unknown, in part due to the lack of a true gold standard. Other possible reasons for the lower estimates of dietary intakes from the ASA24-Kids relate to differences in the time periods covered by the two methods and the different types of memory needed for each method. Responses to the DSQ rely on participants' generic memory, which provides general information about usual intake over the reference time period. By contrast, 24-hour recalls rely on specific shorter term memory to provide detailed information about particular intakes and behaviors [42].

The second assumption, that the ASA24-Kids as a self-administered method produces no additional bias over an interviewer-administered 24-hour recall, may be of concern. Unlike dietary interviewers, study children are not trained to navigate the software and identify foods that best match their intakes. One study showed that when children between the ages of 9 and 11 years reported their own dietary intakes over the past 24 hours, the ASA24-Kids was less accurate than the interviewer-administered AMPM [6]. However, other studies have shown that among computer-literate English-speaking adults, the ASA24 performed similarly to the AMPM [7, 8]. In this study, parent or adult proxies were available to assist children aged 9–11 years, but were instructed by the FDC to provide assistance *only* if asked by the child. More consistent and active assistance from parents about the foods eaten at home and portion sizes may be needed to improve accuracy. However, the lack of an in-person interviewer in the ASA24-Kids may also confer some advantages such as a possible reduction in social desirability bias. Smith et al. found that, among fourth-grade children, reporting accuracy decreased with social desirability when 24-hour recalls were administered in person by interviewers [43].

There are many methods used to compare performance of and agreement between dietary assessment methods. A key strength of this study was the use of measurement error modelling utilizing structural equation modeling to remove the within-person variation in food/nutrient intakes from recalls to estimate usual intake. This method made the estimates derived from the DSQ, designed to measure *usual* intake over a month, and those derived from up to two days of 24-hour recalls more comparable to each other. From this modelling approach, we then derived deattenuated correlations to examine the agreement between reported intake and estimated usual intake as they are a more useful and rigorous assessment than the traditional Spearman or Pearson correlation coefficients and kappa statistics, which do not adjust for intra-individual variation. The derived attenuation factors, which express the amount of potential bias due to measurement error in an exposure-outcome relationship, were also useful in assessing which dietary outcome variables would be candidates for correction of measurement error. We observed a wide range of attenuation factors, $\lambda = 0.01–1.02$. While it is true that as the attenuation factor gets further from 1 it becomes increasingly important to adjust measures of association between observed dietary intakes and outcomes of interest for measurement error, as the attenuation factor gets closer to zero, adjusted estimates become overinflated, making adjusting for error less desirable. Thus, among children 9–11 years old, intakes of total added sugars (among both sexes), whole grains (among girls), and dairy (among boys) may not be good candidates for measurement error correction. Similarly, it may not be advisable to correct for measurement error for intakes of total added sugars among overweight children, or for total added sugars, fruits and vegetables, and fiber among African American children.

Conclusions

The importance of understanding the extent of measurement error in the dietary intake estimates used in the HCS, as measured by the DSQ, is fundamental to interpreting the results of associations between community policies and programs and child dietary outcomes. This study found higher deattenuated correlations and attenuation factors, overall, for intakes estimates of sugars from SSBs, dairy, and fruits and vegetables (foods often targeted in obesity prevention community policies and programs). Based on comparison with intake estimates derived from up to two ASA24-Kids recalls, our findings suggest that the DSQ may be an acceptable tool to measure key obesity-related dietary behaviors of interest among children for the purposes of studies like the HCS. However, further study exploring the assumptions made in using the ASA24-Kids as a reference method is warranted. In addition, our results suggest that measurement error modelling and regression calibration are viable methods for future studies to correct for measurement error within the DSQ for most of the food groups/nutrients among most of the strata examined in this study, which would otherwise lead to underestimating the magnitude of associations between nutrition exposures and outcomes of interest.

Abbreviations

ASA24: Automated Self-Administered 24-hour Recall; ASA24-Kids: Automated Self-Administered 24-Hour Recalls for Children; DSQ: Dietary screener questionnaire; FDC: Field data collector; HCS: Healthy Communities Study; NCI: National Cancer Institute; NHANES: National Health and Nutrition Examination Survey; SSBs: Sugar-sweetened beverages

Acknowledgments

We thank Patricia Wakimoto at UC Nutrition Policy Institute, for assisting with training and quality control/oversight of the interviewers/data collection and data processing; and Shelly Mandel at UC Nutrition Policy Institute for assisting with data processing.

Funding

The Healthy Communities Study was funded by the National Heart, Lung, and Blood Institute, in collaboration with the *Eunice Kennedy Shriver* National Institute of Child Health and Development, the National Institute of Diabetes and Digestive and Kidney Disorders, the National Cancer Institute, and the National Institutes of Health (NIH) Office of Behavioral and Social Sciences Research; DHHS, under Contract No. HHSN268201000041C.
The content is solely the responsibility of the authors and does not necessarily represent the official views of the NIH or the U.S. government. No financial disclosures were reported by the authors of this paper.

Authors' contributions

All authors read and approved the final manuscript.

Competing interests

The authors declare that they have no competing interests.

Author details

[1]Nutrition Policy Institute, University of California, Agriculture and Natural Resources Division, 2115 Milvia Street, Third floor, Berkeley, CA 94704, USA. [2]Risk Factor Assessment Branch, Epidemiology and Genomics Research Program, Division of Cancer Control and Population Sciences, National Cancer Institute, Rm. 4E124, 9609 Medical Center Drive, MSC 9763, Bethesda, MD 20892, USA. [3]Division of Cardiovascular Sciences, National Heart, Lung, and Blood Institute, 6701 Rockledge Drive, Suite 10018, Bethesda, MD 20892, USA. [4]Battelle, 505 King Ave, Columbus, OH 43201, USA.

References

1. Thompson FE, Subar AF. Dietary assessment methodology. In: Coulston AM, rock CL, Monsen ER, editors. Nutrition in the Prevention and Treatment of Disease, Elsevier; 2013. p. 5–46.
2. Ritchie LD, Wakimoto P, Woodward-Lopez G, Thompson FE, Loria CM, Wilson DK, et al. The healthy communities study nutrition assessments: child diet and the school nutrition environment. Am J Prev Med. 2015 Oct; 49(4):647–52. https://doi.org/10.1016/j.amepre.2015.06.016.
3. National Cancer Institute (NCI). Dietary screener questionnaire in the NHANES 2009–10. http://epi.grants.cancer.gov/nhanes/dietscreen/. Updated October 15, 2015. Accessed July 12, 2016.
4. Woodward-Lopez G, Ritchie LD, Gerstein D, Crawford PB. Obesity: dietary and developmental influences. Boca Raton: CRC Press; 2006. https://doi.org/10.1201/9781420008920
5. Dietary Screener Questionnaire (DSQ) in the NHANES 2009–10: Dietary Factors, Food Items Asked, and Testing Status for DSQ. http://epi.grants.cancer.gov/nhanes/dietscreen/evaluation.html. Updated January 4, 2016. Accessed 12 July 2016.
6. Diep CS, Hingle M, Chen TA, Dadabhoy HR, Beltran A, Baranowski J, et al. The automated self-administered 24-hour dietary recall for children, 2012 version, for youth aged 9 to 11 years: a validation study. J Acad Nutr Diet 2015 Oct;115(10):1591–1598. doi: https://doi.org/10.1016/j.jand.2015.02.021. Epub 2015 Apr 14.
7. Kirkpatrick SI, Subar AF, Douglass D, Zimmerman TP, Thompson FE, Kahle LL, et al. Performance of the automated self-administered 24-hour recall relative to a measure of true intakes and to an interviewer-administered 24-h recall. Am J Clin Nutr 2014 Jul;100(1):233–240. doi: https://doi.org/10.3945/ajcn.114.083238. Epub 2014 Apr 30.
8. Thompson FE, Dixit-Joshi S, Potischman N, Dodd KW, Kirkpatrick SI, Kushi LH, et al. Comparison of Interviewer-Administered and Automated Self-Administered 24-Hour Dietary Recalls in 3 Diverse Integrated Health Systems. Am. J. Epidemiol. doi:https://doi.org/10.1093/aje/kwu467 Epub May 10, 2015.
9. John LV, Gregoriou M, Pate RR, Fawcett SB, Crawford PB, Strauss WJ, et al. Operational implementation of the healthy communities study: how communities shape Children's health. Am J Prev Med. 2015 Oct;49(4):631–5. https://doi.org/10.1016/j.amepre.2015.06.019.
10. Fawcett SB, Collie-Akers V, Schultz J, Kelley M. Measuring community programs and policies and their intensity in the healthy communities study. Am J Prev Med. 2015 Oct;49(4):636–41. https://doi.org/10.1016/j.amepre.2015.06.027.
11. Sroka CJ, McIver KL, Sagatov RD, Arteaga SS, Frongillo EA. Weight status measures collected in the healthy communities study: protocols and analyses. Am J Prev Med. 2015 Oct;49(4):642–6. https://doi.org/10.1016/j.amepre.2015.07.001.
12. Strauss WJ, Sroka CJ, Frongillo EA, Arteaga SS, Loria CM, Leifer ES, et al. Statistical design features of the healthy communities study. Am J Prev Med. 2015 Oct;49(4):624–30. https://doi.org/10.1016/j.amepre.2015.06.021.

13. Pate RR, McIver K, Colabianchi N, Richard TP, Jared RP, Dianna CD, et al. Physical activity measures in the healthy communities study. Am J Prev Med. 2015 Oct;49(4):653–9. https://doi.org/10.1016/j.amepre.2015.06.020.
14. Arteaga S, Loria C, Crawford P, Fawcett SB, Fishbein HA, Gregoriou M, et al. The healthy communities study: its rationale, aims, and approach. Am J Prev Med. 2015 Oct;49(4):615–23. https://doi.org/10.1016/j.amepre.2015.06.029.
15. National Cancer Institute (NCI). Dietary screener questionnaire in the NHANES 2009–10: Data Processing & Score Procedures. http://epi.grants.cancer.gov/nhanes/dietscreen/scoring/. Updated October 15, 2015. Accessed July 12, 2016.
16. National Cancer Institute (NCI). Instructions for the Researcher Web site for: ASA24™-2014, ASA24™-Kids-2014, and ASA24™-Canada-2014. https://asa24.nci.nih.gov/researcherSite/assets-r/Researcher_Instructions.pdf#nameddest=DataAnalysisSection8. Updated March 2016. Accessed July 12, 2016.
17. Baranowski T, Islam N, Douglass D, Dadabhoy H, Beltran A, Baranowski J, et al. Food intake recording software system, version 4 (FIRSSt4): a self-completed 24-h dietary recall for children. J Hum Nutr Diet 2014 Jan;27 Suppl 1:66–71. doi: https://doi.org/10.1111/j.1365-277X.2012.01251.x. Epub 2012 May 23.
18. United States Department of Agriculture (USDA). AMPM - USDA Automated Multiple-Pass Method. http://www.ars.usda.gov/Services/docs.htm?docid=7710#what. Updated October 2, 2014. Accessed August 19, 2016.
19. National Cancer Institute (NCI). ASA24™-Kids 2014 and ASA24™-Kids 2012. http://epi.grants.cancer.gov/asa24/respondent/childrens.html?&url=/asa24/respondent/childrens.html. Updated March 29, 2016. Accessed July 12, 2016.
20. National Cancer Institute (NCI). ASA24™. http://epi.grants.cancer.gov/asa24/. Updated July 6, 2016. Accessed July 12, 2016.
21. Conway JM, Ingwersen LA, Vinyard BT, Moshfegh AJ. Effectiveness of the US Department of Agriculture 5-step multiple-pass method in assessing food intake in obese and nonobese women. Am J Clin Nutr. 2003 May;77(5):1171–8.
22. Freedman LS, Carroll RJ, Wax Y. Estimating the relation between dietary intake obtained from a food frequency questionnaire and true average intake. Am J Epidemiol. 1991;134:310–20.
23. Thompson FE, Midthune D, Subar AF, Kahle LL, Schatzkin A, Kipnis V. Performance of a short tool to assess dietary intakes of fruits and vegetables, percentage energy from fat and fibre. Public Health Nutr. 2004 Dec;7(8):1097–105.
24. Thompson FE, Lamphiear DE, Metzner HL, Hawthorne VM, Oh MS. Reproducibility of reports of frequency of food use in the Tecumseh diet methodology study. Am J Epidemiol. 1987 Apr;125(4):658–71.
25. Baranowski T, Islam N, Baranowski J, Martin S, Beltran A, Dadabhoy H, et al. Comparison of a web-based versus traditional diet recall among children. J Acad Nutr Diet 2012 Apr;112(4):527–532. doi: https://doi.org/10.1016/j.jada.2011.10.002. Epub 2012 Feb 1.
26. Livingstone M, Robson P, Wallace J. Issues in dietary intake assessment of children and adolescents. Br J Nutr. 2004;92(Suppl 2):S213–22.
27. Freedman LS, Commins JM, Moler JE, Arab L, Baer DJ, Kipnis V, et al. Pooled results from 5 validation studies of dietary self-report instruments using recovery biomarkers for energy and protein intake. Am J Epidemiol 2014 Jul 15;180(2):172–188. doi: https://doi.org/10.1093/aje/kwu116. Epub 2014 Jun 10.
28. Burrows TL, Martin RJ, Collins CE. A systematic review of the validity of dietary assessment methods in children when compared with the method of doubly labeled water. J Am Diet Assoc 2010 Oct;110(10):1501–10. doi: https://doi.org/10.1016/j.jada.2010.07.008. Review.
29. Magarey A, Watson J, Golley RK, Burrows T, Sutherland R, McNaughton SA, et al. Assessing dietary intake in children and adolescents: considerations and recommendations for obesity research. Int J Pediatr Obes 2011 Feb;6(1):2–11. doi: https://doi.org/10.3109/17477161003728469. Epub 2010 Sep 28.
30. Freisling H, van Bakel MM, Biessy C, May AM, Byrnes G, Norat T, et al. Dietary reporting errors on 24 h recalls and dietary questionnaires are associated with BMI across six European countries as evaluated with recovery biomarkers for protein and potassium intake. Br J Nutr 2012 Mar;107(6):910–920. doi: https://doi.org/10.1017/S0007114511003564. Epub 2011 Jul 27.
31. Kristal AR, Feng Z, Coates RJ, Oberman A, George V. Associations of race/ethnicity, education, and dietary intervention with the validity and reliability of a food frequency questionnaire: the Women's Health Trial Feasibility Study in Minority Populations. Am J Epidemiol. 1997;146(10):856–69 Erratum in: Am J Epidemiol 1998 Oct 15;148(8):820.
32. Mochari H, Gao Q, Mosca L. Validation of the MEDFICTS dietary assessment questionnaire in a diverse population. J Am Diet Assoc. 2008 May;108(5):817–22. https://doi.org/10.1016/j.jada.2008.02.021.
33. Mayer-Davis EJ, Vitolins MZ, Carmichael SL, Hemphill S, Tsaroucha G, Rushing J, et al. Validity and reproducibility of a food frequency interview in a multi-cultural epidemiology study. Ann Epidemiol. 1999 Jul;9(5):314–24.
34. Tucker KL, Bianchi LA, Maras J, Bermudez OI. Adaptation of a food frequency questionnaire to assess diets of Puerto Rican and non-Hispanic adults. Am J Epidemiol. 1998 Sep 1;148(5):507–18.
35. Champagne CM, Delany JP, Harsha DW, Bray GA. Underreporting of energy intake in biracial children is verified by doubly labeled water. J Am Diet Assoc. 1996;96:707–9.
36. Jaceldo-Siegl K, Knutsen SF, Sabaté J, Beeson WL, Chan J, Herring RP, et al. Validation of nutrient intake using an FFQ and repeated 24 h recalls in black and white subjects of the Adventist health Study-2 (AHS-2). Public health Nutr. 2010;13(6):812–9. https://doi.org/10.1017/S1368980009992072 Erratum in: Public Health Nutr 2011 Nov;14(11):2079–80.
37. Jaceldo-Siegl K, Fan J, Sabaté J, Knutsen SF, Haddad E, Beeson WL, et al. Race-specific validation of food intake obtained from a comprehensive FFQ: the Adventist health Study-2. Public health Nutr. 2011;14(11):1988–97. https://doi.org/10.1017/S1368980011000735 Erratum in: Public Health Nutr. 2012 Nov;15(11):2165–6.
38. Subar AF, Kipnis V, Troiano RP, Midthune D, Schoeller DA, Bingham S, et al. Using intake biomarkers to evaluate the extent of dietary misreporting in a large sample of adults: the observing protein and energy nutrition (OPEN) study. Am Journal of Epidemiol. 2003;158:1–13.
39. Tran KM, Johnson RK, Soultanakis RP, Matthews DE. In person vs telephone-administered multiple-pass 24-hour recalls in women: validation with doubly labeled water. J Am Diet Assoc. 2000;100:777–80 783.
40. Kipnis V, Subar AF, Midthune D, Freedman LS, Ballard-Barbash R, Troiano RP, et al. Structure of dietary measurement error: results of the OPEN biomarker study. Am J Epidemiol. 2003;158:14–21.
41. Park Y, Dodd KW, Kipnis V, Thompson FE, Potischman N, Schoeller DA, et al. Comparison of self-reported dietary intakes from the automated self-administered 24-h recall, 4-d food records, and food-frequency questionnaires against recovery biomarkers. Am J Clin Nutr. 2018;107(1):80–93. https://doi.org/10.1093/ajcn/nqx002.
42. Smith AF. Cognitive psychological issues of relevance to the validity of dietary reports. Eur J Clin Nutr. 1993;47(Suppl 2):S6–18 Review.
43. Smith AF, Baxter SD, Hitchcock DB, Finney CJ, Royer JA, Guinn CH. Cognitive ability, social desirability, body mass index and socioeconomic status as correlates of fourth-grade children's dietary-reporting accuracy. Eur J Clin Nutr 2016 Sep;70(9):1028–1033. doi: https://doi.org/10.1038/ejcn.2016.43. Epub 2016 May 25.

14

Higher dietary magnesium intake is associated with lower body mass index, waist circumference and serum glucose in Mexican adults

Analí Castellanos-Gutiérrez[1], Tania G. Sánchez-Pimienta[1], Alicia Carriquiry[2], Teresa H. M. da Costa[3] and Ana Carolina Ariza[4*]

Abstract

Background: Obesity and diabetes mellitus (DM) are public health concerns in Mexico of top-level priority due to their high prevalence and their growth rate in recent decades. The accumulation of adipose tissue leads to an unbalanced release of pro-oxidant factors, which causes cellular damage and favors the development of comorbidities. Recent evidence suggests that oxidative stress also promotes the accumulation of adipose tissue and the development of insulin resistance. The objective of this study is to evaluate the association between usual intake of antioxidant nutrients, specifically vitamins A, C, E and magnesium with body mass index (BMI), waist circumference (WC) and serum glucose concentrations in a representative sample of Mexican adults.

Methodology: We analyzed data on diet, BMI, WC and serum glucose from the Mexican National Health and Nutrition Survey 2012. Analysis included 20- to 65-year-old adults without a known diagnosis of DM ($n = 1573$). Dietary information was obtained using the five-step multiple-pass method developed by the United States Department of Agriculture and adapted to the Mexican context. Nutrient usual intake distributions were estimated using the Iowa State University method, through the "Software for Intake Distribution Estimation" (PC-Side) v.1.02. Associations were analyzed using multivariate regression models.

Results: Higher dietary magnesium intake was associated with lower markers of adiposity, so that an increase in 10 mg per 1000 kcal/day of magnesium was associated with an average decrease in BMI of 0.72% (95% CI: -1.36, – 0.08) and 0.49 cm (95% CI: -0.92, – 0.07) of WC. Additionally, in women with normal glucose concentrations, an increase in magnesium intake was associated with an average decrease in serum glucose by 0.59% (95% CI: -1.08, – 0.09).

Conclusion: The results suggest that magnesium intake is associated with lower BMI, WC and serum glucose in Mexican population. However, more studies are required to elucidate the nature of this association.

Keywords: Obesity, Magnesium, Glucose, Mexico, Adult

* Correspondence: carolina.ariza@insp.mx
[4]National Council of Science and Technology (CONACYT) - Center for Nutrition and Health Research, National Institute of Public Health, Cuernavaca, Morelos, Mexico

Background

Obesity and its comorbidities, including diabetes mellitus (DM), are public health concerns worldwide. In the last decades, they received top-level priority due to their high prevalence and speed of growth [1]. In Mexico, in the year 2016, the estimated prevalence of overweight and obesity in adults was 72.5%, showing a marked increase from a prevalence of 56% in the year 2000 [2, 3]. Furthermore, unpublished data estimated that in 2012, 22% of the Mexican adult population were glucose intolerant, and 13% of women and 14% of men had DM [S. Villalpando, personal communication, January 2018].

The accumulation of adipose tissue favors the presence of systemic oxidative stress (OS), which can be a trigger for the development of alterations in glucose metabolism [4–8]. However, recent evidence suggests that this mechanism may also occur inversely, where OS can favor the accumulation of adipose tissue. It has been observed that treatment with antioxidant nutrients prevents in vitro formation of adipocytes from pre-adipocytes [9], and in animal models prevents the excessive accumulation of adipose tissue associated with diet [10, 11]. In addition, OS causes a disruption in the production of cytokines [4], which together with a high production of reactive oxygen species (ROS), decreases glucose uptake in muscular and adipose tissue [6, 7] and decreases insulin secretion in pancreatic beta cells [8].

Antioxidant nutrients mitigate the damage caused by OS through different mechanisms. Vitamin A inhibits lipid peroxidation by trapping free radicals in cell membranes [12], regulates leptin mRNA in adipose tissue and also exerts an inhibitory effect on adipogenesis [13]. Vitamin C is a redox catalyst that neutralizes ROS [14], while vitamin E in its alfa-tocopherol form reacts with ROS produced in lipid peroxidation, protecting the cell membranes [15, 16]. Magnesium is involved in energy metabolism since intracellular adenosine triphosphate (ATP) is in the form of ATP-Mg [17] and it is also a cofactor of several antioxidant enzymes, including superoxide dismutase (SOD), one of the most important antioxidant enzymes [17, 18].

According to the results from the 2012 Mexican National Health and Nutrition Survey (ENSANUT) there is a high prevalence of inadequate intake of several nutrients with antioxidant function including vitamin A, C, E and magnesium, in the adult Mexican population [19, 20]. However, this prevalence has not been characterized by body weight status or serum glucose concentrations in this population. Additionally, since previous studies have shown a relationship between antioxidant nutrients intake, adiposity and insulin resistance [10, 21–26], the objective of this study is to evaluate the association between dietary intake of vitamins A, C, E, magnesium, and body mass index (BMI), waist circumference (WC), and serum glucose concentrations in a representative sample of 20- to 65-year-old Mexican adults.

Methods

Study design

The ENSANUT 2012 is a population-based multistage probabilistic survey representative of the Mexican population at a national, regional and state level, for urban and rural areas. The main objective of the survey was to quantify the distribution of health and nutrition parameters among the Mexican population as well as their determinants. Information from 96,031 individuals belonging to 50,528 randomly selected households was collected by face-to-face interviews carried out between October 2011 and May 2012. The complete methodology has been previously described elsewhere [27].

Participants

For this study, we considered 20- to 65-year-old nonpregnant nonlactating participants with diet, serum glucose, and anthropometric information ($n = 1739$). Pregnant or lactating women were not included because their nutritional needs and body composition are different from the rest of the women. We excluded from the analysis subjects with low weight ($n = 14$), defined as a BMI < 18.5 kg/m^2, or with known diagnosis of DM ($n = 152$). The final study sample included 1573 participants. Reporting was conducted in accordance with the STROBE statement [see Additional file 1].

Diet

Detailed diet information was obtained with a 24-h dietary recall applied by trained personnel to a randomly selected subsample of ~11% ($n = 10,886$) of the total respondents of the ENSANUT 2012 using the five-step multiple-pass method developed by the United States Department of Agriculture (USDA) [28] and adapted to the Mexican context [29]. A second 24-h recall was applied to a ~ 9% ($n = 981$) random subsample. For this study, 9.3% ($n = 162$) of the 1573 participants answered a second 24-h recall. Interviews were performed between Monday and Sunday, and repeated measurements were obtained on non-consecutive days with an average of 2.4 (± 1.2) days between each other. The detailed methodology for the collection of dietary information is described elsewhere [29].

Intake of vitamins A, C, E and magnesium were estimated using the food composition table compiled by the National Institute of Public Health (INSP) of Mexico [30]. Nutrient intake values higher than 1.5 times the 99th percentile were considered excessive, for vitamin A ($n = 8$), vitamin C ($n = 9$), vitamin E ($n = 4$), and magnesium ($n = 3$), and were replaced with random values between the 95th percentile and 1.5 times de 99th percentile of a uniform distribution.

Anthropometric measurements

Information on weight, height and waist circumference measurements were obtained by trained and standardized personnel using conventional and internationally accepted protocols [31, 32]. Height values between 1.3 and 2.0 m, and BMI values below 58 kg/m^2 were considered as valid data. All observations in the eligible sample were valid data. BMI categorization was based on the criterion proposed by the World Health Organization (WHO) [33]. The WC cut-off points used are the ones proposed by the International Diabetes Federation (IDF) (94 cm in men and 80 cm in women) [34].

Serum glucose

Serum glucose concentrations were analyzed in a sample of venous blood drawn from the antecubital vein and obtained after a minimum 8-h fast. It was collected in tubes without anticoagulant and was centrifuged in situ. Samples were stored in cryovials, placed in liquid nitrogen and stored at − 70 °C until assay. Measurements were performed at the laboratory of the Center for Nutrition and Health Research, INSP using an automatized glucose oxidase method performed in an Abbot ARCHITECT Analyzer.

Categorization was performed using the cut-off points proposed by the American Diabetes Association (ADA), which establish that concentrations between 40 and < 100 mg/dL are normal, 100 to < 126 mg/dL indicate glucose intolerance, and ≥ 126 mg/dL indicate DM [35]. To improve precision on the estimates for the prevalence of inadequate intake of nutrients, we combined categories of glucose intolerance and DM into one category of impaired glucose intolerance (serum glucose ≥100 mg/dL).

Physical activity

Physical activity was measured using the validated short form of the International Physical Activity Questionnaire (IPAQ-SF), which includes 9 items that collect information about frequency, duration and intensity of physical activity [36, 37]. An individual estimate of minutes per week of moderate physical activity was obtained adding the reported time spent doing moderate activity and two times the reported time doing vigorous activity. Based on the WHO recommendations for physical activity [38], participants were categorized as active (≥ 300 min per week), moderately active (150 to < 300), and inactive (< 150 min per week).

Statistical analysis

Nutrient usual intake distributions were estimated using the Iowa State University (ISU) method, through the "Software for Intake Distribution Estimation" (PC-Side) v.1.02. This method eliminates the effect of day-to-day variability in intake of each person, which results in a more accurate estimate of the prevalence of nutrient inadequacy. Intakes below the estimated average requirement (EAR) [39, 40] established by the Institute of Medicine of the United States [41–43] were considered to be inadequate.

Differences in prevalence of inadequate intake of nutrients between men and women and between groups defined by BMI, WC and serum glucose were analyzed performing Z-tests. Null hypotheses were rejected at an α level of 0.05 and Bonferroni corrections for multiple comparisons were applied for BMI groups.

The association between usual nutrient intake and adiposity was evaluated using multivariate multiple regression models, with BMI and WC as outcome variables, and adjusted for sex, age, physical activity and energy intake (kcal/day). The association between nutrient intake and serum glucose was evaluated using multiple regression and adjusted for sex, age, energy intake and BMI. Since BMI and serum glucose did not follow a normal distribution they were transformed to a logarithmic scale. The method used to adjust for energy intake was a multivariate model of nutrient density [44], which considers nutrient density and total energy intake as predictors. Nutrient density is defined as units of the nutrient per kcal of total energy intake.

Nutrient and energy intake for each person were adjusted by measurement error using the ISU method to obtain the best linear unbiased predictor (BLUP) of each person's intake using PC-Side. Nutrient density was estimated from the ratio of the adjusted values of nutrient intake to energy intake and then multiplied by 100 to improve interpretability. These estimates as well as the BLUPs for energy intake were used in the regression models in place of the unobservable usual intakes.

The descriptive statistics of the study sample and the regression models to evaluate association were fitted using the Data Analysis and Statistical Software STATA v. 13.0. For the multivariate regression and all analysis using PC-Side we considered the sampling weight of each individual. For the descriptive statistics and the multiple regression analysis we considered the sampling weight, sampling strata and primary sample unit to adjust for the complex survey design of the ENSANUT.

Results

Characteristics of the study population are shown in Table 1. Our study sample included 1573 subjects, 46% male and 54% female, who together represent more than 37.5 million Mexican adults between the ages of 20 to 65 years. The observed prevalence of overweight was 39% while obesity was 30%, the latter being higher in women (38%) than in men (21%). Serum glucose concentrations compatible with alterations in glucose metabolism were observed in 28% of individuals (24% with glucose intolerance and 4% with DM).

Table 1 Anthropometric characteristics and serum glucose concentrations of 20- to 65-year-old Mexican adults[a]

	Men	Women	Total	N[b]
	n (%)	n (%)	n (%)	
Age (years)				
20–29	149 (31)	197 (22)	346 (27)	9,984,522
30–39	158 (23)	304 (30)	462 (26)	9,942,045
40–49	142 (21)	217 (25)	359 (23)	8,677,882
50–65	190 (25)	216 (23)	406 (24)	8,992,607
BMI				
Normal weight	216 (38)	222 (24)	438 (31)	11,582,022
Overweight	273 (41)	349 (38)	622 (39)	14,805,842
Obese	150 (21)	363 (38)	513 (30)	11,209,192
WC (cm)				
< 94 (men)	344 (56)	146 (17)	490 (35)	13,130,382
< 80 (women)				
≥ 94 (men)	295 (44)	788 (83)	1083 (65)	24,466,675
≥ 80 (women)				
Serum glucose (mg/dL)				
40 - < 100	481 (76)	638 (68)	1119 (72)	26,893,750
100 - < 126	136 (20)	249 (27)	385 (24)	9,061,962
≥ 126	22 (4)	47 (5)	69 (4)	1,641,345
Total	639 (100)	934 (100)	1573 (100)	37,597,056

[a]Values are unweighted *n* and weighted percentages. Data are from the Mexican National Health and Nutrition Survey 2012
[b]Expanded *n*

Nutrient intake information from the total sample (consumers and non-consumers) was used to obtain results. The observed prevalence of inadequate intake of nutrients with antioxidant function was 56% for vitamin A, 29% for vitamin C, 94% for vitamin E and 16% for magnesium (Fig. 1). We did not observe any significant difference between men and women. The mean and percentiles of the estimated usual intake of each nutrient in men and women are presented in an additional table [see Additional file 2].

There were no significant differences in the prevalence of inadequate intake between strata of BMI, WC, and serum glucose for any of the analyzed nutrients (Table 2). However, we did observe that the prevalence of inadequate intake of vitamins A and C tended to be lower among persons with higher BMI; in the case of magnesium, the association between BMI and intake appeared to be negative (Table 2).

A negative association was observed between the intake of magnesium and markers of adiposity, so that an increase of 10 mg per 1000 kcal/day of magnesium was associated with an average decrease in BMI of 0.72% (95% CI: -1.36, − 0.08) and 0.49 cm (95% CI: -0.92, − 0.07) of WC, adjusting by sex, age and energy intake (Table 3). Additionally, an increase in magnesium intake was also associated with an average decrease in serum glucose concentrations of 0.38% (95% CI: -0.74, − 0.02) only in individuals with normal glucose concentrations; when stratifying by sex, this association was only statistically significant in women (− 0.59, 95% CI: -1.08, − 0.09). There were no statistically significant associations between the intake of vitamins A, C, E, and BMI, WC, and serum glucose concentrations.

Discussion

This study analyzed the association between the dietary intake of nutrients with antioxidant function and markers of adiposity and serum glucose concentrations in Mexican adults 20 to 65 years of age. Increased magnesium intake was associated with lower BMI and lower WC. Additionally, increased magnesium intake was associated with lower serum glucose concentrations in individuals with normal glucose. To the best of our knowledge, this is the first study to describe the

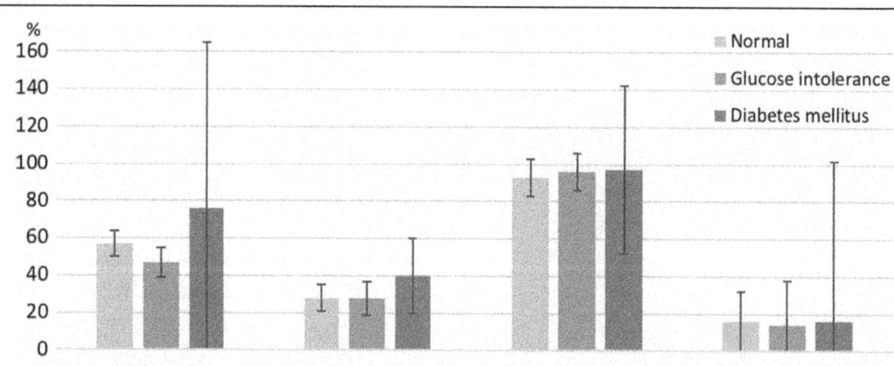

Fig. 1 Prevalence of inadequate intake of antioxidant nutrients in Mexican adults by serum glucose concentrations[1.] [1]Analysis include 20- to 65-year-old adults. Data are from the Mexican National Health and Nutrition Survey 2012. Normal: 40 to < 100 mg/dL, glucose intolerance: 100 to < 126 mg/dL, diabetes mellitus: ≥126 mg/dL

Table 2 Prevalence of inadequate intake of antioxidant nutrients in 20- to 65-year-old Mexican adults[a]

	n	Vitamin A		Vitamin C		Vitamin E		Magnesium	
		%	SE	%	SE	%	SE	%	SE
BMI									
Normal weight	438	64	19	30	9	91	13	14	26
Overweight	622	54	16	28	11	95	11	15	27
Obese	513	52	4	27	7	95	13	20	16
WC (cm)									
< 94 (men)	490	65	16	28	9	90	14	16	31
< 80 (women)									
≥ 94 (men)	1083	53	4	28	7	95	9	16	14
≥ 80 (women)									
Serum glucose (mg/dL)									
40 - < 100	1119	57	7	28	7	93	10	16	16
≥ 100	454	49	5	29	8	96	11	15	22

[a]Values are percentages and standard error (SE). Data are from the Mexican National Health and Nutrition Survey (ENSANUT) 2012

prevalence of inadequate intake of nutrients with antioxidant function by BMI, WC and serum glucose categories and to evaluate the association between its intake and markers of adiposity and glucose metabolism in this population.

In line with previous reports in Mexican population [45], the prevalence of abdominal obesity in our sample was 65%, being particularly high in women (83%). Mexico has one of the highest reported prevalence of abdominal obesity in adults compared to other countries, such as the United States with 56% (46% in men and 65% in women) [46], Brazil with 30% (20% in men and 38% in women) [47], and China with 37% (28% in men and 46% in women) [48]. In Mexican women, this prevalence has risen from 83% in 2012 [45], to 88% in 2016 [2]. This results highlight the magnitude of the problem of obesity as a public health concern in Mexico.

We did not find significant differences in the prevalence of inadequate intake of nutrients among strata of BMI or WC. These results are in line with the findings of a study involving 580 Mexican women from rural communities, where it was observed that, despite the fact that overweight and obese women reported higher energy intake compared to normal weight women, their intake of vitamins A, C and E did not differ significantly between them [49]. In contrast, a cross-sectional study of 18,177 American adults reported a higher prevalence of inadequate intake of several nutrients, including vitamins A, C, E and magnesium, in obese and overweight adults compared to non-obese [50]. This contrast could be explained because in this study we did not take into account the intake of dietary supplements, hence, total nutrient intake may be underestimated, particularly in normal weight individuals since supplement users are more likely to also have a healthier diet [51]. However, the discrepancies could also be explained by a lack of statistical power in this study sufficient to detect significant differences due to a smaller sample size or a greater variance in the usual intake distribution for the Mexican adults.

Consistent with our findings, other studies have also reported an inverse association between magnesium intake and markers of adiposity. A prospective study following 4637 young American adults found an inverse association between magnesium intake and WC [52]. Additionally, a cross-sectional study involving 11,686 American women found an inverse association between magnesium intake and BMI [53]. However, clinical studies evaluating the effect of magnesium supplementation on the accumulation of adipose tissue are still lacking. In animal models, it has been observed that magnesium supplementation prevents the accumulation of adipose tissue associated with diet [22]. The mechanism that explains this association is not yet fully understood. While one of the functions of magnesium is its antioxidant effect through enzymatic mechanisms, the role of OS in the development of obesity is still unclear.

Furthermore, several studies have reported that a lower magnesium intake is associated with an increased risk of insulin resistance [23, 52-54]. A prospective study that followed more than fifty thousand men and women from the United States over a period of 12–18 years

Table 3 Association between the intake of antioxidant nutrients, BMI, WC and glucose concentrations in Mexican adults[a]

Nutrient intake[d] (× 100 kcal/d)	BMI[b] (%)			WC[b] (cm)			Glucose[c] (%)		
	β	IC 95%		β	IC 95%		β	IC 95%	
Vitamin A (RAE)	−0.06	− 0.41	0.28	− 0.04	−0.28	0.20	−0.04	− 0.24	0.16
Vitamin C (mg)	0.36	−0.72	1.45	0.32	−0.39	1.02	−0.01	−0.58	0.56
Vitamin E (mg)	−0.32	−29.86	29.22	−10.22	−29.78	9.34	6.77	−13.70	27.24
Magnesium (mg)	−0.72*	− 1.36	−0.08	− 0.49*	− 0.92	−0.07	− 0.38*	− 0.74	−0.02

[a]Data are from the Mexican National Health and Nutrition Survey (ENSANUT) 2012. BMI: body mass index, WC: waist circumference, RAE: retinol activity equivalent
[b]Total sample (n = 1573). Multivariate regression analysis; adjusted by sex, age, physical activity and energy intake
[c]Only individuals with normal serum glucose concentrations (< 100 mg/dL) (n = 1119). Multiple regression analysis; adjusted by sex, age, energy intake, and BMI
[d]Nutrient intake per 100 kcal of energy intake = (nutrient intake / energy intake) × 100
*$p < 0.05$

found an inverse association between magnesium intake and the risk of developing DM [23]. A recent review identified seven randomized controlled studies (conducted between 1989 and 2014) that evaluated the effect of magnesium supplementation on fasting plasma glucose in prediabetic patients [55]: five studies reported a decrease in fasting plasma glucose after supplementation, while two studies reported no changes. In this study, the association between magnesium intake and serum glucose was only observed in women with normal glucose concentrations. An explanation as to why this association was not observed in glucose intolerants and diabetics could be that in DM, renal excretion of magnesium is increased [56], therefore diabetics may need a higher intake of magnesium to achieve the same concentrations as non-diabetics. The discrepant results between men and women are similar to the findings from a cohort of Japanese adults, in which during a follow-up of 10 years, a higher intake of magnesium was associated with a significantly reduced risk of DM only in women [57]. While the explanation is still not clear, there is evidence that women tend to have lower blood magnesium concentrations than men [58, 59], and thus would be more likely to be deficient and present adverse consequences, including a disrupted glucose metabolism. Additionally, the metabolic pathways involved in the association between magnesium and glucose metabolism may be different between men and women and might be attributed, at least in part, to differences in body composition, such as muscle mass.

This study has several strengths. The data are representative of the Mexican population 20 to 65 years of age. Diet was assessed using the five-step multiple-pass 24-h recall, which more accurately quantifies nutrient intake compared to other dietary assessment instruments [60]. Finally, we used cutting edge statistical methods to estimate usual intake of nutrients, allowing a better estimation of the prevalence of inadequate intake in the groups we considered, by adjusting the distribution of observed intake for within-person variability. However, the standard errors of the quantile estimates obtained using the ISU methodology were approximated using Taylor linearization which only considered the weighting of each individual on the survey and did not consider the strata and the primary sample unit to adjust for the complex survey design of the ENSANUT.

As is the case with any study that relies on self-reported food intake, one limitation is the potential reporting bias that exists with any instrument used to assess diet. It is well known that obese people have a tendency to underreport energy [61], but it is not well understood whether this underreporting is uniform across all dietary components [62, 63]. Since nutrient intake depends on the type of food consumed and not only on the amount of energy consumed, it is still unknown how under-reporting affects the report of specific nutrients. In addition, since this is an observational cross-sectional study, it is not possible to establish causality, for which longitudinal randomized trials are required to confirm these results.

Methods to estimate usual intake distributions rely heavily on the proportion of the variance in intake that is attributable to within-person variability. Most nationwide food consumption surveys (including ENSANUT) collect a second recall on a sub-sample of persons, which affects the precision of the within-person estimates. In our case, the estimated within-person variance in magnesium and vitamin A intake in males was implausibly high, and this had an effect on the accuracy in the prevalence of inadequate intake in these groups. However, a separate analysis using nutrient intake only from the first 24-h recall showed that the direction of the association was maintained and the effect size was attenuated but still significant [see Additional file 3].

Understanding the effect of the intake of a specific nutrient on some health outcome has important biological limitations because diet is a complex entity and there is high correlation and interaction between different nutrients or conditions that can affect their bioavailability. However, considering these limitations, it is striking to observe a strong association between magnesium intake and BMI, WC, and serum glucose concentrations.

On the other hand, we did not observe an association between intake of the rest of the analyzed nutrients and the conditions we considered. The high prevalence of inadequate intake observed, particularly for vitamins A and E, indicates that it is likely that we will observe a high proportion of individuals with deficiencies in the population. Therefore, a possible explanation for the lack of association between intake and health response could be the existence of a threshold above which these nutrients begin to affect the accumulation of adipose tissue and alterations in glucose metabolism. In addition, obese individuals may require a higher intake of antioxidants to achieve the same serum concentrations as normal weight individuals [64] as an increased OS is associated with increased metabolic utilization of antioxidant factors [65, 66]. Finally, the characteristics of vitamin A and E in the diet have to be considered. Vitamin A is a lipid-soluble vitamin found in specific food types that can be consumed sporadically; and oil, an important source of vitamin E, is difficult to quantify. Thus, these nutrients are not fully represented with only two non-consecutive days of intake observations [39, 41, 42]. Furthermore, magnesium may have an effect on adiposity and serum glucose concentrations through other mechanisms not involved in OS, since in addition to its antioxidant function, it is also involved in energy metabolism [17].

Conclusion

The results of this study suggest that increased dietary magnesium intake is associated with lower BMI and WC. In women without impaired glucose metabolism, it is also associated with lower serum glucose concentrations. These results highlight the importance of an adequate dietary magnesium intake. However, more studies are needed to elucidate the nature of this association.

Additional files

Additional file 1: Table S1. STROBE-nut: An extension of the STROBE statement for nutritional epidemiology. STROBE and STROBE-nut recommendations, and page(s) number(s) of the manuscript were information on each item can be found.

Additional file 2: Table S2. Distribution of usual intake of antioxidant nutrients in 20- to 65-year-old Mexican adults. Mean and percentiles of usual intake of vitamins A, C, E, and magnesium in men and women.

Additional file 3: Table S3. Association between intake of antioxidant nutrients, BMI, WC and glucose concentrations in 20- to 65-year-old Mexican adults. Association between intake of antioxidant nutrients, BMI, WC and glucose concentrations, using information from one 24-h recall.

Abbreviations

ATP: Adenosine Triphosphate; BLUP: Best Linear Unbiased Predictor; BMI: Body Mass Index; CONACYT: National Council of Science and Technology; DM: Diabetes Mellitus; EAR: Estimated Average Requirement; ENSANUT: National Health And Nutrition Survey; IDF: International Diabetes Federation; INSP: National Institute Of Public Health; ISU: Iowa State University; OS: Oxidative Stress; PC-Side: Software For Intake Distribution Estimation; ROS: Reactive Oxygen Species; SOD: Superoxide Dismutase; USDA: United States Department Of Agriculture; WC: Waist Circumference; WHO: World Health Organization

Acknowledgments

Not applicable.

Funding

CONACYT contributed with travel expenses for ACG to work with AC and THM at ISU for a period of six weeks.

Authors' contributions

ACA conceived the study; ACA, ACG, and TGSP designed the study; ACG wrote the first draft of the manuscript and analyzed data; AC, THM and TGSP contributed to the data analysis; ACA, TGSP, AC, and THM reviewed the manuscript. All authors read and approved the final manuscript.

Competing interests

All authors declare that they have no competing interests.

Author details

[1]Center for Nutrition and Health Research, National Institute of Public Health, Mexico. Av. Universidad 655, Col. Santa María Ahuacatitlán. Cerrada los pinos y caminera. C.P, 62100 Cuernavaca, Morelos, Mexico. [2]Department of Statistics, Iowa State University, Ames, Iowa 50011, USA. [3]Department of Nutrition, School of Health Science, University of Brasilia, Brasilia - DF, CEP 70910-900, Brazil. [4]National Council of Science and Technology (CONACYT) - Center for Nutrition and Health Research, National Institute of Public Health, Cuernavaca, Morelos, Mexico.

References

1. Trends in adult body-mass index in 200 countries from 1975 to 2014. A pooled analysis of 1698 population-based measurement studies with 19.2 million participants. Lancet. 2016;387(10026):1377–96.
2. Instituto Nacional de Salud Pública. Encuesta Nacional de Salud y Nutrición de Medio Camino 2016. Informe de resultados, vol. 68-72. México; 2016. p. 46.
3. Barquera Simón, Campos-Nonato Ismael, Hernández-Barrera Lucía, Pedroza Adolfo, Rivera-Dommarco Juan A. Prevalencia de obesidad en adultos mexicanos, 2000–2012. Salud pública Méx. 2013;55 Suppl 2:S151-S160.
4. Furukawa S, Fujita T, Shimabukuro M, Iwaki M, Yamada Y, Nakajima Y, et al. Increased oxidative stress in obesity and its impact on metabolic syndrome. J Clin Investig. 2004;114(12):1752–61.
5. Matsuda M, Shimomura I. Increased oxidative stress in obesity: implications for metabolic syndrome, diabetes, hypertension, dyslipidemia, atherosclerosis, and cancer. Obesity Research & Clinical Practice. 2013;7(5): e330–41.
6. Maddux B, See W, Lawrence J, Goldfine A, Goldfine I, Evans J. Protection against oxidative stress--induced insulin resistance in rat L6 muscle cells by micromolar concentrations of -lipoic acid. Diabetes. 2001;50(2):404–10.
7. Rudich A, Tirosh A, Potashnik R, Hemi R, Kanety H, Bashan N. Prolonged oxidative stress impairs insulin-induced GLUT4 translocation in 3T3-L1 adipocytes. Diabetes. 1998;47(10):1562–9.
8. Matsuoka T, Kajimoto Y, Watada H, Kaneto H, Kishimoto M, Umayahara Y, et al. Glycation-dependent, reactive oxygen species-mediated suppression of the insulin gene promoter activity in HIT cells. J Clin Investig. 1997;99(1): 144–50.
9. Cho K. lipoic acid inhibits adipocyte differentiation by regulating pro-adipogenic transcription factors via mitogen-activated protein kinase pathways. J Biol Chem. 2003;278(37):34823–33.
10. Sen Simmons R. Maternal antioxidant supplementation prevents adiposity in the offspring of Western diet-fed rats. Diabetes. 2010;59(12):3058–65.
11. Berniakovich I, Trinei M, Stendardo M, Migliaccio E, Minucci S, Bernardi P, et al. p66Shc-generated oxidative signal promotes fat accumulation. J Biol Chem. 2008;283(49):34283–93.
12. Palozza P, Krinsky N. β-Carotene and α-tocopherol are synergistic antioxidants. Arch Biochem Biophys. 1992;297(1):184–7.
13. Jeyakumar SVajreswari A. Vitamin a as a key regulator of obesity & its associated disorders: evidences from an obese rat model. Indian J Med Res. 2015;141(3):275.
14. Padayatty S, Katz A, Wang Y, Eck P, Kwon O, Lee J, et al. Vitamin C as an antioxidant: evaluation of its role in disease prevention. J Am Coll Nutr. 2003;22(1):18–35.
15. Herrera E, Barbas C. Vitamin E: action, metabolism and perspectives. J Physiol Biochem. 2001;57(1):43–56.
16. Traber M, Atkinson J. Vitamin E, antioxidant and nothing more. Free Radic Biol Med. 2007;43(1):4–15.
17. Morais J, Severo J, Santos L, de Sousa Melo S, de Oliveira Santos R, de Oliveira A, et al. Role of magnesium in oxidative stress in individuals with obesity. Biol Trace Elem Res. 2016;176(1):20–6.
18. Insel P, Ross D, McMahon K, Bernstein M. Discovering nutrition. 4th ed. Burlington, MA, USA: Jones & Bartlett Learning; 2003.
19. Pedroza-Tobías A, Hernández-Barrera L, López-Olmedo N, García-Guerra A, Rodríguez-Ramírez S, Ramírez-Silva I, Villalpando S, Carriquiry A, Rivera JA. Usual vitamin intakes by Mexican population. J Nutr. 2016;146(Suppl):1866S–73S.
20. Sanchez-Pimienta T, Lopez-Olmedo N, Rodriguez-Ramirez S, Garcia-Guerra A, Rivera J, Carriquiry A, et al. High prevalence of inadequate calcium and Iron intakes by Mexican population groups as assessed by 24-hour recalls. J Nutr. 2016;146(9):1874S–80S.
21. Hosseini B, Saedisomeolia A, Allman-Farinelli M. Association between antioxidant intake/status and obesity: a systematic review of observational studies. Biol Trace Elem Res. 2016;175(2):287–97.
22. Devaux S, Adrian M, Laurant P, Berthelot A, Quignard-Boulangé A. Dietary magnesium intake alters age-related changes in rat adipose tissue cellularity. Magnes Res. 2016;29(4):175–83.
23. Lopez-Ridaura R, Willett W, Rimm E, Liu S, Stampfer M, Manson J, et al. Magnesium intake and risk of type 2 diabetes in men and women. Diabetes Care. 2003;27(1):134–40.
24. Moctezuma-Velázquez C, Gómez-Sámano M, Cajas-Sánchez M, Reyes-Molina D, Galindo-Guzmán M, Meza-Arana C, et al. High dietary magnesium intake is significantly and independently associated with higher insulin sensitivity

in a Mexican-mestizo population: a brief cross-sectional report. Rev Investig Clin. 2017;69(1).
25. Gao M, Zhao Z, Lv P, Li Y, Gao J, Zhang M, et al. Quantitative combination of natural anti-oxidants prevents metabolic syndrome by reducing oxidative stress. Redox Biol. 2015;6:206–17.
26. Sales C, Santos A, Cintra D, Colli C. Magnesium-deficient high-fat diet: effects on adiposity, lipid profile and insulin sensitivity in growing rats. Clin Nutr. 2014;33(5):879–88.
27. Romero-Martínez M, Shamah-Levy T, Franco-Nunez A, Villalpando S, Cuevas-Nasu L, Gutierrez JP, Rivera-Dommarco JA. National Health and nutrition survey 2012: design and coverage. Salud Publica Mex. 2013;55(Suppl 2): S332–40 (in Spanish).
28. Blanton CA, Moshfegh AJ, Baer DJ, Kretsch MJ. The USDA automated multiple-pass method accurately estimates group total energy and nutrient intake. J Nutr. 2006;136:2594–9.
29. López-Olmedo N, Carriquiry AL, Rodríguez-Ramírez S, Ramírez-Silva I, Espinosa-Montero J, Hernández-Barrera L, Campirano F, Martínez-Tapia B, Rivera JA. Usual intake of added sugars and saturated fats is high while dietary fiber is low in Mexican population. J Nutr. 2016;146(Suppl):1856S–65S.
30. Instituto Nacional de Salud Pública. Bases de datos del valor nutritivo de los alimentos. Compilación del Instituto Nacional de Salud Pública. Cuernavaca,México: Instituto Nacional de Salud Publica; 2012.
31. Lohman TG, Roche AF, Martorell R. Anthropometric standardization reference manual. Champaign, IL: Human Kinetics Publishers; 1988.
32. Habicht JP. Standardization of quantitative epidemiological methods in the field. Bol Oficina Sanit Panam. 1974;76(5):375–84.
33. WHO. Physical status: The use and interpretation of anthropometry. Report of a WHO expert committee. WHO technical report series 854. Geneva: World Health Organization; 1995.
34. Zimmet P, Alberti K. Introduction: globalization and the non-communicable disease epidemic. Obesity. 2006;14(1):1–3.
35. Diagnosis and Classification of Diabetes Mellitus. Diabetes Care 2010; 34(Supplement_1): S62.
36. Craig CL, Marshall AL, Sjostrom M, Bauman AE, Booth ML, Ainsworth BE, et al. International physical activity questionnaire: 12-country reliability and validity. Med Sci Sports Exerc. 2003;35(8):1381–95.
37. Medina C, Barquera S, Janssen I. Validity and Reliability of the International Physical Activity Questionnaire Among Mexicans. Kingston and National Institute of Public Health. Cuernavaca. Research Report: Queens University; 2012.
38. WHO. Global recommendations on physical activity for health. Switzerland: Geneva; 2010.
39. Shils M, Olson J, Shike M. Modern nutrition in health and disease. Philadelphia: Lea & Febiger; 1994. Criteria of an adequate diet.
40. Carriquiry A. Assessing the prevalence of nutrient inadequacy. Public Health Nutr. 1999;2(01).
41. Dietary reference intakes for vitamin A, vitamin K, arsenic, boron, chromium, copper, iodine, iron, manganese, molybdenum, nickel, silicon, vanadium, and zinc. Washington, D.C.: National Academy Press; 2002.
42. Dietary reference intakes for vitamin C, vitamin E, selenium, and carotenoids. Washington, D.C.: National Academy Press; 2000.
43. Dietary reference intakes for calcium, phosphorus, magnesium, vitamin D, and fluoride. Washington. D.C.: National Academy Press; 1999.
44. Willet WC, Howe GR, Kushi LW. Adjustment for total energy intake in epidemiologic studies. Am J Clin Nutr l997:65(suppl):1220S–8S.
45. Barquera S, Campos-Nonato I, Hernández-Barrera L, Pedroza A, Rivera-Dommarco JA. Prevalence of obesity in Mexican adults, 2000–2012. Salud Pública Méx. 2013;55(2):S151–60.
46. Beltrán-Sánchez H, Harhay MO, Harhay MM, McElligott S. Prevalence and trends of metabolic syndrome in the adult US population, 1999–2010. J Am Coll Cardiol. 2013;62(8):697–703. https://doi.org/10.1016/j.jacc.2013.05.064.
47. Linhares RS, Horta BL, Gigante DP, Dias-da-Costa JS, Olinto MTA. Distribution of general and abdominal obesity in adults in a city in southern Brazil. Cad Saúde Pública. 2012;28(3):438–47. https://doi.org/10.1590/S0102-311X2012000300004.
48. Xi B, Liang Y, He T. Secular trends in the prevalence of general and abdominal obesity among Chinese adults, 1993–2009. Obes Rev. 2012;13(3): 287–96. https://doi.org/10.1111/j.1467-789X.2011.00944.
49. García O, Ronquillo D, Caamaño M, Camacho M, Long K, Rosado J. Zinc, vitamin a, and vitamin C status are associated with leptin concentrations and obesity in Mexican women: results from a cross-sectional study. Nutrition & Metabolism. 2012;9(1):59.
50. Agarwal S, Reider C, Brooks J, Fulgoni V. Comparison of prevalence of inadequate nutrient intake based on body weight status of adults in the United States: an analysis of NHANES 2001–2008. J Am Coll Nutr. 2015;34(2): 126–34.
51. Sebastian RS, Cleveland LE, Goldman JD, Moshfegh AJ. Older adults who use vitamin/mineral supplements differ from nonusers in nutrient intake adequacy and dietary attitudes. J Am Diet Assoc. 2007;107:1322–32.
52. He K. Magnesium intake and incidence of metabolic syndrome among young adults. Circulation. 2006;113(13):1675–82.
53. Song Y, Ridker P, Manson J, Cook N, Buring J, Liu S. Magnesium intake, C-reactive protein, and the prevalence of metabolic syndrome in middle-aged and older U.S. women. Diabetes Care. 2005;28(6):1438–44.
54. Park S, Kim S, Bae Y. Relationship between serum calcium and magnesium concentrations and metabolic syndrome diagnostic components in middle-aged Korean men. Biol Trace Elem Res. 2011;146(1):35–41.
55. Mooren F. Magnesium and disturbances in carbohydrate metabolism. Diabetes Obes Metab. 2015;17(9):813–23.
56. Pham PC, Pham PA, Pham SV, Pham PT, Pham PM, Pham PT. Hypomagnesemia: a clinical perspective. Int J Nephrol Renovasc Dis. 2014;7:219–30.
57. Konishi K, Wada K, Tamura T, Tsuji M, Kawachi T, Nagata C. Dietary magnesium intake and the risk of diabetes in the Japanese community: results from the Takayama study. Eur J Nutr. 2015;56(2):767–74.
58. Sheehan JP. Magnesium deficiency and diabetes mellitus. Magnes Trace Elem. 1991–1992;10:215–9.
59. Ryschon TW, Rosenstein DL, Rubinow DR, Niemela JE, Elin RJ, Balaban RS. Relationship between skeletal muscle intracellular ionized magnesium and measurements of blood magnesium. J Lab Clin Med. 1996;127:207–13. https://doi.org/10.1016/S0022-2143(96)90080-3.
60. Schatzkin A, Kipnis V, Carroll R, Midthune D, Subar A, Bingham S, et al. A comparison of a food frequency questionnaire with a 24-hour recall for use in an epidemiological cohort study: results from the biomarker-based observing protein and energy nutrition (OPEN) study. Int J Epidemiol. 2003; 32(6):1054–62.
61. Orcholski L, Luke A, Plange-Rhule J, Bovet P, Forrester T, Lambert E, et al. Under-reporting of dietary energy intake in five populations of the African diaspora. Br J Nutr. 2015;113(03):464–72.
62. Lafay L, Mennen L, Basdevant A. Does energy intake underreporting involve all kinds of food or only specific food items? Results from the Fleurbaix Laventie Ville Santé (FLVS) study. Int J Obes Relat Metab Disord. 2000;24(11):1500–6.
63. Suchanek P, Poledne R, Hubacek JA. Dietary intake reports fidelity–fact or fiction? Neuro Endocrinol Lett. 2011;32(Suppl 2):29–31.
64. Vioque J, Weinbrenner T, Asensio L, Castelló A, Young I, Fletcher A. Plasma concentrations of carotenoids and vitamin C are better correlated with dietary intake in normal weight than overweight and obese elderly subjects. Br J Nutr. 2007;97(05):977.
65. Weinbrenner T, Schröder H, Escurriol V, Fito M, Elosua R, Vila J, Marrugat J, Covas M-I. Circulating oxidized LDL is associatedwith increased waist circumference independent of body mass index in men and women. Am J Clin Nutr. 2006;83(1):30–5.
66. Saedisomeolia A, Wood LG, Garg ML, Gibson PG, Wark PA. Supplementation of long chain N-3 polyunsaturated fatty acids increase the utilization of lycopene in cultured airway epithelial cells. J Food Lipids. 2008;15(4):421–32.

15

Association between empirically derived dietary patterns with blood lipids, fasting blood glucose and blood pressure in adults - the India migration study

Krithiga Shridhar[1†], Ambika Satija[2†], Preet K. Dhillon[1*], Sutapa Agrawal[1], Ruby Gupta[1], Liza Bowen[3], Sanjay Kinra[3], A. V. Bharathi[4], D. Prabhakaran[1,3,5], K. Srinath Reddy[6], Shah Ebrahim[3] and for the Indian Migration Study group

Abstract

Background: Dietary patterns (DPs) in India are heterogenous. To date, data on association of indigenous DPs in India with risk factors of nutrition-related noncommunicable diseases (cardiovascular disease and diabetes), leading causes of premature death and disability, are limited. We aimed to evaluate the associations of empirically-derived DPs with blood lipids, fasting glucose and blood pressure levels in an adult Indian population recruited across four geographical regions of India.

Methods: We used cross-sectional data from the Indian Migration Study (2005–2007). Study participants included urban migrants, their rural siblings and urban residents and their urban siblings from Lucknow, Nagpur, Hyderabad and Bangalore ($n = 7067$, mean age 40.8 yrs). Information on diet (validated interviewer-administered, 184-item semi-quantitative food frequency questionnaire), tobacco consumption, alcohol intake, physical activity, medical history, as well as anthropometric measurements were collected. Fasting-blood samples were collected for estimation of blood lipids and glucose. Principal component analysis (PCA) was used to identify major DPs based on eigenvalue> 1 and component interpretability. Robust standard error multivariable linear regression models were used to investigate the association of DPs (tertiles) with total cholesterol (TC), low density lipoprotein-cholesterol (LDL-C), high density lipoprotein-cholesterol (HDL-C), triglycerides, fasting-blood glucose (FBG), systolic and diastolic blood pressure (SBP and DBP) levels.

Results: Three major DPs were identified: 'cereal-savoury' (cooked grains, rice/rice-based dishes, snacks, condiments, soups, nuts), 'fruit-vegetable-sweets-snacks' (Western cereals, vegetables, fruit, fruit juices, cooked milk products, snacks, sugars, sweets) and 'animal food' (red meat, poultry, fish/seafood, eggs) patterns. High intake of the 'animal food' pattern was positively associated with levels of TC ($\beta = 0.10$ mmol/L; 95% CI: 0.02, 0.17 mmol/L; p-trend = 0.013); LDL-C ($\beta = 0.07$ mmol/L; 95% CI: 0.004, 0.14 mmol/L; p-trend = 0.041); HDL-C ($\beta = 0.02$ mmol/L; 95% CI: 0.004, 0.04 mmol/L; p-trend = 0.016), FBG: ($\beta = 0.09$ mmol/L; 95% CI: 0.01, 0.16 mmol/L; p-trend = 0.021) SBP ($\beta = 1.2$ mm/Hg; 95% CI: 0.1, 2.3 mm/Hg; p-trend = 0.032); DBP: ($\beta = 0.9$ mm/Hg; 95% CI: 0.2, 1.5 mm/Hg; p-trend = 0.013). The 'cereal-savoury' and 'fruit-vegetable-sweets-snacks' patterns showed no association with any parameter except for a positive association with diastolic blood pressure for high intake of 'fruits-vegetables-sweets-snacks' pattern.

(Continued on next page)

* Correspondence: preet.dhillon@phfi.org
†Equal contributors
[1]Centre for Chronic Conditions and Injuries, Public Health Foundation of India, Gurgaon, Haryana, India

(Continued from previous page)

Conclusion: Our results indicate positive associations of the 'animal food' pattern with cardio-metabolic risk factors in India. Further longitudinal assessments of dietary patterns in India are required to validate the findings.

Keywords: Lipids, Dietary patterns, Animal food, Fasting glucose, Indian migration study, India

Background

Cardiovascular disease (CVD) and type-II diabetes are major noncommunicable diseases (NCDs) accounting for 33.9% of total deaths [1] and 15.7% of all disability-adjusted life years-(DALY's) [2] in 2013 worldwide. Over three-quarters of deaths due to CVD and diabetes occur in low-middle income countries (LMICs) [3] where the probability of dying between ages 30 and 70 years due to NCD is greater than in developed countries (25–30% vs. 10–15%) [3]. Diet is a key modifiable determinant of CVD and type-II diabetes, and potentially influences risk of developing these diseases by modulating blood levels of lipids and fasting glucose as well as blood pressure, important proximal risk factors of CVD and type-II diabetes [4–8].

'Dietary patterns' describe the overall diet; i.e. the varied combinations of foods and nutrients consumed in totality by individuals [9, 10]. Conventionally, nutritional epidemiological studies evaluated associations of individual food components or nutrients with several health outcomes. 'Dietary pattern' studies are relatively a recent approach in nutritional epidemiology studying the cumulative influence of composite diet as a 'whole' on different health outcomes. This approach can better account for any residual confounding by other components or nutrients of diet, and also provides useful evidence for more practical and appropriate dietary recommendations that are likely to succeed in real circumstances [9, 10].

A variety of dietary patterns (DPs) have been evaluated for their effects on CVD risk and mortality and diabetes risk including Dietary Approaches to Stop Hypertension (DASH), prudent and vegetarian diets, as well as regional diets such as the Mediterranean diet, Japanese diet and 'Western' diet [4–8]. Appropriate dietary recommendations are frequently updated based on this evidence [11, 12]. Dietary and culinary cultures are heterogenous in India and there is continued high adherence to indigenous food patterns [13, 14] in spite of the nutrition transition [15]. Evidence from India regarding the role of different dietary patterns on blood lipids, fasting glucose and blood pressure levels is critical given rising death and disability due to cardiovascular disease (leading at 53% increase in deaths and 41.5% increase in pre-mature deaths recorded between years 2005 and 2016) and diabetes (9% increase in disability between years 2005 and 2016) [16]. Diet and associated high blood pressure, fasting glucose and total cholesterol are cited as the leading risk factors of NCDs [16]. However, studies based on Indian dietary patterns are limited to date [9, 10].

We examined the associations of empirically derived indigenous dietary patterns with cardio-metabolic risk factors i.e., blood lipids, fasting blood glucose and blood pressure levels in rural and urban Indians recruited across four geographic regions of the country [Lucknow, North India; Nagpur, Central India; Hyderabad, South-central India and Bangalore, South India] using data from the Indian Migration Study [17, 18].

Methods

Study design and participants

Cross-sectional data from the Indian Migration Study (2005–2007) have been used for this study. The Indian Migration Study (IMS) is a sib-pair study nested within the larger Cardiovascular Disease Risk Factor Study in industrial populations from 10 companies across India [19] with details of the study design and methods reported earlier [17, 18]. In brief, the IMS was carried out in factory settings located in four cities from northern (Lucknow), central (Nagpur), south-central (Hyderabad), and southern (Bangalore) India. Factory workers, who had migrated from rural to urban areas (mean duration of migration 20 years ±5.4SD) and their co-resident spouses, along with a 25% random sample of urban non-migrants and their co-resident spouses were invited to participate in the study. Each migrant and non-migrant participant was asked to identify a sibling residing in a rural or urban area respectively, preferably of the same gender and similar age, who was then again invited to participate. This resulted in drawing of rural and urban dwelling siblings from 18 states across India. Of the 7594 migrant and non-migrant factory workers and their co-resident spouses and rural or urban siblings eligible for the study, 7102 (94%) agreed to complete the clinical examination. The final sample included 3537 sib-pairs (7074 participants) who completed the field work and 7067 respondents were included in the analyses as seven participants did not complete their clinical examination and/or some section of questionnaires.

Description of predictor variables

An interviewer–administered questionnaire was used to collect information on diet, tobacco consumption, alcohol intake, physical activity and medical history in the local language. Anthropometric and physical measurements and fasting blood samples for measurement of blood lipid profiles and glucose levels were collected from participants. Standard of Living Index (SLI) was derived using a sub-set of questions on socio-economic position such as quality of house (kutcha (low quality)/ semi-pucca (partly low quality)/pucca (high quality)), toilet facilities, land ownership, sources of lighting and drinking water and possession of household articles (a total of 14 items). Physical activity was assessed in the past month for occupational, recreational, commuting and other common daily activities [20]. The frequency and average duration was collected for each activity to calculate metabolic equivalent tasks (METs), where 1 MET is equivalent to expending 1 kcal/kg/h, which corresponds to the resting metabolic rate of sitting quietly [20].

Dietary assessment

Diet was assessed using a validated interviewer-administered semi-quantitative food frequency questionnaire (FFQ) [21]. The FFQ collected information on portion size and frequency of 184 commonly consumed food items over the last 1 year. Standard portion size (e.g., tablespoon, ladle, and bowl) and frequency (daily, weekly, monthly, yearly/never) were recorded with the use of visual aids. A single FFQ was designed to cover dietary patterns across the four main regions of the study. Recipes were collected to generate databases of the food group composition of each food item across the four regions, and to calculate average daily food group intake. Nutrient databases were used to calculate the macro and micro-nutrient content of each recipe using Indian food composition tables [22] and the United States Department of Agriculture nutrient database (USDA, Release No. 14) [23] or McCance and Widdowson's Composition of Foods, [24] were used where nutrient values were unavailable from the Indian food composition tables. Total energy, protein, fat, fibre, iron, calcium, zinc, folate, vitamin C and B12 intakes were calculated. A sub-sample was re-interviewed after completion of the FFQ (1–2 months, $n = 185$ and 12 months later, $n = 305$), yielding kappa coefficients = 0.26–0.71, [21] which are similar to reliability estimates from other studies [25, 26]. Three 24-h recalls were implemented in a sub-sample of participants ($n = 530$, 53.9% male) to validate the FFQ. The energy adjusted spearman correlation coefficients for macro-nutrients ranged from 0.43 (fibre) to 0.52 (fats) based on comparisons of FFQ with 24-h recalls [21]. For the present study FFQ responses were complete for 7067 participants, 182 food items (2 food items, *bhagar* and *kesari bhath*, from the grains and sweets categories respectively, were removed due to a high number of missing values) were classified into 30 food groups on the basis of nutrient and culinary similarities (some individual foods such as plain rice, tea and coffee were retained as separate food groups), for identification of dietary patterns. The details have been published elsewhere [9].

Body mass index (BMI)

A digital personal scale (Beurer Model PS16, Ulm, Germany) accurate to 0.1 kg and stadiometer accurate to 1 mm (Leicester height measure (Chasmors Ltd. London UK) were used by trained personnel to record weight and height respectively of the participants in light indoor clothes without shoes [27].

Blood pressure

Blood pressure was measured on the right upper arm with the participant in the sitting position after a rest of 5 min. Two readings were taken using an appropriate-sized cuff connected to a digital device (model M5-I; Omron-Matsusaka Company, Matsusaka City, Japan). Hypertension included doctor-diagnosed disease and/or a systolic BP ≥ 140 mmHg or a diastolic BP ≥ 90 mmHg at the time of the interview. Diabetes included doctor-diagnosed disease and/or a fasting plasma glucose criterion of 7.0 mmol/l.

Biological outcome variables' assessment

Ten ml of fasting (> 8 h) blood sample was collected by trained phlebotomists at the field sites, centrifuged at 2500 rpm for 15 min to separate serum or plasma. After processing (within an hour of collection), samples were stored at -20 °C in deep freezers for two to 3 weeks at field sites, after which they were transported to the laboratory at the All India Institute of Medical Sciences (AIIMS), New Delhi where they were stored at -80 °C ultra low deep freezer for bio-chemical analyses. Serum high density lipoprotein cholesterol level was measured directly using the elimination method, total cholesterol level was measured using an enzymatic endpoint method, triglyceride level was measured using GPO-PAP method, and glucose was measured using the GOD-PAP method using kits from Randox Laboratory Ltd. (Crumlin City, United Kingdom). LDL-C was calculated using Friedewald formula [28]. LDL-C was calculated for participants with TG levels < 400 mg/dl. For participants with TG levels≥400 mg/dL ($N = 50$) LDL-C levels were treated as missing. As part of local internal quality control, duplicate assays were performed and evaluated by AIIMS. The cardiac-biochemistry laboratory was part of external quality assurance program (RIQAS) from Randox.

Statistical analysis

Principal components analysis (PCA) was used to identify major dietary patterns (DPs). The details of the statistical methods have been published in our earlier work

[9]. Principal components generated were rotated by an orthogonal rotation (varimax) to increase interpretability. An eigenvalue cut-off > 1, scree plot and component interpretability were used to decide the number of components to retain, which were labelled on the basis of meaningful interpretation of component loadings and previous literature. Component scores were then generated for each retained component for use in the final analysis, as follows: the intake of each food group (per day average consumption in g) was weighted by its appropriate component loading on a principal component, and all weighted intakes were then summed to obtain a component score for that principal component, for each individual. Thus, we identified three major dietary patterns in this population: 'cereal-savoury' 'fruit-vegetable-sweets-snacks' and 'animal food' patterns. Final analysis for lipid outcomes was based on 7067 participants aged 18 years and above. For further analysis on fasting blood glucose outcome, known diabetics ($n = 486$, 6.9%) were excluded as diagnosis with diabetes may change glucose levels and also dietary habits. Thus, this analysis was based on 6581 participants aged 18 years and above.

One-way ANOVA and Chi-square tests were used for descriptive analysis. Robust standard error multivariable linear regression models adjusting for age, sex, standard of living index (SLI) (continuous), education (categories; no formal education, primary school, secondary school and beyond secondary school), geographical region (Lucknow, Nagpur, Hyderabad and Bangalore), migration status (urban, rural and urban migrant), BMI (continuous), tobacco use (categories), alcohol consumption (categories), energy intake (continuous), physical activity (total METS), regular use of any medication (yes/no) were used to investigate the association of different dietary patterns (using tertiles as cut-off) with total cholesterol (TC), low density lipoprotein-cholesterol (LDL-C), high density lipoprotein-cholesterol (HDL-C), triglycerides (TG), fasting blood glucose (FBG) and blood pressure (systolic and diastolic) levels at the significance level of 5%. All statistical analyses were conducted using STATA software version 10 (Stata-Corp.2009.Stata Statistical Software: Release 10. StataCorp LP).

Results

Characteristics of the dietary patterns

Additional file 1: Table S1 shows the component loadings of food groups on the three major dietary patterns (DPs) identified. There were 7 components which met the eigenvalue > 1 criterion; of these only the first 3 were considered for further analysis on the basis of the scree plot and their interpretability. When we visually examined the scree plot, we observed a sharp drop after the first three components, after which the curve became substantially shallower (data not shown). In addition, when we examined the contributions of individual food groups to the various components, the interpretability of the last four components in terms of what kind of composite dietary patterns they represented was unclear; i.e. they didn't seem to represent cohesive dietary patterns with clear interpretability. Together, the first 3 components explained 28.6% of the total variance.

Component 1 loaded positively on whole/refined grains cooked with other food items, plain rice, rice-based dishes, coffee, nuts, snacks, condiments and soups, and negatively on potato, other vegetables (i.e., other than green leafy vegetables), and cooked milk products. Due to its positive loading on three cereal-groups, and on savoury foods such as nuts, snacks, and condiments, this component was termed the 'cereal-savoury foods' dietary pattern (Additional file 1: Table S1a).

Component 2 loaded positively on western cereals (e.g., corn/cereal flakes, bread/toast/rolls/buns, pizza/burger and noodles/macaroni/pasta), other vegetables (e.g., carrots, beet root, gourds, capsicum etc.), fruit, fruit juices, cooked milk products, snacks, condiments, sugars, sweets, and negatively on coffee. As this component loaded positively on fruits, snacks and sweets, and was the only component of the three to load on vegetables, it was termed the 'fruit-veg- sweets-snacks' dietary pattern (Additional file 1: Table S1a).

Component 3 loaded positively on all animal-food groups (red meat, poultry, fish/seafood, eggs, and other foods made with mutton/chicken) except other non-vegetarian food (organ meats, rabbit), the dairy-based categories and fats; hence it was termed the 'animal food' dietary pattern (Additional file 1: Table S1a).

Sample characteristics

Sample characteristics by geographical region are summarized in Table 1. The mean age of participants was 40.8 (±10.3) years, with 41.6% female, 32.3% urban residents, 9% being illiterate, and 10.4%, 14.0% and 16.1% who were current tobacco smokers, tobacco chewers and alcohol drinkers respectively. Nagpur had the highest proportion of tobacco chewers (28.9%) while Hyderabad had the highest proportion of smokers (12.8%) and alcohol users (31.6%). Across the four regions, the prevalence of hypertension ranged from 5.9 to 33.4% and the prevalence of diabetes ranged from 1.6 to 13.3%. Overall, the average BMI was 23.8 (±4.5) kg/m2 and the average amount of physical activity expressed in total Metabolic Equivalent Tasks (METS) was 38.8(±4.6) hr./week. Sample characteristics according to dietary patterns (lowest and highest tertiles) are summarized in Additional file 1: Table S1b. The 'cereal-savoury' and 'animal food' patterns were consumed more in the Southern regions of Hyderabad and Bangalore and the

Table 1 Socio-demographic and lifestyle characteristics* of the Indian Migration Study participants by different geographical regions ($N = 7067$)

%/ mean(SD)	Lucknow $N = 2000$	Nagpur $N = 1640$	Hyderabad $N = 1995$	Bangalore $N = 1432$	Total $N = 7067$
Age (years)	43.8(8.5)	29.5(6.4)	44.7(9.1)	43.9(8.6)	40.8(10.3)
Gender					
Male	61.5	62.9	52.8	56.3	58.3
Female	38.5	37.0	47.2	43.7	41.6
Illiterate	7.0	2.0	19.7	5.2	9.0
Standard of living index[a]	22.7(6.4)	17.8(5.2)	19.2(6.9)	20.0(5.8)	20.0(6.4)
Migrant Status					
Rural	28.6	28.9	33.6	27.3	29.8
Migrants	28.6	29.0	33.6	27.4	29.8
Urban	41.0	28.9	19.2	43.1	32.3
Smoking					
Never	86.7	92.0	84.3	86.3	87.2
Former	1.8	1.5	2.8	3.2	2.3
Current	11.4	6.4	12.8	10.4	10.4
Tobacco Chewing					
Never	80.7	69.3	90.5	95.2	83.8
Former	2.6	1.7	1.9	2.2	2.1
Current	16.6	28.9	7.5	2.5	14.0
Alcohol					
Never	86.5	88.5	64.8	87.1	80.7
Former	2.6	2.3	4.4	2.7	3.1
Current	10.8	9.2	31.6	10.1	16.1
Diabetes [b]					
No	86.7	97.4	88.7	86.8	89.8
Yes	13.3	1.6	11.1	12.5	9.8
Hypertension[b]					
No	70.6	93.8	66.5	72.8	75.2
Yes	29.4	5.9	33.4	27.0	24.6
Systolic blood pressure mm/Hg	123.4 (17.2)	113.8 (11.7)	127.3 (18.9)	123.1 (17.3)	122.2 (17.4)
Diastolic blood pressure mm/Hg	77.3 (10.7)	73.0 (8.7)	81.6 (11.3)	79.2 (10.9)	77.9 (10.9)
Physical activity METS[c] hr./week	38.7(4.0)	40.2(5.0)	37.9(4.7)	38.7(4.3)	38.8(4.6)
BMI[d] kg/m^2	24.4(4.4)	20.9(3.3)	24.6(4.4)	25.0(4.3)	23.8(4.5)
Dietary patterns in tertiles					
Cereal-savoury foods pattern					
T1	89.6	33.1	0.9	0.07	33.3
T2	9.4	57.9	49.1	16.6	33.3
T3	0.9	8.9	49.9	83.3	33.3
Fruits-vegetables-sweets-snacks pattern					
T1	20.3	17.2	53.1	42.2	33.3
T2	41.2	34.3	26.3	30.9	33.3
T3	38.4	48.3	20.5	26.8	33.3

Table 1 Socio-demographic and lifestyle characteristics* of the Indian Migration Study participants by different geographical regions ($N = 7067$) *(Continued)*

%/ mean(SD)	Lucknow $N = 2000$	Nagpur $N = 1640$	Hyderabad $N = 1995$	Bangalore $N = 1432$	Total $N = 7067$
Animal food pattern (fish-red meat-egg-poultry)					
T1	51.4	39.7	15.4	25.7	33.3
T2	34.9	33.0	34.8	29.4	33.3
T3	13.7	27.2	49.7	44.9	33.3
Biomarker levels [mean (±SD)]					
Fasting blood glucose mmol/l	5.7 (1.8)	4.8 (0.9)	5.1 (0.8)	5.5 (1.7)	5.3 (1.4)
Total cholesterol mmol/l	4.7 (1.1)	4.4 (1.1)	4.8 (1.1)	4.9 (1.1)	4.7 (1.1)
Low-density lipoprotein cholesterol mmol/l	2.8 (0.9)	2.7 (0.9)	2.9 (1.0)	3.1 (0.9)	2.9 (0.9)
High-density lipoprotein cholesterol mmol/l	1.2 (0.2)	1.1 (0.2)	1.1 (0.2)	1.1 (0.2)	1.2 (0.2)
Triglycerides mmol/l	1.5 (0.8)	1.3 (0.6)	1.5 (0.8)	1.5 (0.9)	1.5 (0.8)

*p-values for difference in means or proportions are from ANOVA for continuous data and Chi-square test of significance for categorical data (we found a $p < 0.0001$ for all comparisons between the regions)
[a]Standard of Living Index (SLI) distribution is 1–36 (Median 23, IQR =17–27)
[b]Hypertension included doctor-diagnosed disease and/or a systolic BP ≥ 140 mmHg or a diastolic BP ≥ 90 mmHg at the time of the interview. Diabetes included doctor-diagnosed disease and/or a fasting plasma glucose criterion of > 7.0 mmol/l [33]
[c]*METS* Metabolic Equivalent Tasks
[d]*BMI* Body Mass Index

'fruit-vegetable-sweets-snacks' pattern was largely consumed in Lucknow (North) and Nagpur (Central).

Association of dietary patterns with blood lipids, fasting glucose and blood pressure

Multivariable adjusted linear association of major dietary patterns with blood lipids, fasting glucose and systolic and diastolic blood pressure using robust standard error are presented in Table 2. The 'cereal-savoury foods' and 'fruits-vegetables-sweets-snacks' patterns did not show any association with blood lipids and fasting glucose levels. Higher intake of 'fruits-vegetables-sweets-snacks' pattern was positively associated with diastolic blood pressure (β coefficient T3 vs T1 1.2 mm/Hg; 95% CI: 0.8, 1.2 mm/Hg; p-trend = 0.014). Higher intake of 'animal food' pattern ('fish-red meat-egg-poultry') was positively associated with total cholesterol, LDL-C, HDL-C, fasting blood glucose (FBG) as well as with systolic and diastolic blood pressure (SBP and DBP) levels (β coefficient T3 vs T1 - TC: 0.10 mmol/L; 95% CI: 0.02, 0.17 mmol/L; p-trend = 0.013; LDL-C: 0.07 mmol/L; 95% CI: 0.004, 0.14 mmol/L; p-trend = 0.041; HDL-C: 0.02 mmol/L; 95% CI: 0.004, 0.04 mmol/L; p-trend = 0.016; FBG: 0.09 mmol/L; 95% CI: 0.01, 0.16 mmol/L; p-trend = 0.021; SBP: 1.2 mm/Hg; 95% CI: 0.1, 2.3 mm/Hg; p-trend = 0.032; DBP: 0.9 mm/Hg; 95% CI: 0.2, 1.5 mm/Hg; p-trend = 0.013) (Table 2).

Sensitivity analyses

'Fruits-vegetables-sweets-snacks' pattern was found to be highly variable across different regions of India in terms of component loadings for individual food components (based on our earlier work [9] in the same study population); and there were fewer number of participants in certain categories of the cereal-savoury pattern ($N = 19$ in the highest tertile in Lucknow; $N = 19$ in Hyderabad and $N = 1$ in Bangalore in the lowest tertile) making any sensitivity analysis less meaningful for these patterns. In addition, these dietary patterns showed overall no associations with risk parameters except for a solitary positive association between intake of the 'fruits-vegetables-sweets-snacks' pattern and diastolic blood pressure. Thus, we restricted this analysis to 'animal food' pattern which was the most consistent pattern in terms of component loadings across all regions of India [9].

We conducted sensitivity analyses to evaluate if there were differences in associations of the 'animal food' pattern with cardio-metabolic risk factors based on regions (Lucknow, Nagpur, Bangalore and Hyderabad), locations (urban/ urban migrant/ rural) and standard of living index (SLI; low, medium and high). We also did sensitivity analyses examining the associations of daily consumption of individual animal foods (fish, red meat, egg and poultry in tertiles) with blood lipids, fasting blood glucose and blood pressure, further adjusting for the cereal-savoury foods and fruits-vegetables-sweets-snacks patterns as an attempt to increase the understanding of individual components of 'animal food' dietary pattern in India. Although attenuated, the associations were in similar direction, across regions (Additional file 1: Table S2a), locations (Additional file 1: Table S2b) and SLI (Additional file 1: Table S2c) with few interactions between the 'animal food' pattern and regions, locations or SLI. Nevertheless, there were significant interactions

Table 2 Multivariable-adjusted linear associations[a] (beta co-efficient, 95% confidence interval) of major dietary patterns with cardio-metabolic risk factors in the Indian Migration Study participants ($N = 7067$)

Food patterns Tertiles	Total cholesterol mmol/L		LDL-C mmol/L		Triglycerides mmol/L		HDL-C mmol/L
	Age, sex adjusted	Fully adjusted[a]	Age, sex adjusted	Fully adjusted[a]	Age, sex adjusted	Fully adjusted[a]	Age, sex adjusted
Cereal savoury food pattern							
TI	Ref	Ref	Ref	Ref	Ref	Ref	Ref
T2	−0.03 (−0.09, 0.03)	−0.05 (− 0.15, 0.04)	0.04 (− 0.01, 0.10)	− 0.03 (− 0.12, 0.05)	0.01 (− 0.02, 0.05)	− 0.009 (− 0.06, 0.04)	− 0.07 (− 0.09, − 0.06)
T3	0.12 (0.05, 0.19)	− 0.009 (− 0.13, 0.12)	0.19 (0.13, 0.25)	0.001 (− 0.11, 0.11)	0.09 (0.04, 0.14)	0.01 (− 0.06, 0.1)	−0.10 (− 0.12, − 0.09)
p-trend	0.001	0.946	< 0.0001	0.880	< 0.0001	0.540	< 0.0001
Fruit-veg-sweet-snack pattern							
TI	Ref	Ref	Ref	Ref	Ref	Ref	Ref
T2	0.06 (−0.002, 0.13)	0.02 (−0.05, 0.1)	0.03 (− 0.03, 0.08)	0.01 (− 0.05, 0.08)	0.03 (− 0.01, 0.07)	0.02 (− 0.02, 0.07)	0.02 (0.008, 0.03)
T3	0.04 (− 0.02, 0.11)	−0.02 (− 0.11, 0.07)	0.01 (− 0.05, 0.07)	−0.01 (− 0.09, 0.06)	0.02 (− 0.02, 0.06)	−0.02 (− 0.08, 0.03)	0.01 (0.002, 0.03)
p-trend	0.209	0.604	0.715	0.661	0.341	0.472	0.025
Animal food pattern (Fish-red meat-egg-poultry)							
TI	Ref	Ref	Ref	Ref	Ref	Ref	Ref
T2	0.004 (−0.06, 0.06)	0.01 (−0.05, 0.08)	0.006 (−0.05, 0.06)	0.002 (− 0.05, 0 .06)	0.02 (− 0.01, 0.07)	0.02 (− 0.03, 0.06)	−0.01 (− 0.02, 0.003)
T3	0.17 (0.10, 0.24)	0.10 (0.02, 0.17)	0.15 (0.09, 0.1)	0.07 (0.004, 0.14)	0.11 (0.06, 0.16)	0.04 (−0.01, 0.09)	−0.02 (− 0.03, − 0.006)
p-trend	< 0.0001	0.013	< 0.0001	0.041	< 0.0001	0.181	0.005

Table 2 Multivariable-adjusted linear associations[a] (beta co-efficient, 95% confidence interval) of major dietary patterns with cardio-metabolic risk factors in the Indian Migration Study participants ($N = 7067$) *(Continued)*

Food patterns Tertiles	HDL-C mmol/L	Fasting glucose[b] mmol/L		Systolic blood pressure mm/Hg		Diastolic blood pressure mm/Hg	
	Fully adjusted[a]	Age, sex adjusted	Fully adjusted[a]	Age, sex adjusted	Fully adjusted[a]	Age, sex adjusted	Fully adjusted[a]
Cereal savoury food pattern							
TI	Ref	Ref	Ref	Ref	Ref	Ref	Ref
T2	− 0.01 (− 0.03, 0.01)	−0.37 (− 0.46, − 0.29)	0.007 (− 0.07, 0.08)	1.8 (0.8, 2.7)	0.1 (−1.1,1.3)	1.9 (1.2, 2.5)	− 0.1 (− 0.9, 0.7)
T3	−0.02 (− 0.04, 0.007)	−0.30 (− 0.40,-0.21)	−0.01 (− 0.11, 0.08)	1.3 (0.3, 2.3)	−0.7 (−2.4, 0.9)	2.5 (1.9, 3.2)	− 0.9 (− 1.9, 0.2)
p-trend	0.153	< 0.0001	0.745	Ref	Ref	Ref	Ref
Fruit-veg-sweet-snack pattern							
TI	Ref	Ref	Ref	Ref	Ref	Ref	Ref
T2	−0.0001 (− 0.01, 0.01)	0.06 (− 0.01, 0.05)	−0.01 (− 0.08, 0.06)	−0.7 (−1.7, 2.0)	0.3 (− 0.8, 1.3)	−0.2 (− 0.8, 0.5)	−0.6 (− 0.06, 1.3)
T3	−0.005 (− 0.02, 0.01)	0.03 (− 0.11, 0.03)	−0.06 (− 0.14, 0.02)	−0.3(− 1.2, 0.7)	1.2 (− 0.1, 2.5)	−0.02 (− 0.6, 0.6)	1.2 (0.8, 1.2)
p-trend	0.624	0.331	0.143	0.555	0.067	0.953	0.014
Animal food pattern (Fish-red meat-egg-poultry)							
TI	Ref	Ref	Ref	Ref	Ref	Ref	Ref
T2	0.006 (− 0.008, 0.02)	−0.08 (− 0.17, − 0.001)	0.01 (− 0.05, 0.07)	1.4 (0.5,2.4)	0.5 (− 0.4, 1.5)	1.0 (0.4, 1.6)	0.2 (− 0.4, 0.8)
T3	0.02 (0.004, 0.04)	−0.09 (− 0.18, − 0.009)	0.09 (0.01, 0.16)	2.8 (1.8,3.8)	1.2 (0.1, 2.3)	2.9 (2.3, 3.6)	0.9 (0.2, 1.5)
p-trend	0.016	0.029	0.021	< 0.001	0.032	< 0.001	0.013

[a]Robust standard error adjusted for age (continuous in years), sex (male/female), migration status (rural, urban, urban migrant), site (Lucknow, Nagpur, Hyderabad, Bangalore), SLI (continuous score), education (no formal education, primary school, secondary school and beyond secondary school), BMI (continuous in kg/m^2), total energy (continuous in kcal/day), physical activity (continuous in totalMETS), tobacco (never, past, current), alcohol (never, past, current), use of any regular medication for chronic conditions such as diabetes, hypertension and/or food supplements (yes/no), sib-pair

[b]Analysis excluded known diabetics ($n = 486$)

between the 'animal food' dietary pattern and regions for associations with triglycerides levels (Additional file 1: Table S2a) and the 'animal food' dietary pattern and SLI for associations with fasting blood glucose levels (Additional file 1: Table S2c). High intake of individual 'animal food' components (fish, red meat, poultry and eggs in tertiles) also showed positive associations with the cardio-metabolic risk factors (Additional file 1: Table S3).

Discussion

Across four geographical regions spanning 18 states of India, three major dietary patterns - 'cereals-savoury foods', 'fruit-veg-sweets-snacks' and 'animal food', were identified through principal components analysis (PCA) of dietary intake data in a large cross-sectional study of rural and urban populations. High intake of the 'animal food' pattern was associated with high levels of fasting blood glucose, and total, LDL, and HDL cholesterol as well as systolic and diastolic blood pressure after adjusting for several potential confounders and was consistent in sensitivity analyses. No association was seen for the other largely plant-based dietary patterns except for a solitary positive association with diastolic blood pressure for high intake of 'fruits-vegetables-sweets-snacks' pattern. In a previous analysis with the same IMS data, we found positive associations of the 'animal food' pattern with obesity and abdominal adiposity, in line with our current study [9].

While 'Prudent' (high intake of vegetables, fruit, legumes, whole grains, and seafood), 'Mediterranean' (higher intake of vegetables, legumes, fruits, nuts, whole grains, cheese or yogurt, fish, and monounsaturated relative to saturated fatty acids), and 'DASH' (fruit, vegetables and low fat dairy products) dietary patterns have been found to be inversely associated with cardiovascular diseases and type-II diabetes, the 'Western' dietary pattern characterized by a high intake of processed and red meat, butter and other high-fat dairy products, eggs, and refined grains, has been associated with an increased risk of CVD and type-II diabetes [4, 7, 8].

The three dietary patterns identified here were distinct for our study population and were a blend of healthy and unhealthy aspects of the above mentioned dietary patterns. For example, 'cereals-savoury foods' showed positive loadings for nuts and whole grains but also had positive loadings for refined grains and negative loadings for vegetables; 'fruit-veg-sweets-snacks' pattern showed positive loadings for fruits and vegetables as well as for snacks and sugar. This could have partly attributed to the null associations in general with cardio-metabolic risk factors for these patterns. The positive association of diastolic blood pressure with high intake of 'fruits-vegetables-sweets-snacks' pattern could possibly be attributed to snacks which tend to have a high salt content.

The 'animal food' pattern in our study, the only consistent dietary pattern across all regions and locations of our study population, was a blend of components of prudent (fish) and western (red meat, eggs) dietary patterns and was positively associated with cardio-metabolic risk factors. This was further confirmed in sensitivity analyses where we stratified by regions, locations and SLI. We also found positive associations with cardio-metabolic risk factors for high intake of individual components such as red meat, eggs, poultry and fish. Several potential mechanisms through which the 'animal food' patterns could have influenced cardio-metabolic risk factors in this population can be proposed, although further studies are required to confirm the findings. For example, imbalance in saturated and unsaturated fat (high saturated fat and low unsaturated fat) and potentially low fibre in the 'animal food' coupled with high salt content in cooked animal food could have influenced blood lipids and blood pressure levels respectively [29]. The positive association of high intake of 'fruits-vegetables-sweets-snacks' with diastolic blood pressure lends some support to this theory as high salt content in snacks could have driven the observed association. A study based on data from India's third National Family Health Survey (NFHS-3) that showed a positive association of fish consumption with diabetes (OR: 2.02; 95% CI, 1.59–2.57) alluded that the pattern of cooking such as deep frying with high amounts of cooking oils could have contributed to the positive findings [30]. A study conducted among South Asians (84% Indian origin) living in the US found high total cholesterol (β: 0.45 mmol/L (95% CI: 0.11 to 0.78 mmol/L)) and LDL-C (β: 0.31 mmol/L (95% CI: 0.02 to 0.61 mmol/L)) with high intake of animal protein pattern [31] similar to our study. They found no association of lipids and glucose levels with any other patterns such as 'fried snacks, sweets, and high-fat dairy' and 'fruits, vegetables, nuts, and legumes' except for an inverse association with HDL-C for high intake of 'fried snacks, sweets, and high-fat dairy' pattern ($p < 0.0001$), although 'fruits, vegetables, nuts, and legumes' pattern was inversely associated with the odds of metabolic syndrome and hypertension and 'fried snacks, sweets, and high-fat dairy' pattern was directly associated with insulin resistance [31].

Indian studies evaluating dietary patterns as they relate with CVD and diabetes risk factors are limited [9, 10, 13, 32, 33]. A study among women in West Bengal found three dietary patterns including 'vegetables fruit and pulses' pattern which was similar to our 'fruit-veg-sweets-snacks' pattern but also had positive loadings for poultry and eggs [32]. This pattern had an inverse association with total cholesterol and LDL-C. In the same study the 'hydrogenated and saturated fat and vegetable oil' pattern was positively associated with BMI, waist circumference and HDL-C but no association was found for red meat and high-fat dairy pattern (which also positively loaded for whole and refined grains and low-fat dairy) with any risk factors [32]. Another study in Delhi, Trivandrum and Mumbai, also found specific regional patterns, such as 'fruit-dairy' and 'vegetables-pulses' in New Delhi, 'pulses-rice' and 'sweets-snacks' in Trivandrum and 'fruits-vegetables' and 'snacks-meat' in Mumbai, though the authors did not evaluate associations with lipid and glucose levels [13]. Previously, IMS investigators found five clusters of people (rice and low diversity; rice and fruit; wheat and pulses; wheat, rice and oils; rice and meat) [33] using latent class analysis (LCA) and these clusters were associated with cardio-metabolic risk factors. We are adding to that by examining the IMS dietary data in a different way, using PCA, which may be more applicable because this population is heterogeneous in terms of dietary consumption and it involved participants from over 18 different regions of India consisting of urban, rural as well as migrant population. We have found differences in food consumption patterns in this population based on regions and locations [34].

Through one of our earlier analyses in this populations based on simple lacto-vegetarian and non-vegetarian patterns we found beneficial associations of vegetarian diet with CVD and diabetes risk factors including blood lipids, fasting glucose and blood pressure [29]. At the same time we also found reduced bio-availability of vitamin B12 with Indian vegetarian diets [35] which could be a predictor for various chronic diseases particularly CVD [36]. A more detailed analysis of dietary patterns is needed to facilitate the evaluation of aggregate effects of different food components and nutrients consumed in the Indian context [9].

In India, although there are important regional differences in DPs [13], the 'animal food' pattern showed considerable consistency across regions, urban-rural locations and standard of living. The quantity and pattern of 'animal food' consumption in India are different from their Western counterparts. For example while the median intake is about 49–65 g/day for meat and 33–34 g/day for fish in the West [37–39], the consumption is only about 20.3(9.6–38.9) g/day for meat and 3.9 (0.5–9.9) g/day for fish in our population. Similarly, the Western 'animal foods' dietary pattern largely includes processed meat, red meat and eggs with high fat foods and refined grains, while in our study the 'animal foods' pattern was consumption of red meat, fish, eggs and poultry [37–39]. Despite these differences, we found positive associations of the 'animal food pattern with cardio-metabolic risk factors in India, potentially implying the role of differing cooking patterns [30], in addition to the components of animal food (e.g., red meat). As quantity of everyday consumption of 'animal food' in India is very less compared to Western counterparts, cooking pattern is a factor that holds clinical and public health relevance, if proven by further studies, for potential interventions.

In this study, we used a validated 184-item semi-quantitative food frequency questionnaire (FFQ) to capture the wide range of diets consumed across four different regions of India, and obtained fasting blood samples for measurement of biochemical markers. We used data reduction techniques to identify composite dietary patterns in India. The cross-sectional study design and possible measurement error in dietary intake are the major limitations of the study with potential impact on the study results, which should be interpreted with caution. However, the large, diverse and heterogeneous nature of this study population and their diets and consistency of associations across several sensitivity analyses for 'animal food' pattern, are strengths of the study. Future nutrition research in India should replicate these findings in prospective studies and evaluate specific public health dietary interventions (e.g., lower consumption of certain animal food components, modification of cooking patterns etc.).

Conclusion

High intake of the 'animal food' dietary pattern was positively associated with cardio-metabolic risk factors in India. Our findings possibly indicate that cooking pattern is partly driving the association. Given the cross-sectional nature of this study, comprehensive longitudinal evaluations of diet are needed to better understand and validate the findings to devise potential means of interventions for combatting NCDs in India which could have large public health impact in this population.

Additional file

Additional file 1: Table S1 (a): Component loadings for the 3 main dietary patterns (DPs) identified using principal components analysis (PCA) of FFQ data from the Indian Migration Study*. **Table S1(b):** Socio-demographic and lifestyle characteristics of the Indian Migration study participants in the first (T1) and third (T3) tertiles of the three dietary patterns (N=7067). **Table S2 (a):** Multivariable-adjusted linear associations* (beta co-efficient, 95% confidence interval) of 'animal food' pattern with cardio-metabolic risk factors by four different regions of the Indian Migration Study. **Table S2 (b):** Multivariable-adjusted linear associations* (beta co-efficient, 95% confidence interval) of 'animal food' pattern with cardio-metabolic risk factors by different locations of the Indian Migration Study. **Table S2 (c):** Multivariable-adjusted linear associations* (beta co-efficient, 95% confidence interval) of 'animal food' pattern with cardio-metabolic risk factors by different standard of living (SLI) of the Indian Migration Study.**Table S3:** Multivariable adjusted* associations (beta co-efficient, 95% confidence interval) of daily consumption of individual animal food components in tertiles (fish /red meat/poultry/eggs) with cardio-metabolic risk factors of the Indian Migration Study participants (N=7067).

Abbreviations

BMI: Body mass index; CVD: Cardiovascular disease; DALY: Disability adjusted life years; DASH: Dietary approaches to stop hypertension; DP: Dietary pattern; FFQ: Food frequency questionnaire; HDL-C: High density lipoprotein-cholesterol; IMS: Indian migration study; LDL-C: Low density lipoprotein-cholesterol; LMIC: Low middle income countries; METs: Metabolic equivalent tasks; NCD: Noncommunicable disease; PCA: Principal component analysis; SLI: Standard of living Index; TC: Total cholesterol; TG: Triglycerides and FBG-fasting blood glucose; USDA: United States Department of Agriculture

Acknowledgements
Not applicable

Funding
This work was funded by Wellcome Trust project grant GR070797MF. Wellcome Trust had no role in the design, data collection, analysis or publication of the manuscript. Dr. Krithiga Shridhar and Dr. Sutapa Agarwal were supported by a Wellcome Trust Capacity Strengthening Strategic Award Extension phase to the Public Health Foundation of India and a consortium of UK universities (WT084754/Z/08/A). Dr. Ambika Satija was supported by American Heart Association Grant #16POST29660000.

Authors' contributions
KS, AS, PKD analysed and interpreted the data, KS wrote the first draft of the manuscript, AS,PKD, SA, RG, LB, AVB, DP, SK, KSR, SE reviewed contents of the manuscript at different stages and all authors gave final approval for publication.

Competing interests
The authors declare that they have no competing interests.

Author details
[1]Centre for Chronic Conditions and Injuries, Public Health Foundation of India, Gurgaon, Haryana, India. [2]Harvard T. H. Chan School of Public Health, Boston, USA. [3]London School of Hygiene and Tropical Medicine, London, UK. [4]Just Right Obesity Clinic, Bangalore, India. [5]Centre for Chronic Disease Control, Gurgaon, Haryana, India. [6]Public Health Foundation of India, New Delhi, India.

References
1. Mortality GBD and Causes of Death C. Global, regional, and national age-sex specific all-cause and cause-specific mortality for 240 causes of death, 1990-2013: a systematic analysis for the global burden of disease study 2013. Lancet. 2015;385(9963):117–71.
2. DALYs GBD, Collaborators H, Murray CJ, Barber RM, Foreman KJ, Abbasoglu Ozgoren A, Abd-Allah F, Abera SF, Aboyans V, Abraham JP, Abubakar I, Abu-Raddad LJ, Abu-Rmeileh NM, Achoki T, Ackerman IN, Ademi Z, Adou AK, Adsuar JC, Afshin A, Agardh EE, Alam SS, Alasfoor D, Albittar MI, Alegretti MA, Alemu ZA, Alfonso-Cristancho R, Alhabib S, Ali R, Alla F, Allebeck P, Almazroa MA, Alsharif U, Alvarez E, Alvis-Guzman N, Amare AT, Ameh EA, Amini H, Ammar W, Anderson HR, Anderson BO, Antonio CA, Anwari P, Arnlov J, Arsic Arsenijevic VS, Artaman A, Asghar RJ, Assadi R, Atkins LS, Avila MA, Awuah B, Bachman VF, Badawi A, Bahit MC, Balakrishnan K, Banerjee A, Barker-Collo SL, Barquera S, Barregard L, Barrero LH, Basu A, Basu S, Basulaiman MO, Beardsley J, Bedi N, Beghi E, Bekele T, Bell ML, Benjet C, Bennett DA, Bensenor IM, Benzian H, Bernabe E, Bertozzi-Villa A, Beyene TJ, Bhala N, Bhalla A, Bhutta ZA, Bienhoff K, Bikbov B, Biryukov S, Blore JD, Blosser CD, Blyth FM, Bohensky MA, Bolliger IW, Bora Basara B, Bornstein NM, Bose D, Boufous S, Bourne RR, Boyers LN, Brainin M, Brayne CE, Brazinova A, Breitborde NJ, Brenner H, Briggs AD, Brooks PM, Brown JC, Brugha TS, Buchbinder R, Buckle GC, Budke CM, Bulchis A, Bulloch AG, Campos-Nonato IR, Carabin H, Carapetis JR, Cardenas R, Carpenter DO, Caso V, Castaneda-Orjuela CA, Castro RE, Catala-Lopez F, Cavalleri F, Cavlin A, Chadha VK, Chang JC, Charlson FJ, Chen H, Chen W, Chiang PP, Chimed-Ochir O, Chowdhury R, Christensen H, Christophi CA, Cirillo M, Coates MM, Coffeng LE, Coggeshall MS, Colistro V, Colquhoun SM, Cooke GS, Cooper C, Cooper LT, Coppola LM, Cortinovis M, Criqui MH, Crump JA, Cuevas-Nasu L, Danawi H, Dandona L, Dandona R, Dansereau E, Dargan PI, Davey G, Davis A, Davitoiu DV, Dayama A, De Leo D, Degenhardt L, Del Pozo-Cruz B, Dellavalle RP, Deribe K, Derrett S, Des Jarlais DC, Dessalegn M, Dharmaratne SD, Dherani MK, Diaz-Torne C, Dicker D, Ding EL, Dokova K, Dorsey ER, Driscoll TR, Duan L, Duber HC, Ebel BE, Edmond KM, Elshrek YM, Endres M, Ermakov SP, Erskine HE, Eshrati B, Esteghamati A, Estep K, Faraon EJ, Farzadfar F, Fay DF, Feigin VL, Felson DT, Fereshtehnejad SM, Fernandes JG, Ferrari AJ, Fitzmaurice C, Flaxman AD, Fleming TD, Foigt N, Forouzanfar MH, Fowkes FG, Paleo UF, Franklin RC, Furst T, Gabbe B, Gaffikin L, Gankpe FG, Geleijnse JM, Gessner BD, Gething P, Gibney KB, Giroud M, Giussani G, Gomez Dantes H, Gona P, Gonzalez-Medina D, Gosselin RA, Gotay CC, Goto A, Gouda HN, Graetz N, Gugnani HC, Gupta R, Gutierrez RA, Haagsma J, Hafezi-Nejad N, Hagan H, Halasa YA, Hamadeh RR, Hamavid H, Hammami M, Hancock J, Hankey GJ, Hansen GM, Hao Y, Harb HL, Haro JM, Havmoeller R, Hay SI, Hay RJ, Heredia-Pi IB, Heuton KR, Heydarpour P, Higashi H, Hijar M, Hoek HW, Hoffman HJ, Hosgood HD, Hossain M, Hotez PJ, Hoy DG, Hsairi M, Hu G, Huang C, Huang JJ, Husseini A, Huynh C, Iannarone ML, Iburg KM, Innos K, Inoue M, Islami F, Jacobsen KH, Jarvis DL, Jassal SK, Jee SH, Jeemon P, Jensen PN, Jha V, Jiang G, Jiang Y, Jonas JB, Juel K, Kan H, Karch A, Karema CK, Karimkhani C, Karthikeyan G, Kassebaum NJ, Kaul A, Kawakami N, Kazanjan K, Kemp AH, Kengne AP, Keren A, Khader YS, Khalifa SE, Khan EA, Khan G, Khang YH, Kieling C, Kim D, Kim S, Kim Y, Kinfu Y, Kinge JM, Kivipelto M, Knibbs LD, Knudsen AK, Kokubo Y, Kosen S, Krishnaswami S, Kuate Defo B, Kucuk Bicer B, Kuipers EJ, Kulkarni C, Kulkarni VS, Kumar GA, Kyu HH, Lai T, Lalloo R, Lallukka T, Lam H, Lan Q, Lansingh VC, Larsson A, Lawrynowicz AE, Leasher JL, Leigh J, Leung R, Levitz CE, Li B, Li Y, Lim SS, Lind M, Lipshultz SE, Liu S, Liu Y, Lloyd BK, Lofgren KT, Logroscino G, Looker KJ, Lortet-Tieulent J, Lotufo PA, Lozano R, Lucas RM, Lunevicius R, Lyons RA, Ma S, Macintyre MF, Mackay MT, Majdan M, Malekzadeh R, Marcenes W, Margolis DJ, Margono C, Marzan MB, Masci JR, Mashal MT, Matzopoulos R, Mayosi BM, Mazorodze TT, McGill NW, McGrath JJ, McKee M, McLain A, Meaney PA, Medina C, Mehndiratta MM, Mekonnen W, Melaku YA, Meltzer M, Memish ZA, Mensah GA, Meretoja A, Mhimbira FA, Micha R, Miller TR, Mills EJ, Mitchell PB, Mock CN, Mohamed Ibrahim N, Mohammad KA, Mokdad AH, Mola GL, Monasta L, Montanez Hernandez JC, Montico M, Montine TJ, Mooney MD, Moore AR, Moradi-Lakeh M, Moran AE, Mori R, Moschandreas J, Moturi WN, Moyer ML, Mozaffarian D, Msemburi WT, Mueller UO, Mukaigawara M, Mullany EC, Murdoch ME, Murray J, Murthy KS, Naghavi M, Naheed A, Naidoo KS, Naldi L, Nand D, Nangia V, Narayan KM, Nejjari C, Neupane SP, Newton CR, Ng M, Ngalesoni FN, Nguyen G, Nisar MI, Nolte S, Norheim OF, Norman RE, Norrving B, Nyakarahuka L, Oh IH, Ohkubo T, Ohno SL, Olusanya BO, Opio JN, Ortblad K, Ortiz A, Pain AW, Pandian JD, Panelo CI, Papachristou C, Park EK, Park JH, Patten SB, Patton GC, Paul VK, Pavlin BI, Pearce N, Pereira DM, Perez-Padilla R, Perez-Ruiz F, Perico N, Pervaiz A, Pesudovs K, Peterson CB, Petzold M, Phillips MR, Phillips BK, Phillips DE, Piel FB, Plass D, Poenaru D, Polinder S, Pope D, Popova S, Poulton RG, Pourmalek F, Prabhakaran D, Prasad NM, Pullan RL, Qato DM, Quistberg DA, Rafay A, Rahimi K, Rahman SU, Raju M, Rana SM, Razavi H, Reddy KS, Refaat A, Remuzzi G, Resnikoff S, Ribeiro AL, Richardson L, Richardus JH, Roberts DA, Rojas-Rueda D, Ronfani L, Roth GA, Rothenbacher D, Rothstein DH, Rowley JT, Roy N, Ruhago GM, Saeedi MY, Saha S, Sahraian MA, Sampson UK, Sanabria JR, Sandar L, Santos IS, Satpathy M, Sawhney M, Scarborough P, Schneider IJ, Schottker B, Schumacher AE, Schwebel DC, Scott JG, Seedat S, Sepanlou SG, Serina PT, Servan-Mori EE, Shackelford KA, Shaheen A, Shahraz S, Shamah Levy T, Shangguan S, She J, Sheikhbahaei S, Shi P, Shibuya K, Shinohara Y, Shiri R, Shishani K, Shiue I, Shrime MG, Sigfusdottir ID, Silberberg DH, Simard EP, Sindi S, Singh A, Singh JA, Singh L, Skirbekk V, Slepak EL, Sliwa K, Soneji S, Soreide K, Soshnikov S, Sposato LA, Sreeramareddy CT, Stanaway JD, Stathopoulou V, Stein DJ, Stein MB, Steiner C, Steiner TJ, Stevens A, Stewart A, Stovner LJ, Stroumpoulis K, Sunguya BF, Swaminathan S, Swaroop M, Sykes BL, Tabb KM, Takahashi K, Tandon N, Tanne D, Tanner M, Tavakkoli M, Taylor HR, Te Ao BJ, Tediosi F, Temesgen AM, Templin T, Ten Have M, Tenkorang EY, Terkawi AS, Thomson B, Thorne-Lyman AL, Thrift AG, Thurston GD, Tillmann T, Tonelli M, Topouzis F, Toyoshima H, Traebert J, Tran BX, Trillini M, Truelsen T, Tsilimbaris M, Tuzcu EM, Uchendu US, Ukwaja KN, Undurraga EA, Uzun SB, Van Brakel WH, Van De Vijver S, van Gool CH, Van Os J, Vasankari TJ, Venketasubramanian N, Violante FS, Vlassov VV, Vollset SE, Wagner GR, Wagner J, Waller SG, Wan X, Wang H, Wang J, Wang L, Warouw TS, Weichenthal S, Weiderpass E, Weintraub RG, Wenzhi W, Werdecker A, Westerman R, Whiteford HA, Wilkinson JD, Williams TN, Wolfe CD, Wolock TM, Woolf AD, Wulf S, Wurtz B, Xu G, Yan LL, Yano Y, Ye P, Yentur GK, Yip P, Yonemoto N, Yoon SJ, Younis MZ, Yu C, Zaki ME, Zhao Y, Zheng Y, Zonies D, Zou X, Salomon JA, Lopez AD, Vos T. Global, regional, and national disability-adjusted life years (DALYs) for 306 diseases and

injuries and healthy life expectancy (HALE) for 188 countries, 1990-2013: quantifying the epidemiological transition. Lancet. 2015;386(10009):2145–91.
3. WorldHealthOrganization, NCD Status Report-2014. Available at http://www.who.int/nmh/publications/ncd-status-report-2014/en/ Accessed 22 Apr 2015.
4. Medina-RemOn A, Kirwan R, Lamuela-Raventos RM, and Estruch R. Dietary patterns and the risk of obesity, type 2 diabetes mellitus, cardiovascular diseases, asthma, and mental health problems. Crit Rev Food Sci Nutr. 2018; 58(2):262–296.
5. Fraser GE. Vegetarian diets: what do we know of their effects on common chronic diseases? Am J Clin Nutr. 2009;89(5):1607S–12S.
6. Key TJ, Appleby PN, Rosell MS. Health effects of vegetarian and vegan diets. Proc Nutr Soc. 2006;65(1):35–41.
7. Mente A, de Koning L, Shannon HS, Anand SS. A systematic review of the evidence supporting a causal link between dietary factors and coronary heart disease. Arch Intern Med. 2009;169(7):659–69.
8. Srinath Reddy K, Katan MB. Diet, nutrition and the prevention of hypertension and cardiovascular diseases. Public Health Nutr. 2004;7(1A):167–86.
9. Satija A, Hu FB, Bowen L, Bharathi AV, Vaz M, Prabhakaran D, Reddy KS, Ben-Shlomo Y, Davey Smith G, Kinra S, Ebrahim S. Dietary patterns in India and their association with obesity and central obesity. Public Health Nutr. 2015; 18(16):3031–41.
10. Green R, Milner J, Joy EJ, Agrawal S, Dangour AD. Dietary patterns in India: a systematic review. Br J Nutr. 2016;116(1):142–8.
11. National Clinical Guideline, Lipid modification: cardiovascular risk assessment and the modification of blood lipids for the primary and secondary prevention of cardiovascular disease. 2014, Available at https://www.ncbi.nlm.nih.gov/pubmed/25340243 Accessed 25 Jan 2018.
12. National-Institute-for-HealthandCare-Excellance, NICE guidelines [CG181]. 2014, Available at http://www.nice.org.uk/guidance/cg181/chapter/1-recommendations Accesed on 22 Apr 2015.
13. Daniel CR, Prabhakaran D, Kapur K, Graubard BI, Devasenapathy N, Ramakrishnan L, George PS, Shetty H, Ferrucci LM, Yurgalevitch S, Chatterjee N, Reddy KS, Rastogi T, Gupta PC, Mathew A, Sinha R. A cross-sectional investigation of regional patterns of diet and cardio-metabolic risk in India. Nutr J. 2011;10:12.
14. Bansal D, Satija A, Khandpur N, Bowen L, Kinra S, Prabhakaran D, Reddy KS, Ebrahim S. Effects of migration on food consumption patterns in a sample of Indian factory workers and their families. Public Health Nutr. 2010;13(12): 1982–9.
15. Shetty PS. Nutrition transition in India. Public Health Nutr. 2002;5(1A):175–82.
16. Global Burden of Disease Compare available at http://www.healthdata.org/india. Accessed 1 Nov 2017.
17. Lyngdoh T, Kinra S, Shlomo YB, Reddy S, Prabhakaran D, Smith GD, Ebrahim S. Sib-recruitment for studying migration and its impact on obesity and diabetes. Emerg Themes Epidemiol. 2006;3:2.
18. Ebrahim S, Kinra S, Bowen L, Andersen E, Ben-Shlomo Y, Lyngdoh T, Ramakrishnan L, Ahuja RC, Joshi P, Das SM, Mohan M, Davey Smith G, Prabhakaran D, Reddy KS. The effect of rural-to-urban migration on obesity and diabetes in India: a cross-sectional study. PLoS Med. 2010;7(4):e1000268.
19. Reddy KS, Prabhakaran D, Chaturvedi V, Jeemon P, Thankappan KR, Ramakrishnan L, Mohan BV, Pandav CS, Ahmed FU, Joshi PP, Meera R, Amin RB, Ahuja RC, Das MS, Jaison TM. Methods for establishing a surveillance system for cardiovascular diseases in Indian industrial populations. Bull World Health Organ. 2006;84(6):461–9.
20. Sullivan R, Kinra S, Ekelund U, Bharathi AV, Vaz M, Kurpad A, Collier T, Reddy KS, Prabhakaran D, Ebrahim S, Kuper H. Evaluation of the Indian migration study physical activity questionnaire (IMS-PAQ): a cross-sectional study. Int J Behav Nutr Phys Act. 2012;9:13.
21. Bowen L, Bharathi AV, Kinra S, Destavola B, Ness A, Ebrahim S. Development and evaluation of a semi-quantitative food frequency questionnaire for use in urban and rural India. Asia Pac J Clin Nutr. 2012;21(3):355–60.
22. Gopalan C, editor. Nutritive value of Indian foods. Hyderabad: National Institute of Nutrition; 1971.
23. USDA National Nutrient Database for Standard Reference, Release 14. Nutrient Data Laboratory 2001, U.S. Department of Agriculture, Agricultural Research Service. Available at https://www.ars.usda.gov/ Area Home / Nutrient Data / Services / USDA National Nutrient Database for Standard Reference.
24. Welch AAUI, Buss DH, Paul AA, Southgate DAT. McCance and Widdowson's the composition of foods. Cambridge: Royal Society of Chemistry; 1995.
25. Marchioni DM, Voci SM, Lima FE, Fisberg RM, Slater B. Reproducibility of a food frequency questionnaire for adolescents. Cad Saude Publica. 2007; 23(9):2187–96.
26. Parr CL, Veierod MB, Laake P, Lund E, Hjartaker A. Test-retest reproducibility of a food frequency questionnaire (FFQ) and estimated effects on disease risk in the Norwegian women and cancer study (NOWAC). Nutr J. 2006;5:4.
27. Kuriyan R, Petracchi C, Ferro-Luzzi A, Shetty PS, Kurpad AV. Validation of expedient methods for measuring body composition in Indian adults. Indian J Med Res. 1998;107:37–45.
28. Friedewald WT, Levy RI, Fredrickson DS. Estimation of the concentration of low-density lipoprotein cholesterol in plasma, without use of the preparative ultracentrifuge. Clin Chem. 1972;18(6):499–502.
29. Shridhar K, Dhillon PK, Bowen L, Kinra S, Bharathi AV, Prabhakaran D, Reddy KS. Ebrahim S, and Indian migration study G, the association between a vegetarian diet and cardiovascular disease (CVD) risk factors in India: the Indian migration study. PLoS One. 2014;9(10):e110586.
30. Agrawal S, Millett C, Subramanian SV, Ebrahim S. Frequency of fish intake and diabetes among adult Indians. J Am Coll Nutr. 2014;33(3):215–30.
31. Gadgil MD, Anderson CA, Kandula NR, Kanaya AM. Dietary patterns are associated with metabolic risk factors in south Asians living in the United States. J Nutr. 2015;145(6):1211–7.
32. Ganguli D, Das N, Saha I, Biswas P, Datta S, Mukhopadhyay B, Chaudhuri D, Ghosh S, Dey S. Major dietary patterns and their associations with cardiovascular risk factors among women in West Bengal. India Br J Nutr. 2011;105(10):1520–9.
33. Joy EJ, Green R, Agrawal S, Aleksandrowicz L, Bowen L, Kinra S, Macdiarmid JI, Haines A, Dangour AD. Dietary patterns and non-communicable disease risk in Indian adults: secondary analysis of Indian migration study data. Public Health Nutr. 2017:1–10.
34. Bowen L, Ebrahim S, De Stavola B, Ness A, Kinra S, Bharathi AV, Prabhakaran D, Reddy KS. Dietary intake and rural-urban migration in India: a cross-sectional study. PLoS One. 2011;6(6):e14822.
35. Shridhar K, Dhillon PK, Bowen L, Kinra S, Bharathi AV, Prabhakaran D, Reddy KS, Ebrahim S. Nutritional profile of Indian vegetarian diets–the Indian migration study (IMS). Nutr J. 2014;13:55.
36. O'Leary F, Samman S. Vitamin B12 in health and disease. Nutrients. 2010; 2(3):299–316.
37. McCourt HJ, Draffin CR, Woodside JV, Cardwell CR, Young IS, Hunter SJ, Murray LJ, Boreham CA, Gallagher AM, Neville CE. McKinley MC, and young hearts study G, dietary patterns and cardiovascular risk factors in adolescents and young adults: the Northern Ireland young hearts project. Br J Nutr. 2014;112(10):1685–98.
38. Crowe FL, Appleby PN, Travis RC, Key TJ. Risk of hospitalization or death from ischemic heart disease among British vegetarians and nonvegetarians: results from the EPIC-Oxford cohort study. Am J Clin Nutr. 2013;97(3):597–603.
39. Key TJ, Appleby PN, Spencer EA, Travis RC, Roddam AW, Allen NE. Mortality in British vegetarians: results from the European prospective investigation into cancer and nutrition (EPIC-Oxford). Am J Clin Nutr. 2009;89(5):1613S–9S.

16

Association between diet quality, dietary patterns and cardiometabolic health in Australian adults

Katherine M. Livingstone* and Sarah A. McNaughton

Abstract

Background: Diet quality indices score dietary intakes against recommendations, whereas dietary patterns consider the pattern and combination of dietary intakes. Studies evaluating both methodologies in relation to cardiometabolic health in a nationally representative sample are limited. The aim of the present study was to investigate the relationship between diet quality, dietary patterns and markers of cardiometabolic health in Australian adults.

Methods: Dietary data, using two 24-h dietary recalls, were collected from adults in the cross-sectional Australian Health Survey 2011–2013 ($n = 2121$; 46.4 (SE 0.48) years). Diet quality was estimated using the Dietary Guideline Index (DGI). Dietary patterns (DPs), derived using reduced rank regression, were estimated using fiber density, SFA: PUFA and total sugars intake as intermediate markers. Multi-variable adjusted linear regression analyses were used to examine associations between diet quality and DPs and blood biomarkers, body mass index, waist circumference, diastolic and systolic blood pressure and an overall cardiometabolic risk score.

Results: DGI was associated with lower glucose (coef – 0.009, SE 0.004; P-trend = 0.033), body mass index (coef – 0.017, SE 0.007; P-trend = 0.019) and waist circumference (coef – 0.014, SE 0.005; P-trend = 0.008). Two dietary patterns were derived: dietary pattern-1 was characterized by higher intakes of pome fruit and wholegrain bread, while dietary pattern-2 was characterized by higher intakes of added sugars and tropical fruit. Dietary pattern-1 was associated with lower body mass index (coef – 0.028, SE 0.007; P-trend< 0.001) and waist circumference (coef – 0.017, SE 0.005; P-trend = 0.001). There was a trend towards lower cardiometabolic risk score. Dietary pattern-2 was associated with lower HDL-cholesterol (coef – 0.026, SE 0.012; P-trend = 0.028). There was a trend towards lower diastolic blood pressure. No associations with other markers were observed.

Conclusions: Better diet quality and healthier dietary patterns were primarily associated with favorable anthropometric markers of cardiometabolic health. Findings support the need for comparison of whole-diet based methodologies that take into consideration the interactions between foods and nutrients. Longitudinal studies are warranted to better understand causal relationships between diet and cardiometabolic health.

Keywords: Diet quality, Dietary patterns, Reduced rank regression, Cardiometabolic health, Adults

* Correspondence: k.livingstone@deakin.edu.au
Institute for Physical Activity and Nutrition, School of Exercise and Nutrition Sciences, Deakin University, Melbourne Burwood Campus, 221 Burwood Highway, Geelong, Victoria 3125, Australia

Background

Non-communicable diseases, such as diabetes and cardiovascular disease, are responsible for 40 million deaths per year worldwide [1]. The development of these conditions is mediated through complex biological pathways, such as elevated blood pressure and levels of triglycerides (TAG), total and LDL cholesterol and glucose [2]. With the global health burden of poor cardiometabolic health increasing, a better understanding of major modifiable risk factors, including diet, is needed [3–5].

Research to date has focused primarily on the role of single nutrients and foods in relation to cardiometabolic health [3, 6, 7]. However, given that food and nutrient intakes are often correlated, an increasing body of research is investigating whole diet [8] and its impact on disease risk [9–11]. Whole diet analyses have traditionally been based on data-driven techniques, such as factor analysis, or diet quality indices, estimated according to adherence to dietary guidelines. By combining strengths of both methodologies, reduced rank regression (RRR) uses a priori knowledge of markers of disease risk in a posteriori dietary patterns (DP) derivation [12]. RRR is becoming increasingly used in nutritional epidemiology for deriving DPs and evaluating associations with health outcomes [13–16].

Evidence suggests that better adherence to diet quality indices, such as the Alternate Healthy Eating Index (HEI) [17, 18], the Mediterranean diet score [17] and the Dietary Guideline index (DGI) [19], is associated with more favorable levels of many cardiometabolic biomarkers. Findings from a sample of Australian adults showed that a DP, derived using factor analysis and characterized by high consumption of wholegrains and fruit, was associated with higher odds of having a metabolically healthy phenotype [20]. Similarly, in a study of US adults, a RRR-derived DP low in soft drinks and high in wholegrains was inversely associated with TAG [13]. Despite this evidence, few nationally representative studies have compared more than one whole diet measure and few have considered an overall cardiometabolic risk score, nor the moderating effect of body mass index (BMI) [21]. A comparison between diet quality and a novel DP methodologies is needed to strengthen the evidence base for future DP-based policy development [22, 23]. In addition, RRR may better predict risk of disease than purely data-driven DP methodologies [24, 25], yet there is a paucity of research that has examined RRR-derived DPs in relation to cardiometabolic health [26].

Therefore, the aim of this study was to examine the relationship between diet quality, using the DGI, and DPs, using RRR, and markers of cardiometabolic health, including BMI, waist circumference (WC), total, HDL and LDL cholesterol, glycated hemoglobin (HbA1c), glucose, TAG, apolipoprotein B, diastolic and systolic blood pressure and an overall cardiometabolic risk score, in the cross-sectional, nationally representative 2011–2013 Australian Health Survey (AHS) [27].

Methods

Subjects and study design

The 2011–13 AHS is a population-based survey that sampled urban and rural households across all Australian states and territories. The AHS consists of two separate surveys (the National Health Survey [NHS] and the National Nutrition and Physical Activity Survey [NNPAS]) and the National Health Measures Survey (NHMS), a third component in which participants from both surveys were invited to participate [27]. In the NHS and NNPAS, 21,108 private dwellings ($n = 18,355$ after sample loss in the field stage) and 14,363 private dwellings ($n = 12,366$ after sample loss in the field stage) were selected, respectively. Dietary intakes were estimated in the NNPAS using two, 24-h dietary recalls. Of the 9519 dwellings in the first interview, 7735 (63.6%) completed the second dietary recall. Anthropometric and blood pressure measures were collected in the NNPAS on a voluntary basis by trained interviewers during home visits. Of the 30,329 respondents aged ≥ 5 years in the combined sample (NHS and NNPAS), 11,246 (37.1%) participated in the biomedical component (NHMS). Data relating to fasting tests relate to the fasting population only. For the present analysis individuals were excluded if they i) were pregnant and/or breastfeeding ii) only completed one day of dietary recall and iii) had missing data for outcomes and covariates (Fig. 1). A total of 2121 adults (≥ 19 y) were included in the current analysis. Ethics approval for the NHMS was granted by the Australian Government Department of Health and Ageing Departmental Ethics Committee. Further information on the design and methodologies of these surveys are presented elsewhere [27]. Reporting was conducted in accordance with the STROBE statement (Additional file 1: Table S1).

Study measures

Cardiometabolic risk variables

Weight (kg), height (cm) and WC (cm) measurements were assessed on a voluntary basis by trained interviewers using digital scales, a stadiometer and a metal tape respectively. Waist measurements were taken by placing the tape measure across the top of the belly button. For validation purposes, a random 10% of respondents were selected to be measured for height and waist an additional time. If this second measurement varied by more than one cm then a third reading was taken. Weight measurements were only taken once. Subjects were encouraged to remove their shoes and any heavy clothing prior to having measurements taken, although this was not compulsory, and no correction was applied

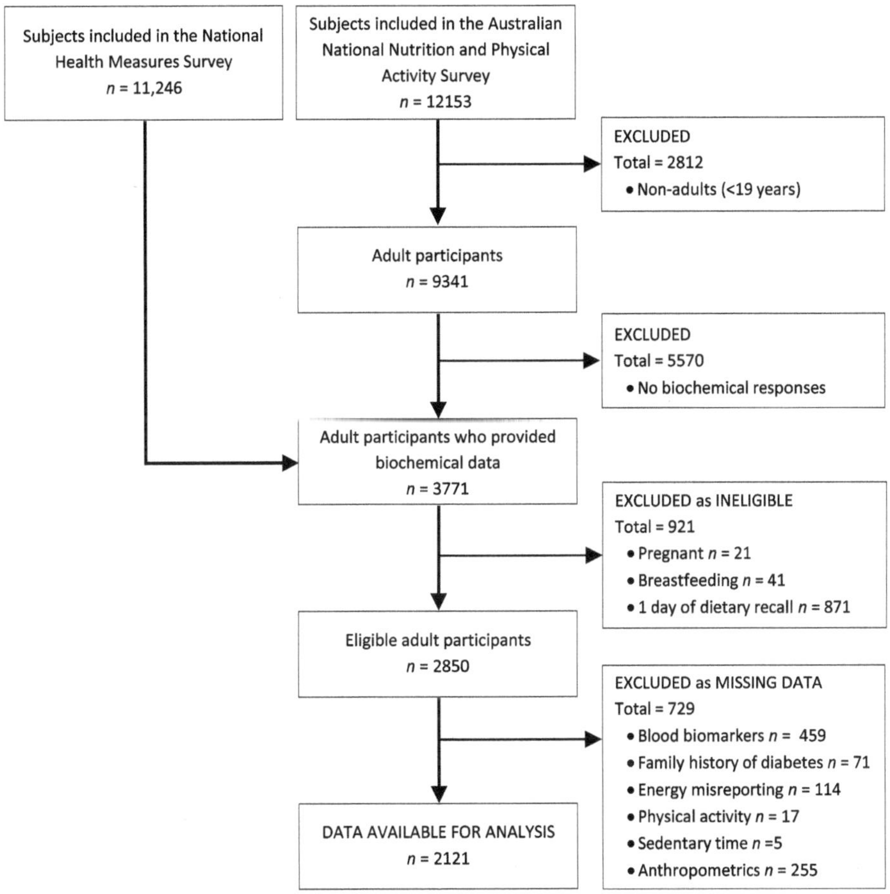

Fig. 1 Flow diagram of subjects included in the cross-sectional analysis of the Australian Health Survey

if they did not. BMI was derived using Quetelet's metric (kg/m^2). Standard cut offs were used to derive BMI and WC categories [28].

LDL cholesterol (mmol/L), TAG (mmol/L) and plasma glucose (mmol/L) were measured from blood samples in individuals who reporting fasting for 8 h or more prior to providing a blood sample [27]. LDL cholesterol was calculated from total cholesterol, HDL cholesterol (mmol/L) and fasting TAG levels using the Friedewald equation [29]. As recommended by the Australian Bureau of Statistics, individuals with a TAG level of ≥ 4.5 mmol/L were treated as missing data for the estimation of LDL-cholesterol [29]. Apolipoprotein B (g/L), HbA1c (mmol/mol) and total and HDL-cholesterol were measured in biological samples without the need for fasting. Abnormal levels of total, HDL- and LDL-cholesterol were defined as ≥ 5.5 mmol/L, < 1.0 mmol/L for males and < 1.3 mmol/L for females and ≥ 3.5 mmol/L, respectively. Abnormal levels of TAG and apolipoprotein B were ≥ 2.0 mmol/L and > 1.3 mmol/L for males and > 1.2 mmol/L for females, respectively. Impaired fasting plasma glucose was defined as > 6.0 mmol/L and < 7.0 mmol/L, while HbA1c levels indicative of increased risk of diabetes was defined as 42–47 mmol/mol [27]. Diabetes prevalence was estimates by self-reported diabetes diagnosed by a doctor. All analyses were conducted by Douglass Hanly Moir (Australia).

Systolic (SBP) and diastolic blood pressure (DBP) measurements were taken on the left arm. Interviewers performed two blood pressure readings using an automated blood pressure monitor. The second reading was used, unless there was a difference greater than 10 mmHg between the readings, in which case a third reading was taken and the second and third readings were averaged. Data on anti-hypertensive and lipid lowering medication were not recorded [27].

An overall cardiometabolic risk score was derived using WC, TAG, HDL-cholesterol, blood pressure (average blood pressure was used as an index for SBP and DBP), and fasting plasma glucose based on an established methodology [30]. Briefly, all variables were normalized (log 10) and standardized (i.e. $z = (\text{value} - \text{mean})/SD$). For HDL-cholesterol, the z-score was multiplied by − 1. All z-scores were then summed to compile the cardiometabolic risk score with units of SD.

Dietary intake

A 24-h dietary recall was used to provide quantitative information on foods and beverages consumed on the day prior to interview based on the in person USDA Automated Multiple-Pass Method [31]. The interview was divided into five phases: quick list description of food and beverages consumed from midnight to midnight the previous day, prompt the respondent to remember any omitted foods, provide information on time and eating occasion, further details (including preparation method and brand names) and a final probe to recall any omitted foods of beverages [27]. A second 24-h recall, via telephone interview, was collected at least 8 days after the first interview. Only participants who completed both recalls were included in the present analysis. Nutrient intakes were derived from the 24-h recalls using the Australian Supplement and Nutrient Database 2011–13 [32]. Information on the following dietary behaviors were collected in the NNPAS survey: type of milk consumed, usual daily intake of fruit and vegetables and use of salt [27].

Dietary guideline index

The DGI is a food-based score designed to reflect the diet quality of individuals according to compliance with the 2013 Australian Dietary Guidelines [33]. Dietary intakes of individuals, based on an average of two 24-h recalls and brief questionnaire items, were scored according to ten recommended dietary components (food variety, fruit, vegetables, cereals [total cereals and proportion that is wholegrains], meat and alternatives [total lean meat and alternatives and proportion that is lean], dairy and alternatives and fluid intake [total beverage and proportion that is water]) and six dietary components that should be limited (discretionary foods, SFA, unsaturated fat, added salt, added sugars and alcohol). Further details are presented in Additional file 2: Table S2 and are available elsewhere [34, 35].

DGI scores ranged between 0 and 130, with a higher score indicating better diet quality. Each item was scored out of 10, with 0 indicating the guideline was not met. Cut-offs used to obtain the maximum score for each component were tailored to age- and sex- specific food-based recommendations outlined in the Australian Dietary Guidelines [36]. Proportionate scores were derived where intakes fell between the maximum and minimum scoring criteria for all items except discretionary foods, saturated and unsaturated fat, salt, sugar and alcohol, which scored either 0 or 10 [34, 37, 38].

Dietary patterns

DPs were determined using RRR is a statistical technique designed to derive DPs that maximize the variation explained by response variables selected based on a priori hypothesis that they are related to the outcome of interest [12]. In the present analyses, fiber density, SFA: PUFA and total sugars intake were selected as response variables. These nutrients were chosen based on evidence from the WHO report on prevention of chronic disease that consumption of dietary fiber, fat and sugars are strongly associated with risk of diabetes and cardiometabolic disease [4, 39]. Recent studies have substantiated the use of these response variables for assessing risk of diabetes [40] and cardiovascular disease [39]. Fiber density was expressed as absolute intake of fiber (g/d) divided by total daily energy intake (MJ). Percentage energy intake from sugars and fat were calculated by dividing energy intake from sugars (kJ) and fat (kJ) respectively by total energy intake (kJ) and then multiplying by 100. SFA:PUFA ratio was expressed as the former divided by the latter.

A total of 48 food groups were created for use as predictors in the RRR analyses (Additional file 3: Table S3) to produce the DPs. Based on the AHS food grouping [27], foods were grouped into the following categories: non-alcoholic beverages (1 group), cereals (7 groups), fats and oils (2 groups), fruit (8 groups), vegetables (8 groups), meat and alternatives (7 groups), dairy (5 groups), soups and sauces (2 groups), snacks and confectionary (4 groups) and alcoholic beverages (3 groups). The number of extracted patterns is dependent on the number of response variables, thus intakes (g/d) of all 48 food groups and the three response variables were used to derive three DPs. These groups were RRR calculated linear functions of food group intakes (dietary patterns) that explained variation in the response variables. A detailed explanation of the RRR methodology can be found elsewhere [12].

To derive a DP score that captured the food groups that contributed most to the RRR pattern, a second, simplified score was derived and used for a sensitivity analysis. This score included food groups with factor loadings greater than > 0.20 [15] and was generated by summing the standardised food group intakes (z-scores) [41]. The simplified score for DP-1 summed positive loadings for pome fruit, wholegrain bread, wholegrain cereals, nuts and seeds, carrots, brassica vegetables, other vegetables, and negative loadings for fruit drinks, high-fat milk, cream, chocolate and non-wholegrain bread. The simplified score for DP-2 summed positive loadings for added sugars, pome fruit, tropical fruit, other fruit, stone fruit and negative loadings for wine and beer and cider. As the third DP explained less than 10% of the variation in response variables it was not further investigated and no sensitivity analysis was conducted.

Covariates

Covariates were identified based on previous literature and via a directed acyclic graph (Additional file 4: Figure S1). Socio-demographic characteristics were collected in the

NNPAS via interviewer-administered questionnaires. Smoking habits were identified as current, ex-smoker and never smoked. Education status was operationalized as low (completed some high-school or less), medium (completed high-school or completed some high-school and/or certificate/diploma) and high (having a University qualification) [42]. Urban or rural location was defined as major city, inner rural or other [43]. Country of birth was operationalized as born in Australia or another English speaking country (Canada, Ireland, NZ, South Africa, UK, USA) and Other. Information on dieting (currently on a diet to lose weight; currently on a diet for health reasons; currently on a diet to gain weight and not currently on a diet) and atypical dietary intake on day of reporting (much more than usual; usual; much less than usual) were collected. Energy misreporting was calculated as the ratio of energy intake to predicted total energy expenditure (using sex and age-specific equations for a range of weight status, using a physical activity (PA) level of "low active" PA level > =1.4 < 1.6) [44]. PA was assessed according to whether participants met recommendations of 150 min of PA per week and 150 min of PA over 5 or more sessions per week. Time spent sedentary (minutes per day) was defined as sitting or lying down (except when sleeping) for various activities, including time spent sitting at work, and time spent sitting while using computers, watching television, and for other leisure activities. Family history of diabetes was assessed (Yes/No).

Statistical analyses

Complete case analysis was used (details of missing data are presented in Fig. 1). Variables were tested for skewness and kurtosis and variables with non-normal distributions, which included BMI, WC, sedentary time and all biomarkers, were logarithmically transformed prior to analysis. Values of logarithmically transformed variables were exponentiated to provide geometric means and SE. DPs identified from RRR were categorized into tertiles. When testing for LDL, TAG and glucose, fasting was required and only fasted data were used. Markers of cardiometabolic health markers were treated as categorical or binary outcome variables for the purpose of descriptive statistics and as continuous variables when evaluating associations with dietary intake. Linear regression analyses were used to test for associations between tertiles of diet quality and DP (independent variables) and markers of cardiometabolic health (dependent variables). Analyses were adjusted in Model 1 for age (continuous), sex, smoking (categorical), physical activity (binary), education (categorical), urban or rural location (categorical), energy misreporting (continuous), dieting (categorical) or atypical dietary intake on day of reporting (categorical) and family history of diabetes (binary). Analyses were further adjusted for BMI (continuous) in Model 2 in order to examine the effect independent of BMI. SAS (version 9; SAS Institute, Cary, NC) was used to derive RRR DPs. Data were analyzed using Stata (version 14; StataCorp., College Station, TX, USA). Survey weightings that were calibrated against population benchmarks (i.e. age, sex and area of usual residence) were used to account for the complex survey design. These weightings were specifically designed by the Australian Bureau of Statistics to account for bias associated with those who volunteered to provide biological samples. $P < 0.05$ was considered statistically significant. No adjustments were made for multiple comparisons given that analyses were pre-defined and methods were comparable with the available literature [17].

Results

A total of 2121 individuals were included in the present analyses (men: $n = 960$; women: $n = 1161$) (Fig. 1). Characteristics of the omitted sample with the analytical sample were broadly similar, although slightly more adults who were middle aged, highly educated and living in major cities were included in the analytical sample (Additional file 5: Table S4). A total of 31% individuals had high total cholesterol, 22% had low HDL-cholesterol, 31% had high LDL-cholesterol, 13% had high triglycerides, 18% had high apolipoprotein B, 6% had impaired fasting plasma glucose and 7% had HbA1c levels indicative of increased risk of diabetes. Five percent of individuals reported having diabetes, while 29% reported having a family history of diabetes.

Dietary patterns

The explained variation in food intakes and response variables and the correlations between response variables and DPs are summarized in Table 1. DP-1 was positively correlated with fiber density ($r = 0.72$) and inversely correlated with SFA: PUFA ($r = -0.53$) and total sugars intake ($r = -0.14$). DP-2 was positively correlated with fiber density ($r = 0.31$), SFA: PUFA ($r = 0.24$) and total sugars intake ($r = 0.72$). As the third DP explained less than 10% of the variation in response variables it was not further investigated.

Food groups with the top 5 positive and negative factor loadings for DP-1 and DP-2 are presented in Table 2. A full list of factor loadings for both DPs is presented in Additional file 6: Table S5. DP-1 was characterized by higher intakes of pome fruit, wholegrain bread, wholegrain cereals, nuts and seeds and carrot and root vegetables and lower intakes of fruit drinks, full-fat milk, cream, chocolate and non-wholegrain bread. DP-2 was characterized by higher intakes of added sugars, pome fruit, tropical fruit, other fruit and stone fruit and low intakes of wines, beers and ciders, wholegrain cereals, fish and fried vegetables (Table 2).

Table 1 Explained variation (%) in food intakes and response variables for each dietary pattern (DP) as assessed using reduced rank regression and correlation coefficient between DP and response variables for cardiometabolic health outcomes ($n = 2121$)[a]

DP	Explained variation (%)					Correlation coefficient[b,c]		
	Food intakes (total)	Responses (total)	Fibre density (g/MJ)	SFA:PUFA	Sugars (%E)	Fibre density (g/MJ)	SFA: PUFA	Sugars (%E)
DP-1	3.94	26.9	50.9	27.5	2.23	0.72***	−0.53***	− 0.26***
DP-2	2.51	21.0	60.0	31.9	51.8	0.30***	0.24***	0.72***
DP-3	2.47	7.99	65.4	46.0	56.3	0.24***	0.36***	−0.20**

[a]*DP* dietary pattern, *SFA* saturated fatty acid, *PUFA* poly-unsaturated fatty acid, *%E* percentage energy
[b]***Denotes correlation coefficient is significant at $P < 0.001$
[c]**Denotes correlation coefficient is significant at $P < 0.01$

Diet quality, dietary patterns and demographic characteristics

As shown in Table 3, those individuals with higher DGI were more highly educated, smoked less and were more physically active. Higher DGI scores were associated with higher DP-1 and DP-2 scores, greater fiber density and lower SFA: PUFA ratios. Participants with higher DP-1 scores were older, more physically active, had higher HbA1c levels and higher SBP, while those with higher DP-2 score smoked less and had lower HDL-cholesterol levels (Additional file 7: Table S6).

Diet quality, dietary patterns and cardiometabolic health

Higher DGI was associated with lower plasma glucose levels, BMI and WC. No other significant associations between DGI and cardiometabolic markers were observed. Following adjustment for BMI, the relationship between DGI and plasma glucose was attenuated but remained significant (Table 4).

Higher DP-1 was associated with lower BMI and WC (Table 5). Higher DP-2 was associated with lower HDL-C. There was a trend towards lower DBP. Following adjustment for BMI, the relationship between DP-2 and HDL-cholesterol was attenuated but remained significant and the association with DBP became significant (Table 6). No associations between DPs and other markers were observed.

Sensitivity analyses

Patterns of significant results remained consistent when associations between simplified DP scores and cardiometabolic health were investigated. Simplified DP-1 was associated with lower BMI (coef − 0.023, SE 0.009; P-trend = 0.012) and WC (coef − 0.014, SE 0.006; P-trend = 0.023) following adjustment for Model 1. Simplified DP-2 was associated with lower HDL-cholesterol (coef − 0.033, SE 0.010; P-trend = 0.001) and DBP (coef − 1.277, SE 0.418; P-trend = 0.003) following adjustment for Model 2.

Discussion

The aim of this study was to investigate the relationship between DPs, diet quality and cardiometabolic health in a nationally-representative sample of Australian adults. Our main findings are that both higher diet quality and a healthier DP (DP1) were primarily associated with favorable anthropometric markers of cardiometabolic health (BMI, WC) independent of numerous potential demographic and health-related confounders. Although effect sizes were small, these findings highlight the consistency of a diet quality and DP methodology to estimate associations with anthropometric markers of cardiometabolic health. Previous studies have independently compared diet quality scores [17] and DP methodologies [20] with markers of cardiometabolic health. However, few studies simultaneously compare multiple measures of overall diet with cardiometabolic health.

Evidence for an association between diet quality and markers of cardiometabolic health is mixed. Consistent with our findings, in a sample of Hispanic adults, higher 2010 Alternative HEI was associated with lower WC and glucose levels [18]. Moreover, studies in Australian adult populations have shown that higher DGI was associated with lower glucose levels [19, 45]. However, given the strength of the association between DGI and glucose levels observed in our study, we cannot discount the possibility of this being a chance finding. In line with a recent cross-sectional study of multiple diet quality scores in US women (predominantly Caucasian) [17], but in contrast with findings for the 2005 HEI (50% Caucasian) [46], diet quality was not associated with total or HDL-cholesterol. Similar inconsistencies are evident for other markers, such as TAG and HbA1c [46]. The inconsistency of associations with markers of cardiometabolic health may be partly attributable to differences in the ethnicity of the sample population [47], given that 80% of our sample were born in Australia or another English speaking country. However, it is likely to largely be due to methodological differences, such as reverse causation given the cross-sectional design, the method of assessing diet quality, choice of covariates and variation in sample sizes and resulting statistical power. To mitigate individual differences in markers, we evaluated an overall cardiometabolic risk score. This score has been used primarily for dietary behaviours [48] rather than patterns and so warrants further investigation.

The role of DPs in relation to cardiometabolic health is mixed, with only a small number of studies utilizing RRR [13, 49–51]. Of these studies, some have used

Table 2 Intakes of response variables and key foods across sex-specific tertiles (T) of dietary pattern ($n = 2121$)[a]

Food groups	Factor loading	Tertile of dietary pattern			*P*-trend[b]
		T1	T2	T3	
DP-1					
Response variables					
Fibre density, g/MJ	–	2.10 ± 0.04	2.75 ± 0.04	3.79 ± 0.06	< 0.001
SFA: PUFA	–	3.55 ± 0.09	2.53 ± 0.06	1.99 ± 0.06	< 0.001
Sugar, %E	–	20.7 ± 0.42	17.7 ± 0.33	18.7 ± 0.37	< 0.001
Direct associations, g/d					
Pome fruit	0.23	51 ± 6	88 ± 11	161 ± 12	< 0.001
Wholegrain bread	0.22	33 ± 5	45 ± 3	82 ± 4	< 0.001
Wholegrain cereals	0.22	31 ± 4	39 ± 3	72 ± 5	< 0.001
Nuts and seeds	0.22	9 ± 1	13 ± 1	29 ± 4	< 0.001
Carrot and root vegetables	0.21	29 ± 3	32 ± 3	72 ± 8	< 0.001
Inverse associations					
Fruit drinks	− 0.24	547 ± 46	283 ± 40	158 ± 17	< 0.001
Full fat milk	− 0.24	447 ± 34	244 ± 20	189 ± 19	< 0.001
Cream	− 0.22	77 ± 8	33 ± 5	20 ± 3	< 0.001
Chocolate	−0.21	23 ± 2	8 ± 1	6 ± 1	< 0.001
Non-wholegrain bread	− 0.20	138 ± 9	108 ± 8	82 ± 6	< 0.001
DP-2					
Response variables					
Fibre density, g/MJ	–	2.52 ± 0.06	2.90 ± 0.05	3.21 ± 0.07	< 0.001
SFA: PUFA	–	2.32 ± 0.07	2.70 ± 0.07	3.07 ± 0.08	< 0.001
Sugar, %E	–	13.9 ± 0.28	18.5 ± 0.37	24.7 ± 0.30	< 0.001
Direct associations, g/d					
Added sugars	0.31	24 ± 2	34 ± 3	53 ± 4	< 0.001
Pome fruit	0.28	52 ± 6	83 ± 8	165 ± 11	< 0.001
Tropical fruit	0.24	45 ± 4	70 ± 6	110 ± 8	< 0.001
Other fruit	0.21	28 ± 3	50 ± 6	77 ± 9	< 0.001
Stone fruit	0.20	18 ± 3	27 ± 4	86 ± 10	< 0.001
Inverse associations, g/d					
Wines	−0.30	281 ± 27	99 ± 13	60 ± 10	< 0.001
Beers and ciders	− 0.30	478 ± 54	187 ± 33	67 ± 13	< 0.001
Non-wholegrain cereals	− 0.19	284 ± 29	200 ± 23	135 ± 13	< 0.001
Fish	− 0.17	70 ± 8	39 ± 5	26 ± 3	< 0.001
Fried vegetables	− 0.15	28 ± 5	21 ± 6	14 ± 3	0.035

[a]*DP* dietary pattern, *SFA* saturated fatty acid, *PUFA* poly-unsaturated fatty acid, *%E* percentage energy; Values represent mean ± SE after adjustment for survey weighting
[b]Linear regression analyses tested for trends across tertiles of dietary pattern. Analyses were adjusted for age and sex

biochemical response variables, such as cholesterol, to derive associations between DPs and markers of cardiovascular health [25] and risk [13]. Associations observed between DP-1, consistent with a 'healthy' DP, and anthropometric outcomes are comparable to other studies [20, 25, 52–54]. In a recent analysis of 10,008 individuals from the Multiethnic Cohort, a RRR-derived DP (using four biomarkers as response variables) and low in fruit drinks and white rice and high in whole grains and fruits was inversely associated with BMI [13]. Few studies have use nutrient intakes as response variables. In a longitudinal study of 2037 Swedish adults, an 'unhealthy' RRR-derived DP characterized by some similar response variables to our study (high dietary energy density, SFA and low fiber-density) was associated with greater adiposity, cholesterol, TAG, SBP and DBP but not with

Table 3 Dietary, demographic and cardiometabolic characteristics of Australian adults across sex-specific tertiles (T) of diet quality ($n = 2121$)[a]

Characteristic	All	Diet quality			*P*-trend[b]
		T1	T2	T3	
Dietary					
DGI	81.8 ± 0.58	67.0 ± 0.49	82.1 ± 0.21	96.2 ± 0.41	< 0.001
Dietary pattern 1	0.07 ± 0.04	− 0.58 ± 0.06	0.07 ± 0.07	0.72 ± 0.06	< 0.001
Dietary pattern 2	0.01 ± 0.04	− 0.31 ± 0.06	0.10 ± 0.05	0.24 ± 0.06	< 0.001
Fibre density, g/MJ	2.87 ± 0.04	2.23 ± 0.04	2.85 ± 0.06	3.54 ± 0.07	< 0.001
SFA: PUFA	2.69 ± 0.05	2.89 ± 0.09	2.72 ± 0.08	2.47 ± 0.07	< 0.001
Sugar, %E	19.0 ± 0.24	18.2 ± 0.40	19.5 ± 0.37	19.4 ± 0.39	0.054
Demographic					
Age, y	46.4 ± 0.48	44.3 ± 1.20	47.1 ± 0.95	47.7 ± 1.29	0.11
Female, %	49.8	47.4	48.5	53.6	0.27
Country of birth (English speaking)	79.8	82.2	78.4	78.9	0.51
Highest level of education					
Low	19.5	22.9	18.5	17.1	0.025
Medium	49.6	51.6	52.0	45.2	
High	30.9	25.5	29.6	37.7	
Smoking, %					
Current smoker	11.9	18.1	11.9	5.81	< 0.001
Former smoker	33.4	37.1	32.6	30.3	
Never smoked	54.7	44.8	55.5	63.9	
Meet PA recommendations, %	50.2	42.8	53.5	54.3	0.036
Sedentary time, min/d	343 ± 5.8	350 ± 10.2	336 ± 11.2	344 ± 8.43	0.64
Cardiometabolic					
HbA1c, mmol/mol	35.6 ± 0.20	35.6 ± 0.32	35.9 ± 0.30	35.4 ± 0.36	0.71
Plasma glucose, mmol/L	5.08 ± 0.02	5.12 ± 0.04	5.12 ± 0.04	5.00 ± 0.04	0.050
Total cholesterol, mmol/L	5.00 ± 0.04	5.00 ± 0.05	5.00 ± 0.07	5.00 ± 0.05	0.88
HDL cholesterol, mmol/L	1.35 ± 0.12	1.35 ± 0.02	1.36 ± 0.02	1.34 ± 0.02	0.57
LDL cholesterol, mmol/L	3.08 ± 0.03	3.07 ± 0.05	3.08 ± 0.06	3.08 ± 0.04	0.72
Triglycerides, mmol/L	1.23 ± 0.02	1.23 ± 0.04	1.20 ± 0.04	1.27 ± 0.04	0.76
Apolipoprotein B, g/L	1.00 ± 0.01	1.00 ± 0.18	1.00 ± 0.02	1.01 ± 0.01	0.29
BMI, kg/m^2	27.0 ± 0.19	27.4 ± 0.34	26.7 ± 0.32	26.8 ± 0.35	0.23
BMI category, %					
Underweight/normal weight	40.4	38.1	39.4	43.7	0.32
Overweight	35.1	33.7	36.4	35.1	
Obese	24.5	28.2	24.2	21.2	
Waist circumference, cm	91.3 ± 0.46	92.6 ± 0.91	91.0 ± 0.90	90.3 ± 0.94	0.14
Systolic blood pressure, mmHg	121 ± 0.58	120 ± 1.11	121 ± 1.10	122 ± 1.18	0.36
Diastolic blood pressure, mmHg	75.6 ± 0.39	75.4 ± 0.75	75.4 ± 0.62	76.0 ± 0.84	0.65
Overall cardiometabolic risk score	− 0.11 ± 0.02	− 0.10 ± 0.04	− 0.11 ± 0.04	− 0.12 ± 0.04	0.69

[a]*BMI* body mass index, *DP* dietary pattern; Education: low (completed some high-school or less), medium (completed high-school or completed some high-school and/or certificate/diploma) and high (having a tertiary qualification). BMI category: underweight/normal weight (BMI < 25 kg/m^2), overweight (25 ≤ BMI < 30 kg/m^2), obese (BMI ≥ 30 kg/m^2); Overall cardiometabolic risk score was based on WC, TAG, HDL-cholesterol, blood pressure (average blood pressure was used as an index for systolic and diastolic blood pressure), and fasting plasma glucose based on an established methodology [30]. Values represent mean ± SE after adjustment for survey weighting. Where transformed for regression analyses, values represent exponentiated geometric mean ± SE

[b]Linear regression analyses (continuous variables) and χ^2 (categorical variables) were used to test for trends across tertiles

Table 4 Multivariable adjusted regression coefficients for cardiometabolic risk markers per sex-specific tertiles (T) of dietary guideline index (DGI) ($n = 2121$)[a]

Characteristic	Tertile of DGI			P-trend[b]
	T1	T2	T3	
HbA1c (mmol/mol)				
Model 1	ref	0.001 (0.008)	− 0.004 (0.010)	0.70
Model 2	ref	0.004 (0.010)	− 0.001 (0.010)	0.90
Plasma glucose (mmol/L)				
Model 1	ref	− 0.004 (0.009)	− 0.024 (0.009)	0.008
Model 2	ref	0.001 (0.009)	−0.019 (0.009)	0.033
Total cholesterol (mmol/L)				
Model 1	ref	−0.001 (0.016)	−0.004 (0.017)	0.82
Model 2	ref	0.004 (0.016)	−0.003 (0.017)	0.98
HDL cholesterol (mmol/L)				
Model 1	ref	−0.003 (0.021)	−0.029 (0.023)	0.20
Model 2	ref	−0.014 (0.020)	−0.041 (0.023)	0.08
LDL cholesterol (mmol/L)				
Model 1	ref	0.008 (0.023)	0.002 (0.025)	0.93
Model 2	ref	0.014 (0.022)	0.009 (0.025)	0.73
Triglycerides (mmol/L)				
Model 1	ref	−0.020 (0.043)	0.025 (0.033)	0.44
Model 2	ref	0.002 (0.041)	0.047 (0.034)	0.17
Apolipoprotein B (g/L)				
Model 1	ref	0.021 (0.024)	0.033 (0.025)	0.20
Model 2	ref	0.030 (0.023)	0.043 (0.025)	0.10
BMI (kg/m^2)				
Model 1	ref	−0.033 (0.015)	−0.033 (0.014)	0.019
Model 2	–	–	–	–
Waist circumference (cm)				
Model 1	ref	−0.022 (0.013)	−0.028 (0.010)	0.008
Model 2	–	–	–	–
Systolic blood pressure (mmHg)				
Model 1	ref	−0.642 (1.153)	0.329 (1.591)	0.83
Model 2	ref	−0.164 (1.120)	0.805 (1.591)	0.61
Diastolic blood pressure (mmHg)				
Model 1	ref	−0.494 (0.834)	−0.076 (1.161)	0.95
Model 2	ref	0.078 (0.765)	0.495 (1.160)	0.67
Overall cardiometabolic risk score				
Model 1	ref	−0.044 (0.050)	−0.030 (0.041)	0.48
Model 2	–	–	–	–

[a]*BMI* body mass index, Values represent regression coefficients and SE. Overall cardiometabolic risk score was based on WC, TAG, HDL-cholesterol, blood pressure (average blood pressure was used as an index for systolic and diastolic blood pressure), and fasting plasma glucose based on an established methodology [30]

[b]Linear regression analyses were used to test for significant differences across tertiles of diet quality score. Analyses were adjusted for Model 1 and Model 2. Model 1 adjusted for age (continuous), sex, smoking (categorical), physical activity (binary), education (categorical), urban or rural location (categorical), energy misreporting (continuous), dieting (categorical) or atypical dietary intake on day of reporting (categorical) and family history of diabetes. Blood biomarkers and blood pressure outcomes were further adjusted for BMI in Model 2

Table 5 Multivariable adjusted regression coefficients for cardiometabolic risk markers per sex-specific tertiles (T) of dietary pattern 1 ($n = 2121$)[a]

Characteristic	Tertile of dietary pattern			P-trend[b]
	T1	T2	T3	
HbA1c (mmol/mol)				
Model 1	ref	0.008 (0.007)	0.004 (0.001)	0.26
Model 2	ref	0.007 (0.010)	0.020 (0.013)	0.13
Plasma glucose (mmol/L)				
Model 1	ref	−0.017 (0.001)	−0.007 (0.010)	0.52
Model 2	ref	−0.010 (0.008)	0.002 (0.010)	0.84
Total cholesterol (mmol/L)				
Model 1	ref	−0.020 (0.016)	−0.022 (0.019)	0.26
Model 2	ref	−0.015 (0.016)	−0.017 (0.019)	0.40
HDL cholesterol (mmol/L)				
Model 1	ref	0.032 (0.021)	0.003 (0.020)	0.93
Model 2	ref	0.017 (0.022)	−0.016 (0.019)	0.37
LDL cholesterol (mmol/L)				
Model 1	ref	−0.035 (0.023)	−0.027 (0.029)	0.37
Model 2	ref	−0.027 (0.024)	−0.016 (0.028)	0.58
Triglycerides (mmol/L)				
Model 1	ref	−0.063 (0.032)	−0.067 (0.036)	0.07
Model 2	ref	−0.031 (0.033)	−0.030 (0.035)	0.41
Apolipoprotein B (g/L)				
Model 1	ref	−0.041 (0.025)	−0.022 (0.028)	0.46
Model 2	ref	−0.027 (0.025)	−0.005 (0.026)	0.88
BMI (kg/m^2)				
Model 1	ref	−0.048 (0.012)	− 0.056 (0.015)	< 0.001
Model 2	–	–	–	–
Waist circumference (cm)				
Model 1	ref	−0.032 (0.009)	−0.035 (0.010)	0.001
Model 2	–	–	–	–
Systolic blood pressure (mmHg)				
Model 1	ref	1.431 (1.132)	0.753 (1.376)	0.61
Model 2	ref	2.132 (1.091)	1.571 (1.286)	0.25
Diastolic blood pressure (mmHg)				
Model 1	ref	0.708 (0.879)	−0.566 (1.024)	0.56
Model 2	ref	1.530 (0.850)	0.394 (1.004)	0.74
Overall cardiometabolic risk score				
Model 1	ref	−0.097 (0.038)	−0.082 (0.042)	0.061
Model 2	–	–	–	–

[a]*BMI* body mass index; Values represent regression coefficients and SE. Overall cardiometabolic risk score was based on WC, TAG, HDL-cholesterol, blood pressure (average blood pressure was used as an index for systolic and diastolic blood pressure), and fasting plasma glucose based on an established methodology [30]

[b]Linear regression analyses were used to test for significant differences across tertiles of dietary pattern score. Analyses were adjusted for Model 1 and Model 2. Model 1 adjusted for age (continuous), sex, smoking (categorical), physical activity (binary), education (categorical), urban or rural location (categorical), energy misreporting (continuous), dieting (categorical) or atypical dietary intake on day of reporting (categorical) and family history of diabetes. Blood biomarkers and blood pressure outcomes were further adjusted for BMI in Model 2

Table 6 Multivariable adjusted regression coefficients for cardiometabolic risk markers per sex-specific tertiles (T) of dietary pattern 2 ($n = 2121$)[a]

Characteristic	Tertile of dietary pattern			P-trend[b]
	T1	T2	T3	
HbA1c (mmol/mol)				
Model 1	ref	−0.003 (0.010)	0.008 (0.009)	0.37
Model 2	ref	−0.004 (0.009)	0.007 (0.009)	0.44
Plasma glucose (mmol/L)				
Model 1	ref	−0.009 (0.008)	−0.007 (0.008)	0.35
Model 2	ref	−0.019 (0.008)	−0.009 (0.007)	0.24
Total cholesterol (mmol/L)				
Model 1	ref	−0.033 (0.018)	−0.009 (0.017)	0.62
Model 2	ref	−0.033 (0.018)	−0.010 (0.017)	0.57
HDL cholesterol (mmol/L)				
Model 1	ref	−0.035 (0.022)	−0.056 (0.024)	0.022
Model 2	ref	−0.034 (0.021)	−0.053 (0.023)	0.028
LDL cholesterol (mmol/L)				
Model 1	ref	−0.023 (0.027)	0.014 (0.026)	0.57
Model 2	ref	−0.024 (0.026)	0.012 (0.025)	0.61
Triglycerides (mmol/L)				
Model 1	ref	−0.063 (0.041)	−0.018 (0.040)	0.69
Model 2	ref	−0.064 (0.042)	−0.024 (0.040)	0.56
Apolipoprotein B (g/L)				
Model 1	ref	−0.026 (0.026)	0.013 (0.025)	0.57
Model 2	ref	−0.026 (0.025)	0.010 (0.023)	0.64
BMI (kg/m^2)				
Model 1	ref	0.001 (0.016)	0.010 (0.014)	0.49
Model 2	–	–	–	–
Waist circumference (cm)				
Model 1	ref	−0.003 (0.012)	0.002 (0.010)	0.84
Model 2	–	–	–	–
Systolic blood pressure (mmHg)				
Model 1	ref	1.885 (1.286)	−0.435 (1.090)	0.67
Model 2	ref	1.871 (1.298)	−0.573 (1.051)	0.57
Diastolic blood pressure (mmHg)				
Model 1	ref	0.275 (0.871)	−1.811 (0.969)	0.07
Model 2	ref	0.258 (0.818)	−1.979 (0.908)	0.033
Overall cardiometabolic risk score				
Model 1	ref	0.002 (0.044)	0.010 (0.046)	0.83
Model 2	–	–	–	–

[a]BMI, body mass index; Values represent regression coefficients and SE. Overall cardiometabolic risk score was based on WC, TAG, HDL-cholesterol, blood pressure (average blood pressure was used as an index for systolic and diastolic blood pressure), and fasting plasma glucose based on an established methodology [30]

[b]Linear regression analyses were used to test for significant differences across tertiles of dietary pattern score. Analyses were adjusted for Model 1 and Model 2. Model 1 adjusted for age (continuous), sex, smoking (categorical), physical activity (binary), education (categorical), urban or rural location (categorical), energy misreporting (continuous), dieting (categorical) or atypical dietary intake on day of reporting (categorical) and family history of diabetes. Blood biomarkers and blood pressure outcomes were further adjusted for BMI in Model 2

CVD endpoints [52]. However, comparability of results was limited as this study was conducted in obese individuals only, who may be more metabolically sensitive to an 'unhealthy' diet [55]. Recent data from a AHS study showed that a 'healthy' DP, derived using factor analysis and characterized by high intakes of wholegrains and fresh fruit and low intakes of take-away foods and soft drinks, was associated with higher odds of having a healthy metabolic profile [20]. Similar findings for a 'healthy' DP were observed in a national longitudinal study in Chinese adults [53] and a representative community sample of Lebanese adults [54] but were mixed in a prospective study of UK males [56]. Our DPs were derived to explain the maximum variation in dietary energy density, SFA: PUFA, and total sugars; it is likely that a DP that explained other nutrient intakes, as well as a DP derived using other methodologies, may show different associations with cardiometabolic health.

Observed associations between DP-2 and cardiometabolic health outcomes requires further investigation. Positive correlations with all response variables resulted in DP-2 food groups that were less consistent with a 'healthy' or 'unhealthy' diet, i.e. DP-2 was high in both added sugar and fruit intake and low in fish, alcohol and non-whole grain cereals. Although other studies have used a ratio of SFA:PUFA [15] and total sugars, [14] the use of a ratio and a lack of specificity of sugar type (added vs natural) may have limited the interpretation of DP-2. Moreover, this may partly explain why we observed inverse associations with both HDL-cholesterol and DBP. Given that RRR derives DPs that best represent the chosen response variables, investigation of alternative response variables is needed to better understand the role of RRR-derived DPs in cardiometabolic heath. In addition, limited RRR research has examined the role of certain individual biomarkers, such as apolipoprotein, which has been linked to better cardiometabolic health using other DP methodologies [57].

Our findings show consistency between two whole-diet based methodologies for identifying associations with anthropometric markers of cardiometabolic health. Foods comprise a complex mixture of nutrients with potentially contrasting associations with cardiometabolic health, thus supporting a whole diet approach. [58] Future studies based on RRR should evaluate the mechanistic role of response variables and the use of comparable methodologies for deriving an overall risk score.

Strengths and limitations

The present study has a number of strengths. This study was conducted in a large, nationally representative survey of Australian adults. Although the generalizability of our sample may have been limited by non-response bias associated with those who volunteered to provide biological samples, our analyses used survey weightings that were specifically designed to account for such bias. Moreover, there was minimal difference in characteristics between the omitted sample and the analytical sample (Additional file 5: Table S4). We derived two whole diet methodologies, which facilitated a comparison between data-driven and dietary adherence-based methodologies within the same population. These scores were derived from two 24-h recalls, thus offering a more accurate estimate of dietary intake than FFQ-based scores [59]. Moreover, the DGI used age and sex-specific cut-offs, thereby increasing the accuracy of diet quality scores across different population groups. A further strength of this study is the evaluation of the role of BMI in the association between diet quality, DPs and cardiometabolic health.

A limitation of this study is its cross-sectional design, which prohibited interpretation of causal relationships. Given that some measures of cardiometabolic health were self-reported, some individuals may have been aware of their poor cardiometabolic health and may have changed their diet as a result. Thus, we cannot discount the possibility of reverse causality. Information on blood pressure or lipid lowering medication was not available and so we were unable to exclude or adjust for this potential confounder. Thus, we cannot discount bias associated with incongruences between blood pressure and lipid data before and after anti-hypertensive and lipid lowering medication use and any associated behavioral changes. While our analyses were adjusted for multiple confounders, including energy misreporting, residual confounding may be a limitation. Moreover, missing data, most notably for biochemical and the second day of dietary recalls, may have introduced bias. Although the timing of 24-h dietary recalls may limit their ability to capture usual intake and seasonal variations in dietary intakes, our use of two 24-h recalls offers an advantage over previous studies based on one day of dietary recall [20] and our research has demonstrated that RRR DPs derived from the average of two days are comparable to those derived using usual intakes [14]. Any seasonal impact on DPs may have influenced smaller food groups, such as stone fruits, but is likely to be minimal in larger food groups, such as brassica vegetables, and in the DGI. Moreover, a seasonal adjustment was also incorporated into the person weights in the NNPAS [27]. Limitations of RRR should also be acknowledged. First, although the food groups are based on AUSNUT 2011–13, the number and definitions of the food groups used in this study may have affected the derived DP. Second, although our choice of response variables was based on published literature the use of different response variables may have resulted in a different DPs. Moreover, RRR derives DPs that closely reflect nutrient intakes or intermediate markers, which may result in DPs less consistent with behavioral patterns compared to factor or cluster analysis. Third, we generated and fitted RRR DP in the same data set. To rule out any effect of over-fitting and to show generalizability of RRR DP, future studies should consider deriving and applying DP in independent data sets. Although we were unable to disaggregate the effect of added sugars from total sugars in our response variable, food group intakes provided information on the foods that characterized the DPs. Prospective studies that consider type 2 diabetes and cardiovascular disease incidence and that compare both diet quality and DP methodologies within the same population are needed.

Implications of findings

Both diet quality and DP methodologies (DP-1) support healthy eating initiates to improve cardiometabolic health that centre on diets rich in fruits, vegetables, wholegrains and lean meats and/or alternatives and low in processed foods and alcohol. Furthermore, this study provides evidence for the comparability of associations between whole diet measures and cardiometabolic health. This evidence is imperative for the effective integration of diet quality and DP research. As a result, the present findings have the potential to inform the design of future DP-based research that aims to evaluate association with cardiometabolic health.

Conclusions

Better diet quality and a healthier DP were primarily associated with favorable anthropometric markers of cardiometabolic health. Findings support the need to compare across multiple whole-diet based methodologies, which take into consideration the interaction between foods and nutrients consumed together. The limited associations observed between diet quality, DPs and biochemical cardiometabolic markers warrants further investigation. Studies that evaluate the role of different response variables and that are longitudinal in design are needed to better understand causal relationships between diet and cardiometabolic health.

Additional files

Additional file 1: Table S1. STROBE-nut: An extension of the STROBE statement for nutritional epidemiology.

Additional file 2: Table S2. Components and scoring methods of the Dietary Guideline Index (DGI).

Additional file 3: Table S3. Food groups used as predictors in the reduced rank regression analyses ($n = 48$)

Additional file 4: Figure S1. Directed acyclic graph (DAG) used to help identify the confounder selection for the statistical analysis.

Additional file 5: Table S4. Characteristics of adults who were omitted from the analytical sample based on only 1 day of 24-h recall and based on missing covariates and those who were included in the analytical sample.

Additional file 6: Table S5. Factor loadings for reduced rank regression dietary patterns.

Additional file 7: Table S6. Demographic and cardiometabolic characteristics of Australian adults across sex-specific tertiles (T) of each dietary pattern ($n = 2121$).

Abbreviations
AHS: Australian Health Survey; BMI: Body mass index; DBP: Diastolic blood pressure; DGI: Dietary guideline index; DP: Dietary pattern; FFQ: Food frequency questionnaire; NHMS: National Health Measures Survey; NNPAS: National Nutrition and Physical Activity Survey; PA: Physical activity; SBP: Systolic blood pressure

Acknowledgements
None

Funding
KML acknowledges support from the Alfred Deakin Postdoctoral Research Fellowship. SAM is supported by an NHMRC Career Development Fellowship Level 2 (ID1104636).

Authors' contributions
The authors' responsibilities were as follows: KML, SM contributed to the research design. KML performed the statistical analysis for the manuscript and drafted the paper. Both authors contributed to a critical review of the manuscript during the writing process. Both authors approved the final version to be published.

Competing interests
None of the authors had a personal or financial conflict of interest.

References
1. World Health Organization. Noncommunicable diseases. http://www.who.int/mediacentre/factsheets/fs355/en/ . Accessed 17 Nov 2017.
2. American Diabetes Association. Management of Dyslipidemia in adults with diabetes. Diabetes Care. 2003;26:s83–6. https://doi.org/10.2337/diacare.26.2007.S83.
3. Hu FB, Manson JE, Stampfer MJ, Colditz G, Liu S, Solomon CG, Willett WC. Diet, lifestyle, and the risk of type 2 diabetes mellitus in women. N Engl J Med. 2001;345:790–7. https://doi.org/10.1056/NEJMoa010492.
4. Diet, Nutrition and the Prevention of Chronic Diseases. Technical Report Series no. 916. http://www.who.int/dietphysicalactivity/publications/trs916/en/ . Accessed 18 Nov 2017.
5. Gakidou E, Afshin A, Abajobir AA, Abate KH, Abbafati C, Abbas KM, Abd-Allah F, Abdulle AM, Abera SF, Aboyans V, et al. Global, regional, and national comparative risk assessment of 84 behavioural, environmental and occupational, and metabolic risks or clusters of risks, 1990-2016: a systematic analysis for the global burden of disease study 2016. Lancet. 2017;390:1345–422. https://doi.org/10.1016/S0140-6736(17)32366-8.
6. Salmerón J, Hu FB, Manson JE, Stampfer MJ, Colditz GA, Rimm EB, Willett WC. Dietary fat intake and risk of type 2 diabetes in women. Am J Clin Nutr. 2001; 73:1019–26.
7. Juan J, Liu G, Willett WC, Hu FB, Rexrode KM, Sun Q. Whole grain consumption and risk of ischemic stroke. Results from 2 prospective cohort studies. Stroke. 2017;48:3203–9. https://doi.org/10.1161/strokeaha.117.018979.
8. Imamura F, Micha R, Khatibzadeh S, Fahimi S, Shi P, Powles J, Mozaffarian D. Dietary quality among men and women in 187 countries in 1990 and 2010: a systematic assessment. Lancet Glob Health. 2015;3:e132–42. https://doi.org/10.1016/S2214-109X(14)70381-X.
9. Milte CM, Thorpe MG, Crawford D, Ball K, McNaughton SA. Associations of diet quality with health-related quality of life in older Australian men and women. Exp Gerontol. 2015;64:8–16. https://doi.org/10.1016/j.exger.2015.01.047.
10. Nanri A, Mizoue T, Shimazu T, Ishihara J, Takachi R, Noda M, Iso H, Sasazuki S, Sawada N, Tsugane S, for the Japan Public Health Center-Based Prospective Study G. Dietary patterns and all-cause, cancer, and cardiovascular disease mortality in Japanese men and women: the Japan public health center-based prospective study. PLoS One. 2017;12:e0174848. https://doi.org/10.1371/journal.pone.0174848.
11. George SM, Ballard-Barbash R, Manson JE, Reedy J, Shikany JM, Subar AF, Tinker LF, Vitolins M, Neuhouser ML. Comparing indices of diet quality with chronic disease mortality risk in postmenopausal women in the Women's Health Initiative observational study: evidence to inform National Dietary Guidance. Am J Epidemiol. 2014;180:616–25. https://doi.org/10.1093/aje/kwu173.
12. Hoffmann K, Schulze MB, Schienkiewitz A, Nöthlings U, Boeing H. Application of a new statistical method to derive dietary patterns in nutritional epidemiology. Am J Epidemiol. 2004;159:935–44. https://doi.org/10.1093/aje/kwh134.
13. Jacobs S, Kroeger J, Schulze MB, Frank LK, Franke AA, Cheng I, Monroe KR, Haiman CA, Kolonel LN, Wilkens LR, et al. Dietary patterns derived by reduced rank regression are inversely associated with type 2 diabetes risk across five ethnic groups in the multiethnic cohort. Curr Dev Nutr. 2017; https://doi.org/10.3945/cdn.117.000620.
14. Livingstone KM, McNaughton S. Dietary patterns by reduced rank regression are associated with obesity and hypertension in Australian adults. Br J Nutr. 2017; https://doi.org/10.1017/S0007114516004505.
15. Sherafat-Kazemzadeh R, Egtesadi S, Mirmiran P, Gohari M, Farahani SJ, Esfahani FH, Vafa MR, Hedayati M, Azizi F. Dietary patterns by reduced rank regression predicting changes in obesity indices in a cohort study: Tehran lipid and glucose study. Asia Pac J Clin Nutr. 2010;19:22–32.
16. Weikert C, Schulze MB. Evaluating dietary patterns: the role of reduced rank regression. Curr Opin Clin Nutr Metab Care. 2016;19:341–6. https://doi.org/10.1097/mco.0000000000000308.
17. Alessa HB, Malik VS, Yuan C, Willett WC, Huang T, Hu FB, Tobias DK. Dietary patterns and cardiometabolic and endocrine plasma biomarkers in US women. Am J Clin Nutr. 2016; https://doi.org/10.3945/ajcn.116.143016.
18. Mattei J, Sotres-Alvarez D, Daviglus ML, Gallo LC, Gellman M, Hu FB, Tucker KL, Willett WC, Siega-Riz AM, Van Horn L, Kaplan R. Diet quality and its association with Cardiometabolic risk factors vary by Hispanic and Latino ethnic background in the Hispanic community health study/study of Latinos. J Nutr. 2016;146:2035–44. https://doi.org/10.3945/jn.116.231209.
19. McNaughton SA, Dunstan DW, Ball K, Shaw J, Crawford D. Dietary quality is associated with diabetes and cardio-metabolic risk factors. J Nutr. 2009;139:734–42. https://doi.org/10.3945/jn.108.096784.
20. Bell L, Edwards S, Grieger J. The relationship between dietary patterns and metabolic health in a representative sample of adult Australians. Nutrients. 2015;7:5295.
21. Frazier-Wood AC, Kim J, Davis JS, Jung SY, Chang S. In cross-sectional observations, dietary quality is not associated with CVD risk in women; in men the positive association is accounted for by BMI. Br J Nutr. 2015;113:1244–53. https://doi.org/10.1017/S0007114515000185.
22. Liese AD, Krebs-Smith SM, Subar AF, George SM, Harmon BE, Neuhouser ML, Boushey CJ, Schap TE, Reedy J. The dietary patterns methods project: synthesis of findings across cohorts and relevance to dietary guidance. J Nutr. 2015;145:393–402. https://doi.org/10.3945/jn.114.205336.
23. Oude Griep LM, Wang H, Chan Q. Empirically-derived dietary patterns, diet quality scores, and markers of inflammation and endothelial dysfunction. Curr Nutr Rep. 2013;2:97–104. https://doi.org/10.1007/s13668-013-0045-3.
24. Manios Y, Kourlaba G, Grammatikaki E, Androutsos O, Ioannou E, Roma-Giannikou E. Comparison of two methods for identifying dietary patterns associated with obesity in preschool children: the GENESIS study. Eur J Clin Nutr. 2010;64:1407. https://doi.org/10.1038/ejcn.2010.168.
25. Nettleton JA, Steffen LM, Schulze MB, Jenny NS, Barr RG, Bertoni AG, Jacobs DR. Associations between markers of subclinical atherosclerosis and dietary patterns derived by principal components analysis and reduced rank regression in the multi-ethnic study of atherosclerosis (MESA). Am J Clin Nutr. 2007;85:1615–25.
26. Rodríguez-Monforte M, Sánchez E, Barrio F, Costa B, Flores-Mateo G. Metabolic syndrome and dietary patterns: a systematic review and meta-analysis of observational studies. Eur J Nutr. 2017;56:925–47. https://doi.org/10.1007/s00394-016-1305-y.
27. Australian Health Survey: Users' Guide, 2011–13, Catalogue No 4363.0.55.001. http://www.abs.gov.au/ausstats/abs@.nsf/Lookup/4363.0.55.001Chapter1002011-13. Accessed 1 Aug 2017
28. World Health Organization.Obesity and overweight. http://www.who.int/mediacentre/factsheets/fs311/en/. Accessed 5 Sept 2017.
29. Friedewald WT, Levy RI, Fredrickson DS. Estimation of the concentration of low-density lipoprotein cholesterol in plasma, without use of the preparative ultracentrifuge. Clin Chem. 1972;18:499–502.
30. Wijndaele K, Healy GN, Dunstan DW, Barnett AG, Salmon J, Shaw JE, Zimmet PZ, Owen N. Increased Cardiometabolic risk is associated with increased TV viewing time. Med Sci Sports Exerc. 2010;42:1511–8. https://doi.org/10.1249/MSS.0b013e3181d322ac.

31. Bliss R. Researchers produce innovation in dietary recall. Agric Res. 2004;52:10–2.
32. AUSNUT 2011–13: Australian Food, Supplement and Nutrient Database. http://www.foodstandards.gov.au/science/monitoringnutrients/ausnut/Pages/about.aspx. Accessed 11 Sept 2017.
33. National Health and Medical Research Council. Australian Dietary Guidelines. Canberra: National Health and Medical Research Council; 2013.
34. Livingstone KM, McNaughton SA. Diet quality is associated with obesity and hypertension in Australian adults: a cross sectional study. BMC Public Health. 2016;16:1037. https://doi.org/10.1186/s12889-016-3714-5.
35. Thorpe M, Milte C, Crawford D, McNaughton S. A revised Australian dietary guideline index and its association with key Sociodemographic factors, health behaviors and body mass index in Peri-retirement aged adults. Nutrients. 2016;8:160.
36. National Health and Medical Research Council. 2013. Educator Guide: Eat for Health. Canberra: National Health and Medical Research Council.
37. Waijers PMCM, Feskens EJM, Ocké MC. A critical review of predefined diet quality scores. Br J Nutr. 2007;97:219–31. https://doi.org/10.1017/S0007114507250421.
38. Wirfält E, Drake I, Wallström P. What do review papers conclude about food and dietary patterns? Food Nutr Res. 2013;57. https://doi.org/10.3402/fnr.v57i0.20523.
39. da Silva BDP, Neutzling MB, Camey S, Olinto MTA. Dietary patterns and hypertension: a population-based study with women from southern Brazil. Cad Saúde Pública. 2014;30:961–71.
40. Johnson L, Mander AP, Jones LR, Emmett PM, Jebb SA. Energy-dense, low-fiber, high-fat dietary pattern is associated with increased fatness in childhood. Am J Clin Nutr. 2008;87:846–54.
41. Schulze MB, Hoffmann K, Kroke A, Boeing H. An approach to construct simplified measures of dietary patterns from exploratory factor analysis. Br J Nutr. 2003;89:409–18. https://doi.org/10.1079/BJN2002778.
42. Australian Standard Classification of Education (ASCED) 2001. http://www.abs.gov.au/AUSSTATS/abs@.nsf/ProductsbyCatalogue/B49672F95CD93ABECA2570B30005BFE1. Accessed 16 Oct 2017.
43. Statistical Geography Volume 1 - Australian Standard Geographical Classification (ASGC) 2006. http://www.abs.gov.au/AUSSTATS/abs@.nsf/Lookup/1216.0Main+Features1Jul%202006?OpenDocument. Accessed 15 Sept 2017.
44. Huang TTK, Roberts SB, Howarth NC, McCrory MA. Effect of screening out implausible energy intake reports on relationships between diet and BMI. Obes Res. 2005;13:1205–17. https://doi.org/10.1038/oby.2005.143.
45. Gopinath B, Rochtchina E, Flood VM, Mitchell P. Diet quality is prospectively associated with incident impaired fasting glucose in older adults. Diabet Med. 2013;30:557–62. https://doi.org/10.1111/dme.12109.
46. Nicklas TA, O'Neil CE, Fulgoni VL. Diet quality is inversely related to cardiovascular risk factors in adults. J Nutr. 2012;142:2112–8. https://doi.org/10.3945/jn.112.164889.
47. Ford ES, Giles WH, Dietz WH. Prevalence of the metabolic syndrome among us adults: findings from the third national health and nutrition examination survey. JAMA. 2002;287:356–9. https://doi.org/10.1001/jama.287.3.356.
48. Smith KJ, Blizzard L, McNaughton SA, Gall SL, Dwyer T, Venn AJ. Takeaway food consumption and cardio-metabolic risk factors in young adults. Eur J Clin Nutr. 2012;66:577–84.
49. Heidemann C, Hoffmann K, Spranger J, Klipstein-Grobusch K, Möhlig M, Pfeiffer AFH, Boeing H. A dietary pattern protective against type 2 diabetes in the European prospective investigation into cancer and nutrition (EPIC)—Potsdam study cohort. Diabetologia. 2005;48:1126–34. https://doi.org/10.1007/s00125-005-1743-1.
50. Liese AD, Weis KE, Schulz M, Tooze JA. Food intake patterns associated with incident type 2 diabetes: the insulin resistance atherosclerosis study. Diabetes Care. 2009;32:263–8. https://doi.org/10.2337/dc08-1325.
51. McNaughton SA, Mishra GD, Brunner EJ. Dietary patterns, insulin resistance, and incidence of type 2 diabetes in the Whitehall II study. Diabetes Care. 2008;31:1343–8. https://doi.org/10.2337/dc07-1946.
52. Johns DJ, Lindroos A-K, Jebb SA, Sjöström L, Carlsson LMS, Ambrosini GL. Dietary patterns, cardiometabolic risk factors, and the incidence of cardiovascular disease in severe obesity. Obesity. 2015;23:1063–70. https://doi.org/10.1002/oby.20920.
53. Li M, Shi Z. Dietary pattern during 1991–2011 and its association with cardio metabolic risks in Chinese adults: the China health and nutrition survey. Nutrients. 2017;9:1218. https://doi.org/10.3390/nu9111218.
54. Nasreddine L, Tamim H, Itani L, Nasrallah MP, Isma'eel H, Nakhoul NF, Abou-Rizk J, Naja F. A minimally processed dietary pattern is associated with lower odds of metabolic syndrome among Lebanese adults. Public Health Nutr. 2017;21:160–71. https://doi.org/10.1017/S1368980017002130.
55. Mathew H, Farr OM, Mantzoros CS. Metabolic health and weight: understanding metabolically unhealthy normal weight or metabolically healthy obese patients. Metabolism. 2016;65:73–80. https://doi.org/10.1016/j.metabol.2015.10.019.
56. Mertens E, Markey O, Geleijnse JM, Givens DI, Lovegrove JA. Dietary patterns in relation to cardiovascular disease incidence and risk markers in a middle-aged British male population: data from the Caerphilly prospective study. Nutrients. 2017;9:75. https://doi.org/10.3390/nu9010075.
57. Chiu S, Bergeron N, Williams PT, Bray GA, Sutherland B, Krauss RM. Comparison of the DASH (dietary approaches to stop hypertension) diet and a higher-fat DASH diet on blood pressure and lipids and lipoproteins: a randomized controlled trial. Am J Clin Nutr. 2016;103:341–7. https://doi.org/10.3945/ajcn.115.123281.
58. Siri-Tarino PW, Chiu S, Bergeron N, Krauss RM. Saturated fats versus polyunsaturated fats versus carbohydrates for cardiovascular disease prevention and treatment. Annu Rev Nutr. 2015;35:517–43. https://doi.org/10.1146/annurev-nutr-071714-034449.
59. Shim J-S, Oh K, Kim HC. Dietary assessment methods in epidemiologic studies. Epidemiol Health. 2014;36:e2014009. https://doi.org/10.4178/epih/e2014009.

17

Dietary patterns and physical activity in the metabolically (un)healthy obese: the Dutch Lifelines cohort study

Sandra N. Slagter[1*], Eva Corpeleijn[2], Melanie M. van der Klauw[1], Anna Sijtsma[3], Linda G. Swart-Busscher[4], Corine W. M. Perenboom[5], Jeanne H. M. de Vries[5], Edith J. M. Feskens[5], Bruce H. R. Wolffenbuttel[1], Daan Kromhout[2] and Jana V. van Vliet-Ostaptchouk[1]

Abstract

Background: Diversity in the reported prevalence of metabolically healthy obesity (MHO), suggests that modifiable factors may be at play. We evaluated differences in dietary patterns and physical activity between MHO and metabolically unhealthy obesity (MUO).

Methods: Cross-sectional data of 9270 obese individuals (30–69 years) of the Lifelines Cohort Study was used. MHO was defined as obesity and no metabolic syndrome risk factors and no cardiovascular disease history. MUO was defined as obesity and ≥2 metabolic syndrome risk factors. Sex-specific associations of dietary patterns (identified by principal component analysis) and physical activity with MHO were assessed by multivariable logistic regression (reference group: MUO). Analyses were adjusted for multiple covariates.

Results: Among 3442 men and 5828 women, 10.2% and 24.4% had MHO and 56.9% and 35.3% MUO, respectively. We generated four obesity-specific dietary patterns. Two were related to MHO, and in women only. In the highest quartile (Q) of *'bread, potatoes and sweet snacks'* pattern, odds ratio (OR) (95% CI) for MHO was 0.52 (0.39–0.70). For the healthier pattern *'fruit, vegetables and fish'*, an OR of 1.36 (1.09–1.71) in Q3 and 1.55 (1.21–1.97) in Q4 was found for MHO. For physical activity, there was a positive association between moderate physical activity and vigorous physical activity in the highest tertile and MHO in women and men, respectively (OR 1.19 (1.01–1.41) and OR 2.02 (1.50–2.71)).

Conclusion: The healthier diet -characterized by *'fruit, vegetables and fish'*- and moderate physical activity in women, and vigorous physical activity in men may be related to MHO. The (refined) carbohydrate-rich *'bread, potatoes and sweet snacks'* dietary pattern was found to counteract MHO in women.

Keywords: Obesity, Metabolic health, Dietary patterns, Physical activity, Lifestyle

Background

Obese individuals are more likely to develop multiple metabolic complications which increase their risk of type 2 diabetes (T2D) and cardiovascular disease (CVD) [1]. However, some obese individuals, called the metabolically healthy obese, show no sign of conditions associated with the metabolic syndrome (MetS), i.e. impaired glucose metabolism, hypertension and dyslipidaemia [2]. Whether metabolically healthy obesity (MHO) is a truly healthy state remains controversial. Meta-analyses have shown that it is not evident that adults with MHO are at increased risk for all-cause mortality [3], but they still have a risk for T2D and CVD that is intermediate between that of healthy normal weight and unhealthy obese adults [4, 5]. Meaning that even without weight loss, the (cardio)metabolic health can be improved in obese individuals. This is an important finding, given the fact that sustained weight loss is difficult [6, 7].

* Correspondence: s.n.slagter@umcg.nl
[1]Department of Endocrinology, University of Groningen, University Medical Center Groningen, HPC AA31, P.O. Box 30001, 9700, RB, Groningen, The Netherlands

Interestingly, the MHO phenotype may be modifiable. Several studies with up to 10 years of follow-up data showed that 43.3–47.6% of subjects with MHO transitioned to metabolically unhealthy obesity (MUO) [8–10]. While the ageing process is an important factor, the BioSHaRE-EU Healthy Obesity Project ($n = 28.077$) reported that even the age-standardized prevalence of MHO highly varied between the European countries, 2–19% among men and 7–28% among women, when the same diagnostic criteria for MHO were used [11]. This suggests that on top of age, sex and possibly genes, lifestyle factors are related to the transition from healthy to unhealthy.

The determinants accounting for the metabolic differences observed between MHO and MUO remain uncertain, and particularly data on the role of diet and physical activity are limited. Previous studies on intake of single foods and/or micro- and macronutrients could not find an association with metabolic health subtypes [12–15]. However, as nutrients interact with each other [16], examination of whole diets may be more suitable to gain insight into the relation between diet and metabolic health within the obese population.

In the study of Cahmi et al. [17], adolescents and women with MHO (19–44 years) had higher scores on the HEI-2005 (Healthy Eating Index), which assesses diet quality in relation to U.S. National Dietary Guidelines (2005), compared to the MUO individuals. While the HEI-2005 is a 'a priori' dietary pattern based on current knowledge about the role of foods, less is known about the role of existing food consumption patterns within the obese population. Factor analysis is a useful tool to examine these habitual 'a posteriori' dietary patterns in a population. Although they do not necessarily represent optimal diets for risk assessment, they are an expression of the way how people eat [15] and are expected to be part of broader lifestyles [16]. Furthermore, they may generate new hypothesis and improve our insight into possibilities for dietary changes for prevention and treatment of metabolic disturbances. A recent systematic review and meta-analysis of observational studies has already shown that 'a posteriori' dietary patterns are associated with MetS in the general adult population [18]. In this study, obesity specific dietary patterns will be investigated in relation to metabolic health.

The aim of this study was to evaluate differences in dietary patterns and physical activity between MHO and MUO in the large population-based Lifelines Cohort Study. More specifically, we aimed to 1) generate obesity-specific dietary patterns and examine their associations with demographic- and other lifestyle factors; and 2) compare the dietary patterns and physical activity between MHO and MUO, taking into account among others demographic characteristics, smoking and alcohol use.

Methods

Subjects

For this study we used a subset of the cross-sectional Lifelines data, collected between 2006 and 2013. Subjects included in the present study had obesity (body mass index (BMI) ≥30 kg/m^2), were of western European origin, and aged 30–69 years ($N = 10{,}771$). In short, Lifelines is a prospective population-based cohort study using a unique three-generation design to study the health and health-related behaviours of 167,729 persons living in the North of The Netherlands. The Lifelines adult population is broadly representative for the adults living in this region [19]. Detailed information on the cohort profile can be found elsewhere [20].

Clinical measures and definitions

Clinical measurements and laboratory methods

Detailed information about the physical examination and biochemical measurements has been published previously [21]. In short, during the first visit measurements of weight, waist circumference, and height (to the nearest 0.5 cm) were performed in light clothing and without shoes. Body weight and height were used to calculate BMI (weight (kg)/height (m)^2). Blood pressure was measured every minute during a period of 10 min with an automated DINAMAP Monitor (GE Healthcare, Freiburg, Germany), the change in blood pressure within that period can be used as a proxy measure of stress. The average of the final three readings confers the traditional measurement after 5–10 min supine rest and was recorded for systolic and diastolic blood pressure. During the second visit, on average two weeks after the first visit, blood samples were drawn after an overnight fast for measurement of plasma glucose (hexokinase method), high density lipoprotein cholesterol (HDL-C) and triglycerides (respectively, colorimetric method and colorimetric UV method, Roche Modular P chemistry analyser, Basel, Switzerland).

Definition of the metabolic health phenotypes

MHO was defined according to the criteria established by the BioSHaRE-EU Healthy Obesity Project [11] this means that subjects with obesity had none of the MetS risk factors, except for waist circumference, according to the revised NCEP ATPIII [22] (using the WHO cut-off of ≥6.1 mmol/L for impaired fasting glucose [23]), and had no previous diagnosis of CVD (defined as self-reported myocardial infarction, stroke, or vascular intervention). MUO was defined as obesity with at least two MetS risk factors, while in 'intermediate' obesity only one MetS risk factor was present. Detailed information can be found in Additional file 1.

Dietary assessment

Food frequency questionnaire

We used a self-administered food frequency questionnaire (FFQ) to assess the intake of 110 food items during the last 4 weeks. An existing validated Dutch FFQ formed the basis for the FFQ used in the Lifelines study [24, 25]. The basic Lifelines FFQ focused on estimates of energy intake and macronutrients, including alcohol intake, and comprised all major food groups. For 46 main food items, frequency of consumption was indicated as 'not this month' or in days per week or month; including the amount (in units or specified portion size) consumed each time. The FFQ also included 37 questions on consumption of sub-items (e.g. $20^{+/}30^{+}$ cheese, 40^{+} cheese, 48^{+} cheese, or cream cheese) for which frequency was specified as never, sometimes, often and (almost) always. After the first visit the FFQ was filled in by the participant at home and handed in, approximately 2 weeks later, at the Lifelines research center during the second visit for fasting venepuncture. To calculate the participants' intake the Dutch food composition table of 2006 (NEVO) was used [26].

To correct for potential under- or over-reporting on the dietary questionnaire, extreme values were identified by the top and bottom 2.5% of daily energy intake (kcal/day) and excluded from the dataset. In total, only 0.05% of the number of servings/food items data was missing, while frequency of consumption had been filled in. Food items with missing data on frequency (0.5%) could not be interpreted and were not included in the calculations.

Dietary patterns in the obese population

Dietary patterns were derived on the basis of principal components analysis (PCA), a type of factor analysis. With PCA, linear combinations of the originally observed variables are formed by grouping together correlated food groups, identifying underlying components, i.e. dietary patterns, within the data. The correlation coefficients defining these linear combinations represent the loading of each food group on the dietary pattern [27].

Individual food items with a similar nutrient profile and culinary use were combined into 58 food groups (Additional file 2). To test the appropriateness of applying PCA on the study sample, the Kaiser-Meyer-Olkin measurement was conducted for testing sampling adequacy and the Bartlett's Test of Sphericity for testing the homogeneity of variances.

Dietary patterns were derived on the basis of consumption (g/day) of each food group, unadjusted for energy intake. Within PCA, orthogonal rotation (varimax option) was used to obtain uncorrelated patterns with greater interpretability, which may be used simultaneously in regression models without affecting collinearity [28]. A dietary pattern was retained if the component Eigenvalue was >1.0, by identification of an inflection point in the Scree plot, and interpretability of the dietary pattern. The dietary patterns were considered stable if the same major patterns were identified in two random halves of the data set and per sex group, e.g. the food groups with significant contributions to the dietary pattern (factor loading >0.3 or <−0.3) were similar.

A dietary pattern score was created for each derived pattern by multiplying the loadings with the corresponding standardized intake of the food (calculating Z-scores for men and women separately), and summing across the food groups for each pattern. Dietary patterns were named according to the foods with the highest loading on the pattern (loadings >0.3).

Physical activity

Physical activity was assessed by the validated SQUASH questionnaire ("Short QUestionnaire to ASsess Health-enhancing physical activity") [29]. Questions included type of activity, frequency, duration and intensity, referring to a normal week in the preceding months. Metabolic equivalent (MET) values were assigned to activities as defined by the Ainsworth' compendium of Physical activities [30]. Activities with a MET value of 4 to <6.5 were classified as moderate, and ≥6.5 as vigorous intensity. For statistical analyses we used: the total minutes of moderate and vigorous physical activity per week, the moderate physical activity score and the vigorous physical activity score. The physical activity scores were calculated by multiplying duration (minutes per week) with the MET value, taking into account the intensity. Subjects with implausible values were excluded if: 1) separate activity categories exceeded plausible values; 2) more than two activity categories of the questionnaire were missing; and/or 3) ≥18 h/day was spent on all activities together (this also included light physical activity (2 to <4 MET)) [31].

Demographic and lifestyle variables

Based on the participants' responses to the self-administered questionnaires, data were assessed on the presence of diabetes mellitus, history of myocardial infarction, stroke or vascular intervention, current medication use, current use of a (self-)prescribed diet (e.g. energy-, fat- or salt restricted diet, prescribed diet for diabetes or high cholesterol, or fiber rich diet), education level and smoking [21]. Missing values on education level (0.6%) and smoking status (0.2%) were imputed, using single point imputation, with age, sex, netto household income and postal code (as a proxy for social economic status) as predictors.

Statistics

All analyses were conducted using IBM SPSS Statistics version 22 (IBM Corporation, Armonk, NY, USA). All data are presented for men and women separately. Study characteristics were expressed as percentage (%), means with standard deviation (SD), or as median with interquartile range in case of non-normally distributed data. Differences between groups were tested by *t*-test for continuous variables or Kruskal-Wallis test when appropriate, and Chi-Square test for categorical variables (applying the Bonferroni method). Multivariable logistic regression was used to determine the associations between MHO, dietary patterns (divided in quartiles) and physical activity scores (moderate physical activity score and vigorous physical activity score divided in tertiles) while adjusting for age (categorical) and BMI (dichotomous) (model 1), then smoking (non-, former-, current smoker), education level (low, middle, high), use of a (self-) prescribed diet (yes/no) and energy intake (continuous) were added to the model (model 2). Alcohol use was not considered in the multivariate logistic regression model, because it was an input variable in the PCA. To test for trends the dietary pattern score (using the median value of each quartile), physical activity score, age and BMI was used as a continuous variable. Subjects with MUO were used as the reference group. A two-sided *P*-value ≤0.05 was considered to be statistically significant.

Results

Prevalence of metabolic health phenotypes

After exclusion of participants with possible under- or over-reporting of energy intake ($N = 532$), implausible physical activity data ($N = 875$), or missing data on clinical measures ($N = 94$), a total of 9270 obese individuals were included in this study (86.1% from the original sample) (Fig. 1). Of those, 3442 were men (37.1%) and 5828 (62.9%) were women. The prevalence of MHO was 10.2% among men and 24.4% among women (MUO: 56.9% vs. 35.3%, respectively) (Table 1). In general, MHO individuals had a lower BMI and waist circumference than MUO subjects (Table 1). MHO decreased in older age groups for both men and women. Most men were defined as MOU, while most women below the age of 50 years were still defined as 'intermediate' obesity (Fig. 2).

Dietary patterns

To validate appropriateness of applying PCA on our study sample, we calculated the Kaiser Meyer Olkin and Barlett's Test of Sphericity values. The observed KMO was 0.73 (should not be lower than 0.5) and the BTS was significant ($P < 0.0001$), indicating homogeneity of variance of the foods consumed. Additional file 3 shows the Scree plot of Eigenvalues for each component, i.e. dietary pattern. The Eigenvalues of the components dropped substantially until the fourth component (Eigenvalues > 1.0). As a result, we retained the 4 components solution explaining 18.7% (5.7%, 4.5%, 4.4% and 4.1%, respectively) of the variations in food intake. PCA conducted on the two random halves of the dataset yielded similar results. The same four major patterns were identified for men and women, although the magnitude of the loadings differed more compared to the derived outcomes in the random halves of the dataset.

Positive loadings of the food groups indicate that it is highly correlated with the corresponding dietary pattern, whereas negative loadings are inversely correlated (detailed description Additional file 4). The first dietary pattern we labeled as the *'savory snacks and sweets'* pattern, the second pattern was labeled as the *'meat and alcohol'* pattern, the third pattern was labeled the *'bread, potatoes and sweet snacks'* pattern and the fourth dietary pattern was labeled as *'fruit, vegetables and fish'* (summary overview Fig. 3). Men with MHO had a higher *'savory snacks and*

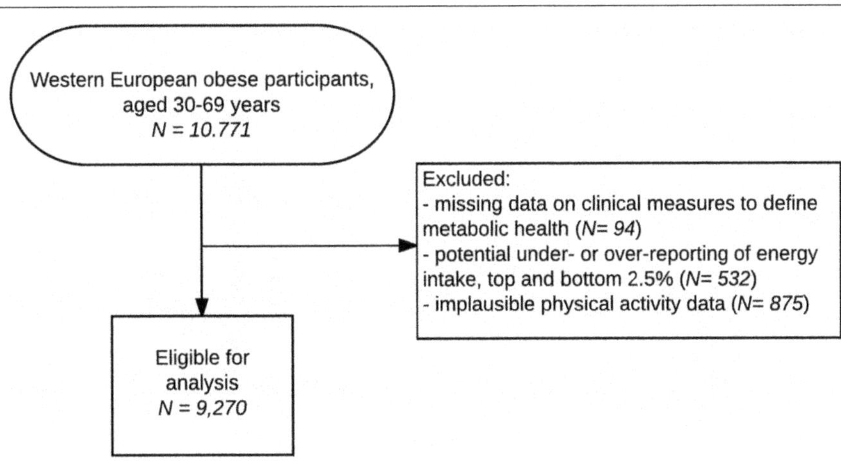

Fig. 1 Flow-chart Dietary patterns and PA in MHO

Table 1 Clinical characteristics according to metabolic health group

	Men			Women		
	MUO	Intermediate	MHO	MUO	Intermediate	MHO
N	1959 (56.9)	1131 (32.9) [b]	352 (10.2) [b]	2058 (35.3)	2348 (40.3) [b]	1422 (24.4) [b]
Age (years)	49.4 ± 9.4	49.6 ± 9.5	45.3 ± 8.6 [b]	50.6 ± 9.4	48.3 ± 9.9 [b]	44.9 ± 8.3 [b]
BMI (kg/m^2)	32.2 [30.9–34.3]	31.8 [30.7–33.4] [b]	31.4 [30.7–32.9] [b]	33.6 [31.5–36.7]	32.8 [31.2–35.4] [b]	32.1 [30.9–34.4] [b]
Waist circumference (cm)	113.0 ± 9.0	111.1 ± 8.2 [b]	108.9 ± 7.2 [b]	108.0 ± 10.7	104.0 ± 9.6 [b]	101.4 ± 8.9 [b]
Systolic BP (mmHg)	139 ± 14	137 ± 14 [b]	122 ± 6 [b]	135 ± 15	131 ± 16 [b]	118 ± 7 [b]
Diastolic BP (mmHg)	81 ± 9	81 ± 9	74 ± 5 [b]	77 ± 9	75 ± 9 [b]	70 ± 6 [b]
Fasting glucose (mmol/L)	5.5 [5.1–6.2]	5.2 [5.0–5.6] [b]	5.2 [4.9–5.5] [b]	5.5 [5.0–6.3]	5.0 [4.7–5.4] [b]	4.9 [4.7–5.2] [b]
HDL cholesterol (mmol/L)	1.02 ± 0.21	1.28 ± 0.25 [b]	1.33 ± 0.20 [b]	1.20 ± 0.27	1.48 ± 0.33 [b]	1.58 ± 0.26 [b]
Triglycerides (mmol/L)	2.04 [1.60–2.72]	1.21 [0.96–1.50] [b]	1.08 [0.85–1.34] [b]	1.76 [1.25–2.21]	1.06 [0.82–1.35] [b]	0.91 [0.72–1.15] [b]
Type 2 diabetes * (%)	10.5	0.6 [b]	0.0	13.3	0.8 [b]	0.0
CVD history (%)	4.7	4.2	0.0	2.7	1.4	0.0
Use of BP lowering drugs	33.0	20.4 [b]	0.0	44.4	24.7 [b]	0.0

Data are presented as mean ± SD or median [interquartile range] or percentage (%). [a] denotes a P ≤ 0.01 and [b] denotes a P ≤ 0.0001 compared to MUO
MHO metabolically healthy obesity, *MUO* metabolically unhealthy obesity, *BMI* body mass index, *BP* blood pressure, *HDL* high-density lipoprotein, *CVD* cardiovascular disease. * Based on known type 2 diabetes and newly-diagnosed type 2 diabetes (defined as a single fasting plasma glucose level ≥ 7.0 mmol/L)

sweets' pattern score than men with MUO. No significant differences were found for the other dietary patterns. Compared to women with MUO, women with MHO had a higher score on the *'savory snacks and sweets'* pattern and the *'fruit, vegetables and fish'* pattern, but lower scores on the *'meat and alcohol'* pattern and the *'bread, potatoes and sweet snacks'* pattern. No differences in total energy intake or the macronutrient intake (% of energy intake) were observed between the three metabolic health phenotypes (Table 2).

Physical activity

Obese men and women with MHO were more moderate-vigorous physically active than subjects with MUO (Table 2). Furthermore, more men with MHO had a vigorous physical activity score in the highest tertile compared to men with MUO (43.8% vs 30.4%, $P < 0.0001$). MHO women had more often a moderate physical activity score in the highest tertile compared to MUO women (36.1 vs 31.2%, $P < 0.01$).

Smoking, alcohol consumption and education level

Fewer subjects with MHO were current smoker or did not use alcohol compared to subjects with MUO. Men and women with MHO were more frequently light-moderate alcohol consumers (≤2 drinks/day). The distribution of education level was not different between the metabolic health subgroups in men. However, women with MHO

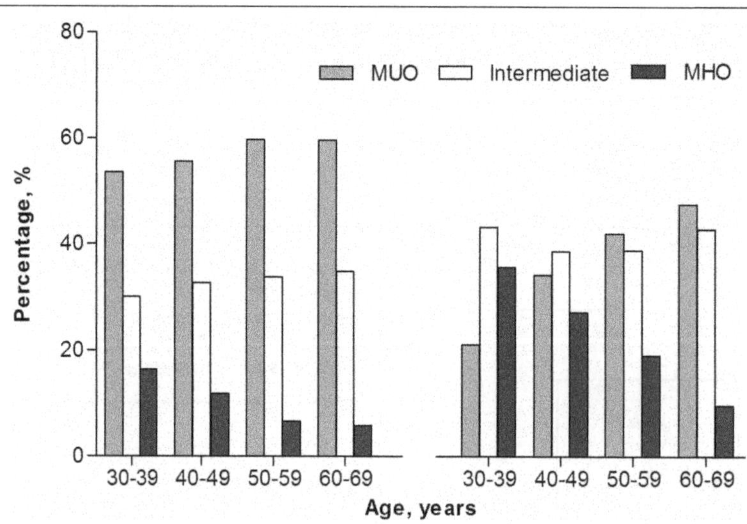

Fig. 2 Percentage of the metabolic health phenotype by age groups (left panel men, right panel women)

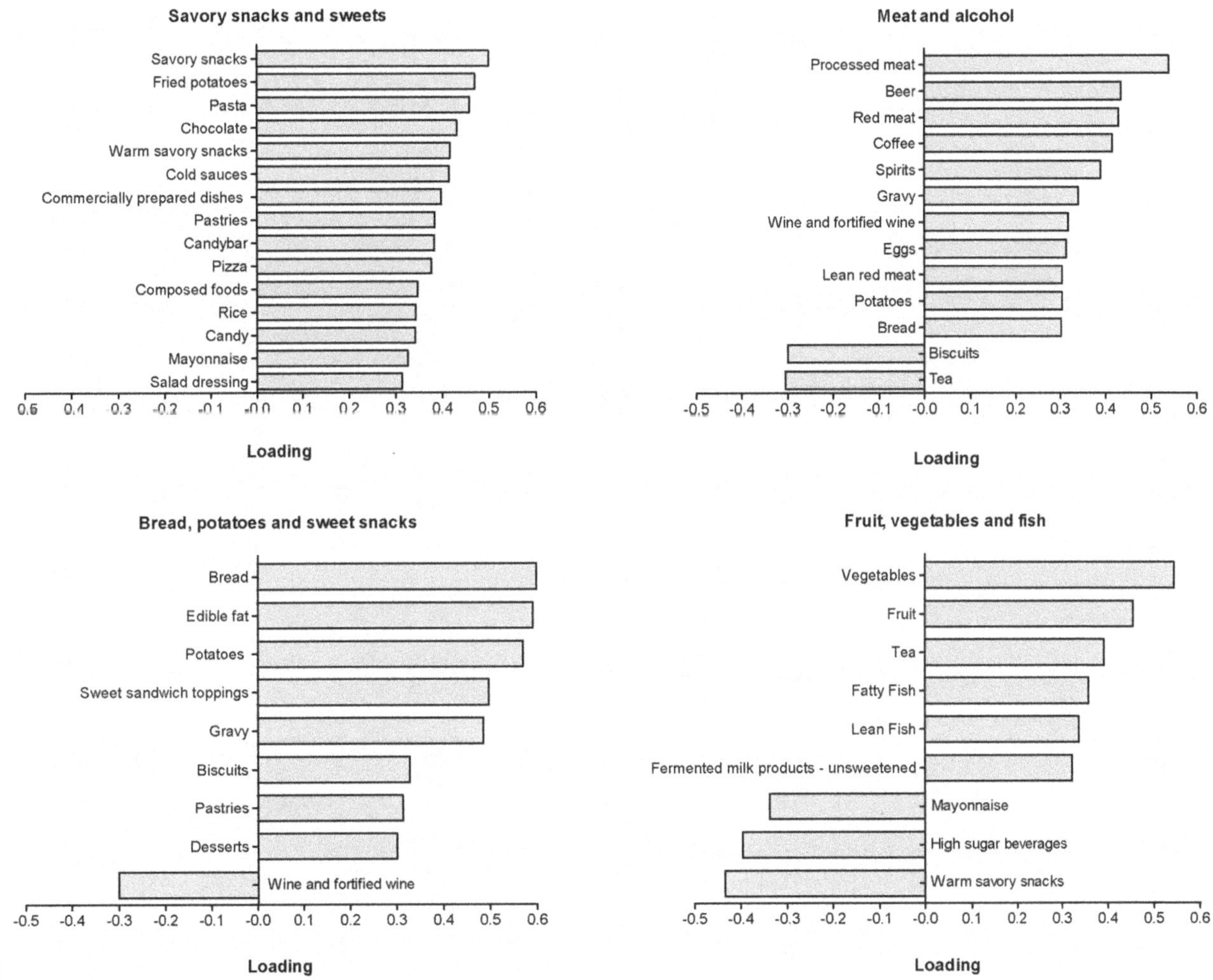

Fig. 3 Summary overview of obesity-specific dietary patterns

were more frequent highly educated (24.8%) compared to women with MUO (13.8%) ($P < 0.0001$) (Table 2).

Demographic, physical activity and other lifestyle characteristics within dietary patterns

Because dietary patterns are part of a broader pattern of lifestyle factors, demographic and lifestyle characteristics are shown by quartiles of dietary pattern scores (Table 3). We also checked the dietary pattern scores across age groups (Additional file 5). Subjects in the highest quartile of the *'savory snacks and sweets'* pattern, were of a younger age, more often metabolically healthy obese, higher educated and had less often a chronic condition (T2D, CVD history, or hypertension) or used a (self-) prescribed diet. At the same time, they were less physically active and more often smokers. Scores on both the *'meat and alcohol'* pattern and the *'bread, potatoes and sweet snacks'* were stable across age groups, but subjects with a high score were less often metabolically healthy obese and less educated compared to subjects with a low score. The *'meat and alcohol'* pattern was, furthermore, characterized by less physical activity, smoking and heavy alcohol use (19.0% consuming >2 drinks/day). In contrast, subjects in the highest quartile of the *'bread, potatoes and sweet snacks'* pattern were more physically active, less often a smoker and drank less alcohol. Older people were more likely to fit the *'fruit, vegetables and fish'* pattern. The pattern was associated with higher education levels, more physical activity, less smokers (although more former smokers) and less alcohol use. However, chronic conditions and use of a (self-) prescribed diet was more prevalent in the highest tertile.

Dietary patterns and physical activity as determinants of MHO

Of the four obesity-specific dietary patterns, two patterns were associated with MHO and in women only.

Table 2 Macronutrient intake, lifestyle factors and education level according to metabolic health phenotype

	Men			Women		
	MUO	Intermediate	MHO	MUO	Intermediate	MHO
N	1959 (56.9)	1131 (32.9) [b]	352 (10.2) [b]	2058 (35.3)	2348 (40.3) [b]	1422 (24.4) [b]
Energy intake (kcal/day)	2072 ± 488	2088 ± 496	2084 ± 492	1724 ± 443	1722 ± 451	1731 ± 465
Protein (% EI)	15.7 ± 2.3	15.6 ± 2.4	15.7 ± 2.5	16.4 ± 2.7	16.5 ± 2.7	16.4 ± 2.7
Plant	6.1 ± 1.0	6.1 ± 1.0	6.2 ± 1.1	6.1 ± 1.0	6.1 ± 0.9	6.1 ± 1.0
Animal	9.5 ± 2.5	9.4 ± 2.6	9.6 ± 2.8	10.4 ± 2.9	10.4 ± 2.8	10.3 ± 2.9
Carbohydrates (% EI)	45.0 ± 6.1	44.9 ± 6.4	45.2 ± 6.3	46.2 ± 6.3	46.0 ± 6.1	45.9 ± 6.2
Mono- and disaccharides	19.6 ± 5.8	19.5 ± 5.5	19.7 ± 5.3	20.6 ± 5.8	20.6 ± 5.4	20.5 ± 5.2
Polysaccharides	25.4 ± 4.8	25.3 ± 4.8	25.4 ± 4.7	25.5 ± 4.4	25.3 ± 4.5	25.3 ± 4.6
Fat (% EI)	36.0 ± 5.1	36.0 ± 5.1	36.0 ± 4.6	35.9 ± 5.4	35.9 ± 5.2	36.1 ± 5.1
Use of (self-) prescribed diet (%)	5.1	4.9	6.6	12.6	12.2	10.6
Dietary pattern score (Z-scores)						
Savory snacks and sweets	−0.06	−0.01	0.38 *	−0.30	−0.01	0.46 [b]
Alcohol and meat	0.02	0.04	−0.23	0.08	0.03	−0.16 [a]
Bread, potatoes and sweet snacks	0.01	0.02	−0.11	0.24	−0.05	−0.25 [b]
Fruit, vegetables and fish	−0.03	0.05	0.00	−0.13	0.03	0.15 [a]
MVPA (min/week)	285 [60–960]	360 [120–999] [a]	360 [140–1337] [a]	230 [60–600]	270 [100–646] [a]	242 [90–720] [a]
Moderate PA score						
T1 'low'	45.7	43.4	41.5	48.0	43.2 [a]	43.1[a]
T2 'middle'	21.1	21.9	23.6	20.8	23.2	20.7
T3 'high'	33.2	34.7	34.9	31.2	33.6	36.1[a]
Vigorous PA score						
T1 'low'	36.1	31.2 [a]	25.9 [a]	36.2	33.6	32.5
T2 'middle'	33.5	33.7	30.4	30.0	31.0	33.1
T3 'high'	30.4	35.1[a]	43.8 [b]	33.8	35.5	34.4
Smoking (%)						
Non	33.4	40.5 [a]	47.7 [b]	41.2	46.8 [a]	49.2 [b]
Former	42.0	41.8	36.6	38.6	38.9	37.9
Current	24.6	17.7 [b]	15.6 [a]	20.2	14.3 [b]	12.9 [b]
Alcohol use (%)						
Non	15.0	9.7 [b]	9.1*	39.2	31.4 [b]	27.8 [b]
≤ 2 drinks	70.4	75.5 [a]	79.3 [a]	58.0	65.4[b]	70.0 [b]
> 2 drinks	14.7	14.8	11.6	2.8	3.2	2.3
Education level (%)						
Low	39.7	39.4	36.4	46.8	40.1[b]	32.2 [b]
Middle	37.8	38.0	41.5	39.3	42.0	43.0
High	22.5	22.5	22.2	13.8	17.9 [a]	24.8 [b]

Data is presented as mean ± SD or median [interquartile range]. * denotes a $P \leq 0.05$, [a] denotes a $P \leq 0.01$, and [b] denotes a $P \leq 0.0001$. *EI* energy intake, *MUO* metabolically unhealthy obesity, *MHO* metabolically healthy obesity, *MVPA* moderate-vigorous physical active, *PA* physical activity. Education level: low (no formal education, only primary school or intermediate vocational education), middle (higher secondary education) or high (higher vocational education and university)

Among women, a higher score on the *'fruit, vegetables and fish'* pattern was associated with a higher OR for MHO (P for trend <0.0001) (Table 4, model 1 and 2). In contrast, higher scores on the *'bread, potatoes and sweet snacks'* pattern was associated with a lower OR for the MHO phenotype (P for trend <0.0001). A higher moderate physical activity score and a higher vigorous physical activity score was associated with a higher OR for MHO in women (P for trend 0.020, model 2) and men (P for trend 0.0001, model 1 and 2), respectively.

Table 3 Demographic, physical activity and other lifestyle characteristics within the first and fourth quartile of the dietary pattern

	Savory snacks and sweets		Meat and alcohol		Bread, potatoes and sweet snacks		Fruit, vegetables and fish	
	Q1	Q4	Q1	Q4	Q1	Q4	Q1	Q4
N	2317	2317	2317	2317	2317	2317	2317	2317
Males (%)	860 (37.1)	860 (37.1)	860 (37.1)	860 (37.1)	860 (37.1)	860 (37.1)	860 (37.1)	859 (37.1)
Age (years), mean ± sd	53.9 ± 9.9	44.2 ± 7.4 [b]	47.9 ± 10.1	48.7 ± 8.9	49.0 ± 9.5	48.4 ± 9.8	44.8 ± 8.1	51.6 ± 9.9 [b]
BMI (kg/m^2), median [IQR]	33.5 [30.9–34.7]	32.6 [31.1–35.3] [a]	32.5 [30.9–34.8]	32.5 [31.0–35.2]	32.4 [30.9–34.8]	32.4 [30.9–34.9]	32.7 [31.1–35.4]	32.3 [30.9–34.6] [b]
Metabolic health (%)								
MUO	46.4	40.1 [b]	42.1	43.8	39.4	44.9 [a]	44.8	41.3
Intermediate	38.6	37.5	36.3	37.9	38.5	37.4	36.7	38.9
MHO	15.0	22.4 [b]	21.7	18.3 [a]	22.1	17.7 [a]	18.5	19.8
Energy intake (kcal/day)	1486 ± 412	2279 ± 411 [b]	1572 ± 449	2191 ± 456 [b]	1504 ± 432	2256 ± 404 [b]	1973 ± 511	1813 ± 490 [b]
MVPA (min/week)	280 [110–720]	255 [90–769]	268 [90–720]	280 [90–780]	250 [75–660]	300 [100–840] [b]	270 [60–960]	290 [120–680]
Moderate PA score	225 [0–1350]	300 [0–2625] [a]	240 [0–2025]	300 [0–1700] [a]	300 [0–1700]	300 [0–2700] [a]	300 [0–3780]	300 [0–1500] [a]
Vigorous PA score	960 [105–2160]	645 [0–1600] [b]	800 [48–1920]	640 [0–1680] [b]	720 [0–1800]	780 [80–1920] [a]	480 [0–1440]	960 [240–2160] [b]
Education level (%)								
Low	52.1	29.8 [b]	37.1	41.4 [a]	32.2	46.9 [b]	47.5	32.8 [b]
Middle	33.4	45.7 [b]	41.1	40.5	40.1	39.4	41.1	38.5
High	14.5	24.5 [b]	21.8	18.1 [a]	27.7	13.8 [b]	11.4	28.6 [b]
Smoking (%)								
Non	38.6	46.3 [b]	54.4	31.3 [b]	38.6	46.6 [b]	39.0	44.2 [a]
Former	45.0	34.0 [b]	34.9	42.8 [b]	42.4	37.5 [a]	30.3	46.7 [b]
Current	16.4	19.7 [a]	10.7	25.9 [b]	19.0	15.9 [a]	30.7	9.1 [b]
Alcohol use (%)								
Non	30.0	23.4 [b]	39.3	14.3 [b]	16.9	32.8 [b]	29.6	22.4 [b]
≤ 2 drinks/day	63.9	68.3*	60.1	66.6 [b]	69.5	64.2 [a]	59.8	71.0 [b]
> 2 drinks/day	6.1	8.2*	0.6	19.0 [b]	13.6	3.0 [b]	10.6	6.6 [b]
(Self-) prescribed diet (%)	18.2	3.9 [b]	11.8	7.0 [b]	15.8	5.2 [b]	3.5	18.9 [b]
Type 2 diabetes (%)	10.3	2.8 [b]	5.6	5.0	4.5	5.4	3.2	6.6 [b]
CVD history (%)	4.4	1.2 [b]	2.2	2.4	2.6	2.8	1.8	3.4 [a]
Use of BP lowering drug (%)	37.3	17.7 [b]	24.3	25.2	25.2	24.5	19.5	29.4 [b]

Data is presented as mean ± SD or median [interquartile range] or percentage (%). * denotes a P ≤ 0.05, [a] denotes a P ≤ 0.01 and [b] denotes a P ≤ 0.0001 compared to Q1 of the same dietary pattern. *BMI* body mass index, *MUO* metabolically unhealthy obesity, *MHO* metabolically healthy obesity, *MVPA* moderate–vigorous physical activity, *PA* physical activity, *CVD* cardiovascular disease, *BP* blood pressure. Education level: low (no formal education, only primary school or intermediate vocational education), middle (higher secondary education) or high (higher vocational education and university)

Table 4 Multivariable-adjusted odds ratios for the associations of dietary patterns and physical activity with metabolically healthy obesity

	Men		Women	
	Model 1	Model 2	Model 1	Model 2
Dietary pattern				
Savory snacks and sweets				
Q1	1	1	1	1
Q2	1.12 (0.78–1.63)	1.18 (0.79–1.73)	**1.26** (1.01–1.57)	1.16 (0.92–1.46)
Q3	**1.46** (1.02–2.09)	**1.57** (1.05–2.36)	1.13 (0.90–1.42)	1.00 (0.77–1.29)
Q4	1.29 (0.88–1.90)	1.41 (0.86–2.30)	**1.43** (1.13–1.81) [a]	1.24 (0.90–1.71)
P for trend	NS	NS	0.045	NS
Meat and alcohol				
Q1	1	1	1	1
Q2	0.89 (0.64–1.23)	0.98 (0.70–1.36)	0.98 (0.80–1.21)	1.05 (0.85–1.30)
Q3	0.78 (0.56–1.09)	0.91 (0.64–1.30)	0.83 (0.67–1.03)	0.88 (0.71–1.10)
Q4	0.72 (0.51–1.02)	0.94 (0.63–1.42)	1.02 (0.82–1.26)	1.14 (0.89–1.46)
P for trend	0.045	NS	NS	NS
Bread, potatoes and sweet snacks				
Q1	1	1	1	1
Q2	0.78 (0.56–1.09)	0.77 (0.54–1.09)	**0.64** (0.52–0.80)	**0.64** (0.51–0.80) [b]
Q3	0.75 (0.54–1.06)	0.76 (0.52–1.10)	**0.66** (0.53–0.81)	**0.66** (0.52–0.83) [a]
Q4	0.92 (0.66–1.28)	0.92 (0.59–1.44)	**0.55** (0.44–0.68)	**0.52** (0.39–0.70) [b]
P for trend	NS	NS	<0.0001	<0.0001
Fruit, vegetables and fish				
Q1	1	1	1	1
Q2	1.03 (0.75–1.44)	1.01 (0.73–1.41)	**1.24** (1.01–1.54)	1.14 (0.91–1.41)
Q3	0.88 (0.62–1.24)	0.83 (0.57–1.18)	**1.55** (1.25–1.92) [b]	**1.36** (1.09–1.71) [a]
Q4	0.96 (0.68–1.36)	0.87 (0.60–1.25)	**1.75** (1.40–2.19) [b]	**1.55** (1.21–1.97) [a]
P for trend	NS	NS	<0.0001	<0.0001
Moderate PA score				
T1 'low'	1	1	1	1
T2 'middle'	1.22 (0.90–1.65)	1.18 (0.87–1.61)	1.10 (0.90–1.34)	1.08 (0.88–1.31)
T3 'high'	1.03 (0.78–1.35)	0.99 (0.75–1.32)	1.15 (0.97–1.36)	**1.19** (1.01–1.41)
P for trend	NS	NS	NS	0.020
Vigorous PA score				
T1 'low'	1	1	1	1
T2 'middle'	1.21 (0.89–1.65)	1.20 (0.88–1.63)	1.17 (0.97–1.40)	1.13 (0.94–1.35)
T3 'high'	**2.11** (1.57–2.83) [b]	**2.02** (1.50–2.71) [b]	**1.21** (1.01–1.45)	1.17 (0.98–1.41)
P for trend	<0.0001	0.0001	NS	NS
Age group				
30–39	1	1	1	1
40–49	0.75 (0.56–1.00)	**0.73** (0.54–0.99)	**0.45** (0.37–0.55)	**0.47** (0.38–0.57)
50–59	**0.36** (0.25–0.53) [b]	**0.36** (0.24–0.53) [b]	**0.22** (0.17–0.28) [b]	**0.22** (0.17–0.28) [b]
60–69	**0.33** (0.21–0.53) [b]	**0.33** (0.21–0.54) [b]	**0.10** (0.07–0.13) [b]	**0.09** (0.07–0.13) [b]

Table 4 Multivariable-adjusted odds ratios for the associations of dietary patterns and physical activity with metabolically healthy obesity *(Continued)*

	Men		Women	
	Model 1	Model 2	Model 1	Model 2
P for trend	<0.0001	<0.0001	<0.0001	<0.0001
BMI group				
30–34.9	1	1	1	
≥ 35	**0.37** (0.24–0.55) [b]	**0.33** (0.22–0.50) [b]	**0.38** (0.32–0.45) [b]	**0.37** (0.31–0.44) [b]
P for trend	<0.0001	<0.0001	<0.0001	<0.0001
Smoking				
Non		1		1
Former		0.77 (0.58–1.00)		0.97 (0.82–1.14)
Current		**0.45** (0.32–0.63) [b]		**0.52** (0.42–0.65) [b]
Education level				
Low		1		1
Middle		0.99 (0.75–1.30)		0.96 (0.82–1.16)
High		0.88 (0.63–1.24)		**1.30** (1.04–1.63)
Use of a (self-) prescribed diet				
No		1		1
Yes		1.42 (0.86–2.36)		**0.68** (0.53–0.87) [a]
Energy intake*		0.84 (0.53–1.33)		0.95 (0.72–1.36)

Data are expressed as odds ratios (95% confidence interval). Reference group is the metabolically unhealthy obese. Values in BOLD indicate a P ≤ 0.05, [a] denotes a P ≤ 0.01 and [b] denotes a P ≤ 0.0001. P for trend test was performed by using for the dietary patterns the median value of each quartile, and a continuous score for physical activity, age and BMI. * Energy intake is given per 1.000 kcal increase. Model 1 (dietary patterns + physical activity): adjusted for age group and BMI group. Model 2 (dietary patterns + physical activity): adjusted for age group, BMI group, smoking, education level, use of a (self)prescribed diet and energy intake

We used the WHO cut-off of ≥6.1 mmol/L for impaired fasting glucose [23]. However, in a subsequent analysis we applied the lower cut-off of ≥5.6 mmol/L for impaired fasting glucose to define metabolic health [32]. This resulted in 196 fewer individuals classified as MHO and 566 more individuals classified as MUO. The observed OR were slightly higher (generally first decimal place increased), for both men and women, using the lower threshold. No new associations were found (data not shown).

Discussion

In this study more than half of the obese men and more than one third of obese women were metabolically unhealthy. Only 10% of men, and 25% of women were metabolically healthy obese. Compared to those with MUO, we found that women with MHO had a healthier diet, rich in fruit, vegetables, fish and unsweetened fermented milk products while avoiding high sugar beverages and, savory- and sweet snackfood. Women with MHO engaged in more intensive moderate physical activity, while men with MHO were characterized by higher engagement in intensive vigorous physical activity.

Consistent with previous data, total intake of energy and macronutrients did not differ between subjects with MHO and subjects with MUO [12–15]. We identified four major obesity-specific dietary patterns of which only two were associated with MHO, and in women only. The *'fruit, vegetables and fish'* pattern was positively associated with MHO, and mainly consisted of foods considered as healthy. Previous studies showed that higher intakes of vegetables and fruit were associated with a lower risk of MetS, CVD [33], and only the latter with lower risk of T2D [34, 35]. Higher scores on the *'fruit, vegetables and fish'* pattern mean higher intake of fish, chicken, unsweetened fermented milk products and low-fat cheese. Both epidemiological and experimental data show that the consumption of dairy products have a beneficial effect on MetS risk factors and are associated with a lower risk of body fat gain and obesity, as well as CVD [36]. Consumption of cheese and fermented dairy product were inversely associated with T2D incidence [37]. The pattern of *'bread, potatoes and sweet snacks'* was inversely associated with MHO in our study. The pattern consists of carbohydrate-rich food products, mainly refined, which are known to have a high glycaemic index and a low fiber content [38]. Indeed, previous studies have reported an inverse association between high glycaemic index diets and HDL-C [39, 40] and a positive association with triglycerides [41] and MetS [42]. Furthermore, higher glycaemic index and low fiber content are relevant aspects related to insulin resistance and impaired glucose tolerance, which are important co-morbidities of MetS [43].

To date, only a few studies examined dietary patterns and metabolic health in obesity specifically. In two studies 'a priori' dietary scores were applied [15, 17]. A study in the US found a higher total score on the HEI-2005 (Healthy Eating Index) in MHO adolescents and adult women compared with metabolically abnormal obese, e.g. MUO [17]. In an Irish cohort study, there was no association between the DASH score (Dietary Approaches to Stop Hypertension)) or the food pyramid score and MHO in adjusted analysis (for sex, age, physical activity, alcohol, smoking and dietary quality) [15]. To the best of our knowledge there is only one study by Bell et al. [44], which used the 'a posteriori' approach like in this study. The authors found that the odds of having a more metabolically healthy profile was 16% greater for every standard deviation increase in the 'healthy' dietary pattern score (including high loadings of whole grains, fresh fruit, dried fruit, legumes and low fat dairy) [44]. The criteria for metabolic health between our study and the one by Bell et al. [44] were different and dietary patterns were in the latter based on a population including non-obese and obese participants. Still, the outcomes of both studies make us hypothesize that without a calorie restricted diet, 'healthy' changes in the dietary pattern may improve metabolic health risk.

Our findings for dietary patterns and MHO were observed for women only. Such a sex difference may reflect differences in physiology, reporting of diet, or the amount consumed of the specific types of foods that contributed strongly to the pattern score [45]. Indeed, higher pattern scores in women also correlated with higher intakes (absolute and/or relative) of the specific foods likely to be associated with metabolic (un)health (Additional file 6).

Increasing one's physical activity has the potential to improve adiposity profile and metabolic risk, even in the absence of weight loss [46]. A more favourable fat distribution, with less visceral fat, was associated with a long-term metabolically healthy profile in obese adults over a period of 10 year, and no excess risk of T2D and CVD [47]. Other studies on physical activity and MHO found that both objectively measured physical activity [48] and self-reported moderate-vigorous physical activity were higher in the MHO group compared to MUO group [49–51]. In the present study, moderate physical activity in women and vigorous physical activity in men was an important feature in the relationship between physical activity and MHO. In general, men engaged in more physical activity compared to women. To illustrate this, within the 'fruit, vegetables and fish' pattern and the 'bread and potatoes' pattern men engaged in more moderate to vigorous physical activity compared to women. At the same time men were also more physical active in the lowest vs. highest quartile of the 'fruit, vegetables and fish' pattern, and more physical active in the highest vs. lowest quartile of the 'bread and potatoes' pattern. This was not seen in women (data not shown). We hypothesize that this results in the stronger positive association between vigorous physical activity and MHO seen in men. Studies using accelerometers will be useful to differentiate physical activity patterns in MHO and MUO separately for men and women.

Our study includes a representative sample of the Dutch population using extensive questionnaires to measure important lifestyle behaviors, and standardized protocols to obtain clinical and biochemical measurements. Another strength of our study is the use of obesity-specific dietary patterns and that it is the largest study on this topic to date.

A limitation of the study includes the use of self-reported data, which are subject to recall bias. Obese individuals tend to underestimate their dietary intake and overestimate their physical activity [52, 53]. However, in our study we only used obese subjects to make comparisons, hence, we ranked individuals into categories which reduces the effect of over- or under-reporting.

PCA is extensively used in nutritional epidemiology and showed reasonable reproducibility and validity using FFQ data [54–57]. It remains, however, a data driven approach. Derived patterns may therefore not be reproducible across studies. Not only the dietary variables can differ across studies, also the process to select the final dietary patterns requires several arbitrary decisions [27]. Yet, it was also found that derived dietary patterns are robust for the subjective factor analytical decisions [58].

Next, we utilized cross-sectional data from which we cannot infer causality. It is, therefore, not possible to rule out reverse causality. Age played an important role within and between the dietary patterns. Furthermore, individuals which experience negative health outcomes, such as having T2D, a CVD history or the knowledge of having dyslipidaemia or hypertension, may have changed their dietary intake and their physical activity. We consider it likely that dietary patterns are not isolated, but part of a broader lifestyle and subject to someone's phase in life. Furthermore, it was not possible to tease apart the influence of obesity duration on the described associations.

In the literature MHO is still defined by the different classification systems that use different methods to measure metabolic abnormalities as well as different cut-off points or set of parameters to define MetS and/or its components. This makes it difficult to compare and interpret findings of studies on MHO. We defined previously a harmonized set of criteria for MHO within an international collaborative project (BioSHaRE-EU Healthy Obesity Project) [11]. The definition is based on the most widely used criteria for MetS (NCEP ATPIII) and also strict regarding metabolic health status (i.e. according to the classification none of the metabolic disturbances may be present (except for waist circumference) and no history of CVD). A major strength of our definition for MHO is that it can be easily applied in clinical practice and it may also have a greater utility to estimate differences in risk for T2D, CVD and mortality. Future work with longitudinal data should be encouraged to examine the influence of (changes in) dietary patterns on developing adverse metabolic outcomes and more ideally to examine the effect on hard endpoints (i.e. T2D, CVD and mortality).

Conclusion

In conclusion, our research showed that key lifestyle behaviors differed between metabolically healthy obese and metabolically unhealthy obese adults aged 30–69 years. Non-modifiable factors like age and sex are important for determining someone's baseline odds for MHO. However, our data suggests that in women, the healthier diet -characterized by *'fruit, vegetables and fish'*- and moderate physical activity, and in men, vigorous physical activity may be related to this favourable obesity state. The (refined) carbohydrate-rich *'bread, potatoes and sweet snacks'* dietary pattern was found to counteract MHO in women. Identification of behavioural lifestyle patterns may help in pinpointing vulnerable subgroups in the obese population and to develop potential strategies improving metabolic health.

Additional files

Additional file 1: Definition for metabolically healthy obesity (MHO), intermediate obesity and metabolically unhealthy obesity. (MUO)

Additional file 2: Detailed information on the food items grouping.

Additional file 3: Scree plot resulting from principal component analysis.

Additional file 4: Loadings of the food groups on the dietary patterns.

Additional file 5: Dietary pattern scores across age groups (left panel men, right panel women).

Additional file 6: Mean intake of food groups highly correlated with the dietary pattern, in men and women.

Abbreviations

BMI: body mass index; BP: blood pressure; CVD: cardiovascular disease; EI: energy intake; FFQ: food frequency questionnaire; HDL: high-density lipoprotein; MET: metabolic equivalent; MetS: metabolic syndrome; MHO: metabolically healthy obesity; MUO: metabolically unhealthy obesity; MVPA: moderate-vigorous physical active; PA: physical activity; PCA: principal component analysis

Acknowledgements

The authors wish to acknowledge the services of the Lifelines Cohort Study, the contributing research centers delivering data to Lifelines, and all the study participants.

Funding

The Lifelines Cohort Study is supported by the Netherlands Organization of Scientific Research NWO (grant 175.010.2007.006), the Ministry of Economic Affairs, the Ministry of Education, Culture and Science, the Ministry for Health, Welfare and Sports, the Northern Netherlands Collaboration of Provinces (SNN), The Province of Groningen, University Medical Center Groningen, the University of Groningen, Dutch Kidney Foundation and Dutch Diabetes Research Foundation. This work was supported by the National Consortium for Healthy Ageing, and funds from the European Union's Seventh Framework program (FP7/2007–2013) through the BioSHaRE-EU (Biobank Standardisation and Harmonisation for Research Excellence in the European Union) project, grant agreement 261433. J.V. van Vliet-Ostaptchouk was supported by a Diabetes Funds Junior Fellowship from the Dutch Diabetes Research Foundation (project no. 2013.81.1673). Lifelines (BRIF4568) is engaged in a Bioresource research impact factor (BRIF) policy pilot study, details of which can be found at: http://www.bioshare.eu/content/bioresource-impact-factor.

Authors' contributions

SNS was the primary investigator. JVvVO, EC, DK and BHRW contributed to the study design. JHMdV, CWMP, LGSB and EJF were involved in the nutritional data validation. AS and SNS performed the data validation of physical activity data. Other essential data validation was performed by SNS. SNS and EC were responsible for the statistical analyses. EC, DK, JVvVO contributed to interpretation of the data and analyses. SNS drafted the manuscript. All authors participated in critical revision of the manuscript for important intellectual content. All authors read and approved the final manuscript.

Competing interests

The authors declare that they have no competing interests.

Author details

[1]Department of Endocrinology, University of Groningen, University Medical Center Groningen, HPC AA31, P.O. Box 30001, 9700, RB, Groningen, The Netherlands. [2]Department of Epidemiology, University of Groningen, University Medical Center Groningen, PO Box 30001, 9700, RB, Groningen, The Netherlands. [3]Lifelines Cohort Study, University of Groningen, University Medical Center Groningen, PO Box 30001, 9700, RB, Groningen, The Netherlands. [4]Department of Paramedical Sciences, University of Groningen, University Medical Center Groningen, PO Box 30001, 9700, RB, Groningen, The Netherlands. [5]Division of Human Nutrition, Wageningen University, PO Box 17, 6700, AA, Wageningen, The Netherlands.

References

1. Mokdad AH, Ford ES, Bowman BA, Dietz WH, Vinicor F, Bales VS, Marks JS. Prevalence of obesity, diabetes, and obesity-related health risk factors, 2001. JAMA. 2003;289(1):76–9.
2. Denis GV, Obin MS. 'Metabolically healthy obesity': origins and implications. Mol Asp Med. 2013;34(1):59–70. https://doi.org/10.1016/j.mam.2012.10.004.
3. Zheng R, Zhou D, Zhu Y. The long-term prognosis of cardiovascular disease and all-cause mortality for metabolically healthy obesity: a systematic review and meta-analysis. J Epidemiol Community Health. 2016;70(10):1024–31. https://doi.org/10.1136/jech-2015-206948.
4. Bell JA, Kivimaki M, Hamer M. Metabolically healthy obesity and risk of incident type 2 diabetes: a meta-analysis of prospective cohort studies. Obesity reviews : an official journal of the International Association for the Study of Obesity. 2014;15(6):504–15. https://doi.org/10.1111/obr.12157.

5. Lassale C, Tzoulaki I, Moons KGM, Sweeting M, Boer J, Johnson L, Huerta JM, Agnoli C, Freisling H, Weiderpass E, Wennberg P, der AD v, Arriola L, Benetou V, Boeing H, Bonnet F, Colorado-Yohar SM, Engstrom G, Eriksen AK, Ferrari P, Grioni S, Johansson M, Kaaks R, Katsoulis M, Katzke V, Key TJ, Matullo G, Melander O, Molina-Portillo E, Moreno-Iribas C, Norberg M, Overvad K, Panico S, Quiros JR, Saieva C, Skeie G, Steffen A, Stepien M, Tjonneland A, Trichopoulou A, Tumino R, van der Schouw YT, WMM V, Langenberg C, Di Angelantonio E, Riboli E, Wareham NJ, Danesh J, Butterworth AS. Separate and combined associations of obesity and metabolic health with coronary heart disease: a pan-European case-cohort analysis. Eur Heart J. 2017; https://doi.org/10.1093/eurheartj/ehx448.
6. Ebbeling CB, Swain JF, Feldman HA, Wong WW, Hachey DL, Garcia-Lago E, Ludwig DS. Effects of dietary composition on energy expenditure during weight-loss maintenance. JAMA. 2012;307(24):2627–34. https://doi.org/10.1001/jama.2012.6607.
7. Kraschnewski JL, Boan J, Esposito J, Sherwood NE, Lehman EB, Kephart DK, Sciamanna CN. Long-term weight loss maintenance in the United States. International journal of obesity (2005). 2010;34(11):1644–54. https://doi.org/10.1038/ijo.2010.94.
8. Achilike I, Hazuda HP, Fowler SP, Aung K, Lorenzo C. Predicting the development of the metabolically healthy obese phenotype. International journal of obesity (2005). 2015;39(2):228–34. https://doi.org/10.1038/ijo.2014.113.
9. Eshtiaghi R, Keihani S, Hosseinpanah F, Barzin M, Azizi F. Natural course of metabolically healthy abdominal obese adults after 10 years of follow-up: the Tehran lipid and glucose study. International journal of obesity (2005). 2015;39(3):514–9. https://doi.org/10.1038/ijo.2014.176.
10. Hamer M, Bell JA, Sabia S, Batty GD, Kivimaki M. Stability of metabolically healthy obesity over 8 years: the English longitudinal study of ageing. European journal of endocrinology / European Federation of Endocrine Societies. 2015;173(5):703–8. https://doi.org/10.1530/eje-15-0449.
11. van Vliet-Ostaptchouk JV, Nuotio ML, Slagter SN, Doiron D, Fischer K, Foco L, Gaye A, Gogele M, Heier M, Hiekkalinna T, Joensuu A, Newby C, Pang C, Partinen E, Reischl E, Schwienbacher C, Tammesoo ML, Swertz MA, Burton P, Ferretti V, Fortier I, Giepmans L, Harris JR, Hillege HL, Holmen J, Jula A, Kootstra-Ros JE, Kvaloy K, Holmen TL, Mannisto S, Metspalu A, Midthjell K, Murtagh MJ, Peters A, Pramstaller PP, Saaristo T, Salomaa V, Stolk RP, Uusitupa M, van der Harst P, van der Klauw MM, Waldenberger M, Perola M, Wolffenbuttel BH. The prevalence of metabolic syndrome and metabolically healthy obesity in Europe: a collaborative analysis of ten large cohort studies. BMC Endocr Disord. 2014;14:9. https://doi.org/10.1186/1472-6823-14-9.
12. Hankinson AL, Daviglus ML, Van Horn L, Chan Q, Brown I, Holmes E, Elliott P, Stamler J. Diet composition and activity level of at risk and metabolically healthy obese American adults. Obesity (Silver Spring, Md). 2013;21(3):637–43. https://doi.org/10.1002/oby.20257.
13. Kimokoti RW, Judd SE, Shikany JM, Newby PK. Food intake does not differ between obese women who are metabolically healthy or abnormal. J Nutr. 2014;144(12):2018–26. https://doi.org/10.3945/jn.114.198341.
14. Kimokoti RW, Judd SE, Shikany JM, Newby PK. Metabolically healthy obesity is not associated with food intake in white or black men. J Nutr. 2015; 145(11):2551–61. https://doi.org/10.3945/jn.115.221283.
15. Phillips CM, Dillon C, Harrington JM, McCarthy VJ, Kearney PM, Fitzgerald AP, Perry IJ. Defining metabolically healthy obesity: role of dietary and lifestyle factors. PLoS One. 2013;8(10):e76188. https://doi.org/10.1371/journal.pone.0076188.
16. FB H. Dietary pattern analysis: a new direction in nutritional epidemiology. Curr Opin Lipidol. 2002;13(1):3–9.
17. Camhi SM, Whitney Evans E, Hayman LL, Lichtenstein AH, Must A. Healthy eating index and metabolically healthy obesity in U.S. adolescents and adults. Prev Med. 2015;77:23–7. https://doi.org/10.1016/j.ypmed.2015.04.023.
18. Rodriguez-Monforte M, Sanchez E, Barrio F, Costa B, Flores-Mateo G. Metabolic syndrome and dietary patterns: a systematic review and meta-analysis of observational studies. Eur J Nutr. 2017;56(3):925–47. https://doi.org/10.1007/s00394-016-1305-y.
19. Klijs B, Scholtens S, Mandemakers JJ, Snieder H, Stolk RP, Smidt N. Representativeness of the LifeLines cohort study. PLoS One. 2015;10(9): e0137203. https://doi.org/10.1371/journal.pone.0137203.
20. Scholtens S, Smidt N, Swertz MA, Bakker SJ, Dotinga A, Vonk JM, van Dijk F, van Zon SK, Wijmenga C, Wolffenbuttel BH, Stolk RP. Cohort profile: LifeLines, a three-generation cohort study and biobank. Int J Epidemiol. 2015;44(4):1172–80. https://doi.org/10.1093/ije/dyu229.
21. Slagter SN, van Vliet-Ostaptchouk JV, Vonk JM, Boezen HM, Dullaart RP, Kobold AC, Feskens EJ, van Beek AP, van der Klauw MM, Wolffenbuttel BH. Combined effects of smoking and alcohol on metabolic syndrome: the LifeLines cohort study. PLoS One. 2014;9(4):e96406. https://doi.org/10.1371/journal.pone.0096406.
22. Executive Summary of The Third Report of The National Cholesterol Education Program (NCEP) Expert Panel on Detection, Evaluation, And Treatment of High Blood Cholesterol In Adults (Adult Treatment Panel III) (2001). Jama 285 (19):2486–2497.
23. Organization WH. Definition and diagnosis of diabetes mellitus and intermediate hyperglycaemia. Geneva, World Health Org: Report of a WHO/IDF consulation; 2006.
24. Siebelink E, Geelen A, de Vries JH. Self-reported energy intake by FFQ compared with actual energy intake to maintain body weight in 516 adults. Br J Nutr. 2011;106(2):274–81. https://doi.org/10.1017/s0007114511000067.
25. Streppel MT, de Vries JH, Meijboom S, Beekman M, de Craen AJ, Slagboom PE, Feskens EJ. Relative validity of the food frequency questionnaire used to assess dietary intake in the Leiden longevity study. Nutr J. 2013;12:75. https://doi.org/10.1186/1475-2891-12-75.
26. Bureau stichting NEVO, NEVO-tabel 2006 (2006). Den Haag: Voedingscentrum,
27. Newby PK, Tucker KL. Empirically derived eating patterns using factor or cluster analysis: a review. Nutr Rev. 2004;62(5):177–203.
28. Tucker KL. Dietary patterns, approaches, and multicultural perspective. Appl Physiol Nutr Metab. 2010;35(2):211–8. https://doi.org/10.1139/h10-010.
29. Wendel-Vos GC, Schuit AJ, Saris WH, Kromhout D. Reproducibility and relative validity of the short questionnaire to assess health-enhancing physical activity. J Clin Epidemiol. 2003;56(12):1163–9.
30. Ainsworth BE, Haskell WL, Herrmann SD, Meckes N, Bassett DR Jr, Tudor-Locke C, Greer JL, Vezina J, Whitt-Glover MC, Leon AS. 2011 compendium of physical activities: a second update of codes and MET values. Med Sci Sports Exerc. 2011;43(8):1575–81. https://doi.org/10.1249/MSS.0b013e31821ece12.
31. Sijtsma A, Sauer PJ, Corpeleijn E. Parental correlations of physical activity and body mass index in young children–he GECKO Drenthe cohort. The international journal of behavioral nutrition and physical activity. 2015;12: 132. https://doi.org/10.1186/s12966-015-0295-0.
32. Grundy SM, Cleeman JI, Daniels SR, Donato KA, Eckel RH, Franklin BA, Gordon DJ, Krauss RM, Savage PJ, Smith SC Jr, Spertus JA, Costa F. Diagnosis and management of the metabolic syndrome: an American Heart Association/National Heart, Lung, and Blood Institute scientific statement. Circulation. 2005;112(17):2735–52. https://doi.org/10.1161/circulationaha.105.169404.
33. Esmaillzadeh A, Kimiagar M, Mehrabi Y, Azadbakht L, FB H, Willett WC. Fruit and vegetable intakes, C-reactive protein, and the metabolic syndrome. Am J Clin Nutr. 2006;84(6):1489–97.
34. Bazzano LA, Li TY, Joshipura KJ, FB H. Intake of fruit, vegetables, and fruit juices and risk of diabetes in women. Diabetes Care. 2008;31(7):1311–7. https://doi.org/10.2337/dc08-0080.
35. Muraki I, Imamura F, Manson JE, Hu FB, Willett WC, van Dam RM, Sun Q. Fruit consumption and risk of type 2 diabetes: results from three prospective longitudinal cohort studies. BMJ (Clinical research ed). 2013;347: f5001. https://doi.org/10.1136/bmj.f5001.
36. Astrup A (2014) Yogurt and dairy product consumption to prevent cardiometabolic diseases: epidemiologic and experimental studies. The American journal of clinical nutrition 99 (5 Suppl):1235s-1242s. doi:https://doi.org/10.3945/ajcn.113.073015.
37. Gijsbers L, Ding EL, Malik VS, de Goede J, Geleijnse JM, Soedamah-Muthu SS. Consumption of dairy foods and diabetes incidence: a dose-response meta-analysis of observational studies. Am J Clin Nutr. 2016;103(4):1111–24. https://doi.org/10.3945/ajcn.115.123216.
38. FB H. Are refined carbohydrates worse than saturated fat? Am J Clin Nutr. 2010;91(6):1541–2. https://doi.org/10.3945/ajcn.2010.29622.
39. Jenkins DJ, Kendall CW, McKeown-Eyssen G, Josse RG, Silverberg J, Booth GL, Vidgen E, Josse AR, Nguyen TH, Corrigan S, Banach MS, Ares S, Mitchell S, Emam A, Augustin LS, Parker TL, Leiter LA. Effect of a low-glycemic index or a high-cereal fiber diet on type 2 diabetes: a randomized trial. JAMA. 2008;300(23):2742–53. https://doi.org/10.1001/jama.2008.808.
40. Maki KC, Rains TM, Kaden VN, Raneri KR, Davidson MH. Effects of a reduced-glycemic-load diet on body weight, body composition, and cardiovascular disease risk markers in overweight and obese adults. Am J Clin Nutr. 2007; 85(3):724–34.
41. Ebbeling CB, Leidig MM, Feldman HA, Lovesky MM, Ludwig DS. Effects of a low-glycemic load vs low-fat diet in obese young adults: a randomized trial.

JAMA. 2007;297(19):2092–102. https://doi.org/10.1001/jama.297.19.2092.
42. Finley CE, Barlow CE, Halton TL, Haskell WL. Glycemic index, glycemic load, and prevalence of the metabolic syndrome in the cooper center longitudinal study. J Am Diet Assoc. 2010;110(12):1820–9. https://doi.org/10.1016/j.jada.2010.09.016.
43. de la Iglesia R, Loria-Kohen V, Zulet MA, Martinez JA, Reglero G, Ramirez de Molina A. Dietary strategies implicated in the prevention and treatment of metabolic syndrome. Int J Mol Sci. 2016;17(11) https://doi.org/10.3390/ijms17111877.
44. Bell LK, Edwards S, Grieger JA. The relationship between dietary patterns and metabolic health in a representative sample of adult Australians. Nutrients. 2015;7(8):6491–505. https://doi.org/10.3390/nu7085295.
45. van Dam RM, Grievink L, Ocke MC, Feskens EJ. Patterns of food consumption and risk factors for cardiovascular disease in the general Dutch population. Am J Clin Nutr. 2003;77(5):1156–63.
46. Swift DL, Johannsen NM, Lavie CJ, Earnest CP, Church TS. The role of exercise and physical activity in weight loss and maintenance. Prog Cardiovasc Dis. 2014;56(4):441–7. https://doi.org/10.1016/j.pcad.2013.09.012
47. Appleton SL, Seaborn CJ, Visvanathan R, Hill CL, Gill TK, Taylor AW, Adams RJ. Diabetes and cardiovascular disease outcomes in the metabolically healthy obese phenotype: a cohort study. Diabetes Care. 2013;36(8):2388–94. https://doi.org/10.2337/dc12-1971.
48. Bell JA, Hamer M, van Hees VT, Singh-Manoux A, Kivimaki M, Sabia S. Healthy obesity and objective physical activity. Am J Clin Nutr. 2015;102(2):268–75. https://doi.org/10.3945/ajcn.115.110924.
49. Camhi SM, Waring ME, Sisson SB, Hayman LL. Must a (2013) physical activity and screen time in metabolically healthy obese phenotypes in adolescents and adults. J Obes. 2013:984613. https://doi.org/10.1155/2013/984613.
50. Gutierrez-Repiso C, Soriguer F, Rojo-Martinez G, Garcia-Fuentes E, Valdes S, Goday A, Calle-Pascual A, Lopez-Alba A, Castell C, Menendez E, Bordiu E, Delgado E, Ortega E, Pascual-Manich G, Urrutia I, Mora-Peces I, Vendrell J, Vazquez JA, Franch J, Girbes J, Castano L, Serrano-Rios M, Martinez-Larrad MT, Catala M, Carmena R, Gomis R, Casamitjana R, Gaztambide S. Variable patterns of obesity and cardiometabolic phenotypes and their association with lifestyle factors in the Di@bet.es study. Nutrition, metabolism, and cardiovascular diseases : NMCD. 2014;24(9):947–55. https://doi.org/10.1016/j.numecd.2014.04.019.
51. Kanagasabai T, Thakkar NA, Kuk JL, Churilla JR, Ardern CI. Differences in physical activity domains, guideline adherence, and weight history between metabolically healthy and metabolically abnormal obese adults: a cross-sectional study. The international journal of behavioral nutrition and physical activity. 2015;12:64. https://doi.org/10.1186/s12966-015-0227-z.
52. Lichtman SW, Pisarska K, Berman ER, Pestone M, Dowling H, Offenbacher E, Weisel H, Heshka S, Matthews DE, Heymsfield SB. Discrepancy between self-reported and actual caloric intake and exercise in obese subjects. N Engl J Med. 1992;327(27):1893–8. https://doi.org/10.1056/nejm199212313272701.
53. Trijsburg L, Geelen A, Hollman PC, Hulshof PJ, Feskens EJ, Van't Veer P, Boshuizen HC, de Vries JH. BMI was found to be a consistent determinant related to misreporting of energy, protein and potassium intake using self-report and duplicate portion methods. Public Health Nutr. 2016:1–10. https://doi.org/10.1017/s1368980016002743.
54. FB H, Rimm E, Smith-Warner SA, Feskanich D, Stampfer MJ, Ascherio A, Sampson L, Willett WC. Reproducibility and validity of dietary patterns assessed with a food-frequency questionnaire. Am J Clin Nutr. 1999;69(2):243–9.
55. Khani BR, Ye W, Terry P, Wolk A. Reproducibility and validity of major dietary patterns among Swedish women assessed with a food-frequency questionnaire. J Nutr. 2004;134(6):1541–5.
56. Liu X, Wang X, Lin S, Song Q, Lao X, IT Y. Reproducibility and validity of a food frequency questionnaire for assessing dietary consumption via the dietary pattern method in a Chinese rural population. PLoS One. 2015;10(7):e0134627. https://doi.org/10.1371/journal.pone.0134627.
57. Newby PK, Weismayer C, Akesson A, Tucker KL, Wolk A. Long-term stability of food patterns identified by use of factor analysis among Swedish women. J Nutr. 2006;136(3):626–33.
58. Balder HF, Virtanen M, Brants HA, Krogh V, Dixon LB, Tan F, Mannisto S, Bellocco R, Pietinen P, Wolk A, Berrino F, Van den Brandt PA, Hartman AM, Goldbohm RA. Common and country-specific dietary patterns in four European cohort studies. J Nutr. 2003;133(12):4246–51.

18

Relative validity of a web-based food frequency questionnaire for Danish adolescents

Anne A. Bjerregaard[1*], Thorhallur I. Halldorsson[1,2], Freja B. Kampmann[3,4,5], Sjurdur F. Olsen[1] and Inge Tetens[6]

Abstract

Background: With increased focus on dietary intake among youth and risk of diseases later in life, it is of importance, prior to assessing diet-disease relationships, to examine the validity of the dietary assessment tool. This study's objective was to evaluate the relative validity of a self-administered web-based FFQ among Danish children aged 12 to 15 years.

Methods: From a nested sub-cohort within the Danish National Birth Cohort, 124 adolescents participated. Four weeks after completion of the FFQ, adolescents were invited to complete three telephone-based 24HRs; administered 4 weeks apart. Mean or median intakes of nutrients and food groups estimated from the FFQ were compared with the mean of 3x24HRs. To assess the level of ranking we calculated the proportion of correctly classified into the same quartile, and the proportion of misclassified (into the opposite quartile). Spearman's correlation coefficients and de-attenuated coefficients were calculated to assess agreement between the FFQ and 24HRs.

Results: The mean percentage of all food groups, for adolescents classified into the same and opposite quartile was 35 and 7.5%, respectively. Mean Spearman's correlation was 0.28 for food groups and 0.35 for nutrients, respectively. Adjustment for energy and within-person variation in the 24HRs had little effect on the magnitude of the correlations for food groups and nutrients. We found overestimation by the FFQ compared with the 24HRs for fish, fruits, vegetables, oils and dressing and underestimation by the FFQ for meat/poultry and sweets. Median intake of beverages, dairy, bread, cereals, the mean total energy and carbohydrate intake did not differ significantly between the two methods.

Conclusion: The relative validity of the FFQ compared with the 3x24HRs showed that the ranking ability differed across food groups and nutrients with best ranking for estimated intake of dairy, fruits, and oils and dressing. Larger variation was observed for fish, sweets and vegetables. For nutrients, the ranking ability was acceptable for fatty acids and iron. When evaluating estimates from the FFQ among Danish adolescents these findings should be considered.

Keywords: Dietary assessment, School-age children, Diet, Dietary intake, Cohort study, Food groups, Nutrients, Diet recall

Background

Dietary intake among adolescents has consistently been associated with later health and disease risk in adult life [1, 2]. Diet-disease associations measured in adolescence are often based on dietary intake estimated from a food frequency questionnaire (FFQ) particularly in largescale studies [2–6]. The FFQ method is often self-administered which is more cost-effective, less intrusive, and less time-consuming for the participants compared with other dietary assessment methods such as multiple 24-h recalls (24HR) and food records [7]. However, prior to assessing diet-disease relationships, the validity of the dietary assessment tool must be examined [8].

Validity refers to the degree to which an assessment method captures true dietary intake [9]. Such assessment requires comparison with 'a gold standard' method which, in reality, is rarely available. Therefore researchers are often left with the option of examining relative validity by comparing one dietary assessment method with another method that has a different error structure [10].

* Correspondence: anne@ssi.dk
[1]Center for Fetal Programming, Department of Epidemiology Research, Statens Serum Institut, Artillerivej 5, 2300 Copenhagen, Denmark

Although a 24HR relies on memory, as does the FFQ, 24HRs are common in relative validity studies using FFQs among adolescents [11, 12]. FFQs are in general considered suitable or valid for ranking adolescents at group level with correlation coefficients ranging from 0.2 to 0.8 [11–14]. In terms of what can be considered as acceptable validity in such studies, Cade et al. suggested a cut-off of 0.40 as an acceptable correlation [15]. However, such an approach has been criticised by others, as a correlation of 0.50 indicates that 75% of the variance in estimates is error, thus increasing the risk of misclassification in association studies [16]. Nevertheless, correlation coefficients are still the main statistical approach in validation studies which ensures the possibility for some comparison across studies. A recent meta-analysis found correlation coefficients above 0.40 for most nutrients in 16 validity studies comparing an FFQ to food record or 24HRs among 13- to 17-year-old adolescents [10]. However, high heterogeneity was also reported in validation studies with administration mode and recall interval as strongest contributors [10]. Other factors which potentially influence validity are the respondent's memory and ability to identify and quantify consumed foods [17, 18]. In addition, compared with validation studies in adults, a higher degree of intrusion and omission among children has been demonstrated [19]. Thus, it is important to evaluate if an FFQ can assess dietary intake and rank adolescents in terms of energy, nutrient, and food intakes. To our knowledge, a web-based FFQ has not previously been validated among Danish adolescents. The aim of this study therefore was to evaluate the relative validity of a web-based FFQ using a nested sub-cohort of adolescents aged 12 to 15 years old, within the Danish National Birth Cohort (DNBC).

Methods

Subjects

The DNBC includes information from 101,042 pregnancies and is described in details elsewhere [20]. In brief, information on participants was recorded through telephone interviews in gestation weeks (GW) 12 and 30, and 6 and 18 months postpartum. Maternal diet was assessed in GW 25 using an extensive FFQ [20]. Additional available offspring data were collected at age 7 and 11.

Data for the present study were obtained in a nested sub-cohort within the DNBC called the Diabetes and Women's Health Study, which ran from May 2012 to April 2014 [21]. In a group of women who had had gestational diabetes (GDM) and a group of women who had had a normal pregnancy, insulin sensitivity, risk of type 2 diabetes, and risk of diabetes in offspring aged 9–15 years were investigated [21]. This sub-cohort provided an opportunity to invite adolescents between 12 to 15 years of age to participate in the validation study. The invited adolescents were offspring of women already in the DNBC cohort. These adolescents were all considered relatively healthy in terms of non-communicable diseases, and no exclusion criteria were applied.

Design

All offspring of mothers participating in the Diabetes and Women's Health Study were invited to fill out a web-based FFQ during their pre-planned clinical visit. After the clinic visit, 178 adolescents were asked to participate in the 24HRs by e-mail (45), phone (12) or hand out at the clinic (121). Follow-up on the invitation was done by e-mail and by phone call approximately 7 days after the invitation was received and 7 days apart. The first 24HR was carried out 4 weeks after the FFQ followed by two recalls 4 weeks apart. Three non-consecutive telephone-based 24HRs were conducted by four trained nutritionists, and each interview took approximately 25 min. In order to make the 24HRs represent weekdays and weekends, a set of three different days were randomly designed. A set of 3 days was distributed to the participants, ensuring equal distribution of all 7 days of the week at group level. Participants were not informed beforehand as to which day the 24HR would be performed. They only received a mobile text message on the day the recall took place, to arrange a suitable time for the conversation. All participants automatically entered into a competition to win one of three Ipads.

The food frequency questionnaire

The web-based self-administered FFQ developed for this study was based on the validated youth/adolescent questionnaire (YAQ) from the Growing Up Today Study [13, 22] which is a follow-up study of children born to women in the Nurses' Health Study 2 (NHS-2). The YAQ was translated into Danish and modified to include typical Danish foods based on the reports National Danish Dietary Habits and Physical activity [23, 24]. The aim of modifying the YAQ was to make sure that the FFQ reflects Danish dietary patterns and thus intake of Danish foods and beverages. We previously evaluated the reproducibility of the FFQ and showed high concordance between two repeated measurements with the FFQ with a Spearman's correlation coefficient for energy of 0.78 [25].

The FFQ included 145 frequency questions on food items clustered into 8 food groups (number of food items in brackets): beverages (18), dairy (8), bread and cereals including butter on bread (14), spread on bread (14), cold and warm dishes (25), side dishes and condiments (18), fruits and vegetables (29), snacks and desserts (20). Frequency scales ranged from "did not drink/ consume the last month" to "2 times or more per day" or "4 times or more per day" and the recall period was 1 month. Portion sizes were predefined for dairy products (bowl), breakfast cereals (bowl), and beverages (glass/bottle), slides of bread, fruits (pc.), selected vegetables (pc.), and cake (pc.), whereas no portion size was given for the remaining items. Portion sizes were based on standard portions developed by the National Food Institute in Denmark [26]. Additional information on food allergy, other foods the participant may wish to avoid and any major changes in food habits during the last month was included in three open-end questions.

Before the FFQ, questions on age, gender, and self-reported height and weight were listed. Following the FFQ, questions on (number of questions in parenthesis); meal habits (15), physical activity (11) and puberty (6) were listed. Finally, the participants were asked to which degree they completed the questionnaire themselves or received help from an adult. Written instruction on how to complete the questionnaire was given at the beginning of the questionnaire together with short examples of answers. Time for filling in the FFQ was approximately 40 min. The FFQ was based on the online html program Limesurvey.

The 24-h recalls

To conduct the 24HRs, a structured interview guide was developed, with questions in a chronological order covering daily meal patterns including promt questions. Dietary intake reported by the participant was reported directly into a pre-coded Danish food record by the interviewer. The pre-coded Danish food record is a semi-closed questionnaire with answer categories for the most commonly consumed dishes according to meal patterns in Denmark as used in the nationally representative survey of Dietary Habits and Physical Activity (DANSDA) in 2011–2013 [27]. Open answers were available in each section if consumed foods were not found in the pre-coded categories. Household measures were used for quantification of portion sizes. After the interview, answers were reviewed orally together with the adolescent to make sure everything he/she had consumed was recorded.

Calculation foods and nutrient intakes from the FFQ and the 24HRs

Frequencies of intake were computed into grams per day using nutrition software Foodcalc v.3 [28]. Nutritional calculations for the FFQ were done based on assumptions of standard portion sizes. The 24HRs were entered into an online registration system (fa.kostvaner.dk, template by cmsimple-styles.com) developed at the Danish National Food Institute (Tue Christensen, personal communication). National food composition tables [29] were used for both the FFQ and the 24HRs.

Statistics

All statistical analyses were performed in the statistical program SAS version 9.4 (SAS Institute, Cary, NC, USA). Participant characteristics were evaluated using descriptive statistics. Age- and gender-specific cut-offs for overweight and obesity among the offspring were based on values provided by the International Obesity Task Force (IOTF) [30]. Parental educational level was retrieved from the maternal FFQ in the DNBC.

We presented median along with 25th and 75th percentile for food groups and nutrients since data were non-normally distributed both before and after log-transformation (except energy percent of macronutrients which were normally distributed). Paired t-test was used to compare differences between the two methods for normally distributed variables while Wilcoxon rank test was used for skewed variables. To compare differences in estimated intake between the two methods the median difference in percentages was calculated according to the formula: ((FFQ - 24HR)/24HR)*100. Misclassification analysis (into quantiles) including weighted Kappa was applied in order to test whether the FFQ ranked adolescents according to magnitude of dietary and nutrient intake by comparison to the mean of the three 24HRs. It has been suggested that at least 50% of subjects should be classified into the same category, no more than 10% should be classified into the opposite category, and Cohen's weighted Kappa should preferably be above 0.4 [31]. Bland-Altman plots were used to elaborate whether the differences between the two methods were constant across the range of measurements, and mean intake was plotted against mean difference [32]. The association between food and nutrient intakes estimated with the two methods was assessed using crude, energy adjusted and de-attenuated Spearman's correlation coefficients. Correlation coefficients were adjusted using the ratio of within- and between-person variation assessed on the basis of the three 24HRs. These de-attenuated correlation coefficients should provide an estimate similar to that obtained with a higher number of 24HRs [9]. Adjustment for energy was performed with the residual method [9].

To estimate the degree of selection as a result of our recruitment strategy we compared characteristics of participants with those who did not wish to participate in the validation study (non-participants). Differences in characteristics of participants born to GDMmothers vs. other offspring participants were also compared. Finally, characteristics of our participants were compared with those in the full source population, i.e. the DNBC 14-year follow-up study. For these comparisons we applied analysis of variance.

Results

The mean age (SD) and body mass index (BMI) for the 124 participants were 13.2 (0.7) years and 19.1 kg/m^2, respectively (Table 1). Among participants, 62% were born to GDMmothers, and 27.4% were overweight or obese (Table 1). The relative validity of the FFQ was evaluated by comparing estimated intake of food groups, energy and nutrients with the average of three 24HRs (Table 2). We found significant difference between the FFQ and the mean of three 24HRs for the majority of food groups. The food groups; fish, fruits, vegetables, and oils and dressing were overestimated by the FFQ when compared with the mean of three 24HRs, whereas meat/poultry and sweets were underestimated by the FFQ. We found no significant difference for beverages, dairy, bread, and cereals. Median difference (%) revealed the smallest differences for beverages (+10%), bread (−10%), and dairy (−5%) and larger differences for fish (+1000%), fruits (+121%), and sweets (−70%) (Table 2).

For nutrients, there were no significant differences in total energy, polyunsaturated fatty acids (PUFA), energy percent (E%) from carbohydrate, dietary fibres, calcium and iron. Protein E% and vitamin C were overestimated, while the remaining nutrients were underestimated by the FFQ in comparison with the three 24HRs. The median differences (%) showed smallest differences (or null for carbohydrate E% and iron) for fat E% (−3%) and calcium (−0.7), whereas the largest degree of under- or overestimation was seen for added sugar (−36%) and vitamin C (+34%) (Table 2).

Consistency between the two methods was also examined using Bland-Altman plots. These plots for beverages, dairy, meat/poultry, vitamin C, and calcium revealed some outliers, but no systematic patterns were observed (exemplified with dairy Fig. 1). For the remaining variables, the plots indicated a tendency towards higher difference between the FFQ and the 24HRs at higher mean intakes. This indicates a higher degree of overestimation and underestimation at higher intakes (exemplified with sweets Fig. 2). The mean difference in intake of e.g. sweets was below zero, confirming an underestimation by the FFQ. The pattern of observations indicated a higher degree of underestimation at higher mean intakes.

Table 1 Participant characteristics ($n = 124$, 52% girls)

	All	Girls	Boys
Age, years (mean, SD)	13.2 (0.7)	13.3 (0.6)	13.2 (0.7)
Height, cm (mean, SD)	165.9 (8.3)	164.7 (7.9)	167.4 (8.5)
BMI[a] (kg/m^2) (mean, SD)	19.1 (7.9)	19.2 (7.9)	19.1 (8.3)
Overweight[a] (%)	13.7	15	12
Obese[a] (%)	13.7	12	15
Born to GDM mothers[b] (%)	62	57	68
Parental educational level (%)			
High level of education	21	26	15
Medium level of education	32.5	29	36
Skilled workers	32.5	30	36
Student	0.8	1.5	0
Unskilled	12	14	11
Unemployed	0.8	0	1.8

BMI body mass index = weight (kg)/height (m)^2 *GDM* gestational diabetes mellitus

[a]Classification by Cole et al. [30]

[b]Adolescents born to mothers with registered gestational diabetes

Misclassification (into the opposite quartile) was below 10% for all food groups and nutrients, except for fish and carbohydrate E% (Table 2). Correct classification ranged from 23% (meat/poultry) to 46% (dairy), while nutrients ranged from 25% (carbohydrate E%) to 45% (monounsaturated fatty acids (MUFA)). Weighted Kappa values ranged from 0.05 (meats/poultry) to 0.43 (dairy) (Table 2).

Spearman's correlation coefficients for food groups ranged from 0.03 (fish) to 0.60 (dairy). Three of the 10 food groups and 5 of the 12 nutrients examined had Spearman's correlations above 0.4. These were dairy, fruits, oils and dressing, saturated fatty acids (SFA), MUFA, PUFA, calcium, and iron (Table 3). For energy, the Spearman's correlation coefficient was 0.38 and the mean correlation coefficient for nutrients was 0.35 (Table 3). De-attenuation improved Spearman's correlation coefficients lightly for most variables, while further adjustment for energy only improved the correlation coefficients for MUFA (from 0.54 to 0.60) (Table 3).

The main reason given for not wishing to participate in this validation study (54 out of 178 invited) was lack of time. When we examined characteristics of participants ($n = 124$) and non-participants ($n = 54$), no substantial differences were found for sex, age, BMI, proportion born to GDM mothers, or parental education. Within our set of participants, we observed no significant differences in dietary intakes between offspring born to GDM and non-GDM mothers for all dietary variables tested except for vegetables (mean difference of: 25 g/d, highest among offspring born to GDM mothers) (data not shown). Overall, minor differences in dietary habits between overweight- and normal-weight participants were found: the mean difference between the FFQ and the 3x24HRs was significantly higher for energy from protein (1.3E%) and significantly lower for carbohydrate (−3.7E%) among overweight children compared with normal weight children (Additional file 1: Table S1). Furthermore, comparing our study population in which GDMmothers are overrepresented (and not participating in the DNBC follow-up, $n = 76$) with the adolescents from the DNBC 14-year follow-up ($n =$ 24,879) we found no significant difference for proportion

Table 2 Relative validity: mean and median intake of food groups, energy and nutrients from FFQ and 3x24HR, percentage difference, and percentage agreement in categories ($n = 124$)

	FFQ		3x24HR		Median diff. %	Classification (%)		
Food groups (g/d)	Median	q1-q3	Median	q1-q3		Same quartile	Opposite quartile	Weighted Kappa
Beverages	1131	648–1273	1032	821–1464	−10	35	9	0.20
Dairy	319	182–636	335	182–521	−4.7	46	6	0.43
Bread	185	109–275	204	146–258	−9	28	7	0.12
Cereals	27	14–50	24	9–52	12	35	6	0.25
Meats/poultry	82*	56–118	107	69–139	−23	23	7	0.05
Fish	11*	6–18	1	0–16	1000	32	18	n.a.
Fruits	126**	52–247	57	9–135	121	43	6	0.32
Vegetables	116*	65–171	91	62–130	27	32	9	0.12
Sweets	17**	10–28	57	24–108	−70	33	4	0.20
Oils & dressing	36*	22–47	26	18–51	38	38	3	0.32
Nutrients	Mean or Median	SD or q1-q3	Mean or Median	SD or q1-q3				
Energy (MJ/d)	7.6	5.7–9.7	8.5	7.0–11.0	−10	36	5	0.26
Protein (E%)	15**	2.7	13	2.5	15	37	6	0.24
Fat (E%)	34*	6.3	35	6.0	−3	34	8	0.24
SFA (g/d)	26**	19–33	33	23–44	−21	40	2	0.34
MUFA (g/d)	24*	16–31	27	20–36	−11	45	2	0.39
PUFA (g/d)	12	8–15	11	9–15	9	36	3	0.29
Carbohydrate (E%)	51	6.5	51	6.0	0	25	14	0.10
Added sugar (g/d)	26**	15–38	41	25–69	−36	31	5	0.23
Dietary fiber (g/d)	21	15–32	18	15–24	16	41	5	0.30
Vitamin C (mg/d)	66**	43–100	49	33–69	34	31	7	0.14
Calcium (mg/d)	867	647–1374	873	672–1229	−0.7	39	6	0.33
Iron (mg/d)	8.3	6.3–12.5	8.3	6.7–10.8	0	40	4	0.29

Variables that reached normality after log-transformation were beverages, dairy, bread, oils & dressing, energy, SFA, MUFA, PUFA, added sugar, dietary fibers, vitamin C, calcium and iron whereas cereals, meat/poultry, fish, fruit, vegetables and sweets did not reach normality after log-transformation
Median difference in percent = median (FFQ-24HR/24HR)*100
FFQ food frequency questionnaire, *24HR*, 24-h recalls, *SFA* saturated fatty acids, *MUFA* monounsaturated fatty acids, *PUFA* polyunsaturated fatty acids
*$p < 0.05$ significantly different from 24HR
**$p < 0.001$ significantly different from 24HR

of girls (47% vs. 52%, $p = 0.10$), parental education ($p = 0.11$), and maternal smoking ($p = 0.13$). However, children in the validation study were significantly younger (7 months, $p < 0.0001$), and were more frequently overweight/obese (16% vs. 9%, $p = 0.03$) compared with the adolescents from the DNBC 14-year follow-up. No significant differences in nutrient intake on a group level were observed across the three 24HRs (data not shown).

Discussion

Comparing dietary intake assessed by the web-based FFQ with that of three 24HRs among Danish adolescents we found that four (fish, fruits, vegetables, and oils and dressing) out of 10 food groups and three (protein E%, dietary fibres, and vitamin C) of the 11 nutrients were overestimated by the FFQ. This is similar to what has often been reported in similar studies in adolescents [13, 33, 34]. Total energy intake did not differ significantly between the two methods which is comparable to what was found in the validation study of the original GUTS questionnaire [13]. However, in the validation study by Rockett et al. mean Pearson correlation coefficients for nutrients were 0.41 compared with 0.35 in our study (Spearman's correlation coefficients). Even though the agreement estimated by the kappa statistics primarily was poor to fair/moderate (ranging from 0.05–0.43 [35]), the ability to rank adolescents according to magnitude of intake was good in the sense that

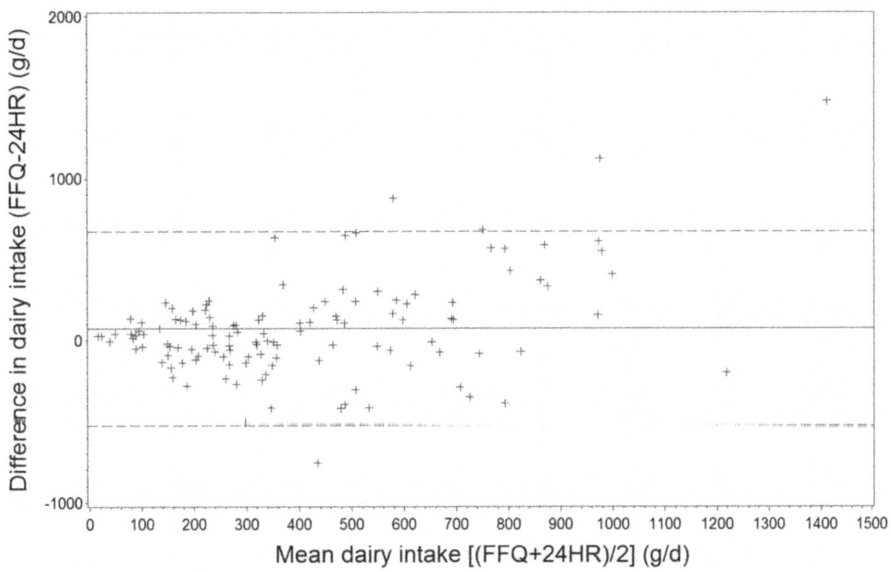

Fig. 1 Bland-Altman plot for dairy intake for the two methods FFQ and mean of three 24HR among participants ($n = 124$). The difference in intake is plottet v. the mean intake from the two methods. ———— represents the mean difference ——— represents the 95% limits of agreement

misclassification (in the opposite quartile) below 10% was seen for most food groups and nutrients, except for fish and carbohydrate E% [31]. Misclassification below 5% was seen for oils and dressing, fatty acids, and iron.

When comparing our results with a validation study performed using a similar FFQ to ours in the Norwegian mother-child cohort, we found a lower level of misclassification into opposite quartile in general. However, it must be noted that the Norwegian study used quintiles [12].

Intake of fish, fruits, and sweets differed significantly between the two methods, with higher intake of fruits and fish and lower intake of sweets in the FFQ relative to the 24HRs. Fish is often rarely consumed and may not be captured by only 3 days of dietary recording, as was also observed in other studies [12]. Even though the three randomly assigned 24HRs covered all 7 weekdays, three 24HRs might not have sufficiently estimated the day-to-day variability [9] of e.g. fish, resulting in large median difference and low correlation between the two

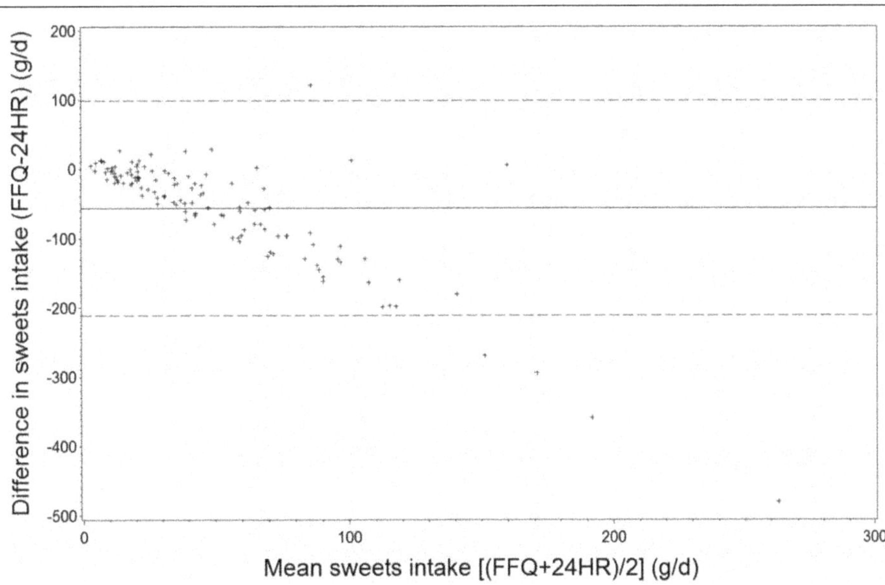

Fig. 2 Bland-Altman plot for sweets intake for the two methods FFQ and mean of three 24HR among participants ($n = 124$). The difference in intake is plottet v. the mean intake from the two methods. ———— represents the mean difference ——— represents the 95% limits of agreement

Table 3 Spearman correlation coefficient between FFQ and 3x24HR ($n = 124$)

	Spearman correlation coefficients *r*		
Food groups (g/d)	crude	De-attenuated	Energy adjusted & de-attenuated
Beverages	0.22*	0.24*	0.24*
Dairy	0.60**	0.69**	0.61**
Bread	0.19*	0.19*	0.19*
Cereals	0.33*	0.35*	0.35*
Meats/poultry	0.16	0.17	0.16
Fish	0.03	0.03	0.03
Fruits	0.40**	0.43**	0.41**
Vegetables	0.13	0.13	0.13
Sweets	0.31*	0.32*	0.31*
Oils & dressing	0.46**	0.48**	0.47**
Nutrients			
Energy (MJ/d)	0.38**	0.54**	
Protein (E%)	0.28	0.32	
Fat (E%)	0.27*	0.28*	
SFA (g/d)	0.51**	0.54**	0.53**
MUFA (g/d)	0.52**	0.54**	0.60**
PUFA (g/d)	0.47**	0.48**	0.47**
Carbohydrate (E%)	0.09	0.09	
Added sugar (g/d)	0.37**	0.38**	0.39**
Dietary fiber (g/d)	0.32*	0.33*	0.33*
Vitamin C (mg/d)	0.21*	0.22*	0.22*
Calcium m(g/d)	0.46**	0.51**	0.51**
Iron (g/d)	0.40*	0*.41	0.41*

De-attenuated, correlation coefficients adjusted for within-person variation using ANOVA to estimate within- and between-person variance and ratio
*$p < 0.05$, significant Spearman correlation
**$p < 0.001$, significant Spearman correlation

methods. Further, a high number of subjects were misclassified in the opposite quartile of intake which was also observed in the study by Overby et al. [12]. According to a Danish study using dietary data from The Danish National Survey of Dietary Habits and Physical Activity 2003–2008, intake of sweets, cakes, and sugar-sweetened beverages among 789 children aged 4–14 years were higher during weekends compared with weekdays [36]. Together with the fact that adolescents were found to be more prone to omit foods compared with adults [19], the lower estimated intake of sweets in the FFQ might be a result of intake during weekends being omitted by the adolescents when completing the FFQ.

The percentage difference in intake between the FFQ and 3x24HRs of 121% for fruits (highest in the FFQ) and a correlation coefficient of 0.13 for vegetables deserves some attention. A relatively large intervention study among 9-10-year-old Danish children ($n = 798$) reported a median (p10, p90) intake of fruits of 126 g/d (38, 244) and a median (p10, p90) intake of vegetables of 126 g/d (54, 227) measured by 7d food records [37]. The level of intake is comparable to the median (p25, p75) intake of fruits estimated with our FFQ; 126 g/d (52–247). Additionally, the Danish study showed a significantly higher consumption during school hours compared with outside school [37]. Further, a study among 96 adolescents aged 11 to 15 years found only 30% match between a 24HR method and direct observations [38]. Therefore, it could be speculated that meals consumed during school hours were omitted during 24HRs and fruits and vegetables were underestimated by the 24HRs. However, since prompt questions were included in the 24HRs to ensure that intake during school hours was captured, intake of fruits may have been overestimated by the FFQ as a consequence of a high number of questions about fruits in the FFQ. Variation in season should, furthermore, also be considered. The FFQ was completed from December to March whereas the 24HRs were conducted between January and June. Thus, there were some overlapping periods at group level. If season had had a substantial impact, we would have expected higher intakes of fruits and vegetables estimated from the 24HRs in the spring. However, median intakes of fruits and vegetables were lower in the 24HRs compared with the FFQ.

The observed disparities in mean intakes of food groups and low percentages classified into same quartile were to some extent expected due to the adolescent study population. Adolescents are known to pay less attention to dietary habits, and their snacking and eating habits tend to be more unstructured compared with those of adults. They may also be less motivated to record their dietary intake and have increased focus on body image, which seems to affect the accuracy of their self-report [39]. These characteristics may result in high within person day-to-day variability among adolescents which seems to attenuate correlation coefficients [9, 14]. This was in particular evident for dairy, energy intake, MUFA, and calcium where Spearman's correlation coefficient increased after de-attenuation which was also reported in the study by Rockett et al. [13]. However, Spearman's correlation coefficients for bread, fish and carbohydrate E% did not improve after de-attenuation. This suggests that intake of bread and fish was reported consistently over time, whereas other intakes varied more among the participating adolescents. De-attenuation improved an already strong correlation coefficient for dairy, indicating some variation between days nevertheless; recall of milk products was rather constant. Studies have reported that adolescents might have some difficulties in combining amount of foods eaten and frequency [18] which could also have contributed to the observed level of inconsistencies across foods and nutrients.

Energy adjustment did not affect level of correlation coefficients substantially in any direction, indicating that intake was not related to systematic errors of under- or over estimation of intake, nor was nutrient intake related to energy intake [9]. Difficulties in reaching strong correlation coefficients among adolescents were presented in a systematic review where only 2 of the 18 validity studies reported mean correlation coefficients above 0.50 [40]. Recall periods of 1 day or 1 week and fewer than 70 food items in the FFQ were assigned as main reasons for stronger correlation coefficients [40]. However, in a recent meta-analysis by Tabacchi et al., correlation coefficients for most nutrients in 16 validity studies were above 0.40, and it was suggested that the number of food items should not exceed 114 [10]. We cannot rule out that the number of food items in our FFQ (145) could be a contributor to the observed overestimation of some food groups. However, the correlation coefficient of e.g. fruits was 0.40. Nonetheless, both similar and stronger correlation coefficients ranging from ~0 to 0.8 have been reported for nutrients and food groups in other validation studies among adolescents [12, 14, 34]. Also in adults, higher correlation coefficients have been observed [41, 42] which could be due to better skills in frequency estimation, better memory of consumed foods, and better knowledge to identify foods compared with those of children [18]. This was to some extent confirmed in a study among 11- to 15-year-old children accordingly to which unfamiliar food terms, unfamiliar measurements, and poor knowledge of food fractions made recording diet problematic using a web-based 24HR [38]. Training of recalling diet among children has previously been suggested by Lu and colleagues in order to improve accuracy [43]. It could therefore be speculated whether training in recalling diet before the actual dietary assessment with an FFQ could increase both motivation and food knowledge among the adolescent population and thereby improve the quality of the results.

This validation study has several strengths. The web-based FFQ was easy to administer and it may increase participant motivation that recording takes less than 1 h, thereby potentially increasing participation rate [44]. The time interval of 4 weeks between the FFQ and the 24HRs seemed adequate to avoid carryover effects from the FFQ to the 24HRs [45]. Three non-consecutive 24HRs were chosen as reference method, because these have been suggested to be sufficient to assess habitual energy intake [46]. Since adolescents seem to have high within-person variation in diet, de-attenuated correlation coefficients were calculated in order to obtain an estimate similar to that gained with a higher number of 24HRs [9]. We ensured high quality of the 24HRs with four trained project team members conducting the interviews. Recalls by telephone have shown to yield results similar to those of face-to-face interviews [47]. Moreover, this method was less expensive and we were able to reach participants from across the country [48]. Furthermore, telephone interviews potentially decreased the correlation between the test and reference method [49]. With the allocation of interview days, we secured representation of all weekdays at group level. Nevertheless, due to adolescents' eating habits, some food items might not have been captured sufficiently. When we report correlation coefficients between the FFQ and the three 24HRs that rely on individual responses to these assessments, the number of days are not equally distributed between study participants. Since the days were randomly allocated this should not bias our estimates.

Limitations of the present study are firstly the different recall periods of the FFQ and the 24HRs. This could potentially increase the differences in observed estimates, as the FFQ was a self-administered long-term recall compared with the interview-based prompted short-term 24HR. Secondly, the 12–15-year age range of both boys and girls may have contributed to the relatively large variability within the study population and thus overall have lowered the level of relative validity. Thirdly, the FFQ and 24HR methods share measurement errors, e.g. both methods rely on memory [50]. Therefore, more objective measures, though also subject to measurement errors, such as observations in school or the double labelled water method, could have added an objective validation perspective of the FFQ tested. Finally, the fact that cohorts are often oversampled with a higher level of socio-economic status, and that 62% of the present study population were born to GDMmothers may render the results of the present study less representative for the Danish adolescent population with respect to e.g. proportion of overweight/obese adolescents [51, 52]. However, comparisons between our participants and the entire DNBC cohort of 14-year-olds (currently participated $n = 24{,}879$) revealed relatively minor differences. In these analyses, the difference in age was relatively small and is due to the recruitment of children younger than 14 years of age, which was necessary to increase sample size in the validation study.

Conclusion

The relative validity of the FFQ compared with the 3x24HRs showed that the ranking ability differed across food groups and nutrients. When considering the classification in quartiles and the Spearman's correlation coefficients together, the relative validity showed that the ranking ability was acceptable for estimated intake of dairy, fruits, oils and dressing, SFA, MUFA and iron. No major misclassification was observed for oils and dressings and fatty acids. Larger variation was seen for fish, sweets, and vegetables, and caution should be taken when interpreting estimation from the FFQ of fish and carbohydrate E%. When evaluating estimates from the web-based FFQ among Danish adolescents these findings should be considered.

Abbreviations

24HRs: 24-h recalls; BMI: Body Mass Index; DNBC: Danish national birth cohort; E%: Energy percent; FFQ: Food frequency questionnaire; GDM: Gestational diabetes mellitus; GUTS: Growing up today study; GW: Gestation week; IOTF: International obesity task force; MUFA: Monounsaturated fatty acids; NHS II: Nurses' health study II; PUFA: Polyunsaturated fatty acids; SD: Standard deviation; SFA: Saturated fatty acids; YAQ: Youth/adolescent questionnaire

Acknowledgments

The authors would like to thank senior researcher Tue Christensen, National Food Institute, Technical University of Denmark, for providing access to the precoded Danish food record, introduction to the program used for entering dietary recalls, and for supervision in data handling. We also want to thank dietician Karin Hess Ygil, National Food Institute, Technical University of Denmark, for helpful support in interpretating of the dietary recalls. Finally, many thanks to BSc students Nynne Dose, Maria Wichmann and Samiha El Halimi for professional data collection and to Samiha El Halimi for detailed check during data entry. The Danish Diabetes Academy is supported by the Novo Nordisk Foundation.

Funding

The study was supported by grants from The Danish Research Council 09-067124 (Center for Fetal Programming), 09-075611; and the Intramural Research Program of The *Eunice Kennedy Shriver* National Institute of Child Health and Human Development, National Institutes of Health (contract # HHSN275201000020C). The funding bodies had no role in the design of the study, collection, analysis, interpretation of data or in writing the manuscript.

Authors' contributions

SFO initiated the validation study and secured funding for it. In coorperation, all authors formulated the research question and design of the study. AAB was responsible for carrying out the study, analysing the data and writing the article. TIH assisted in analysing the data. TIH, FBK and IT assisted interpreting the data and writing the article. TIH, FBK, SFO, and IT critically reviewed the manuscript and all co-authors approved the final version submitted.

Competing interests

The authors declare that they have no competing interests.

Author details

[1]Center for Fetal Programming, Department of Epidemiology Research, Statens Serum Institut, Artillerivej 5, 2300 Copenhagen, Denmark. [2]The Unit for Nutrition Research, Faculty of Food Science and Nutrition, School of Health Sciences, University of Iceland, Sæmundargata 2, 101 Reykjavík, Iceland. [3]Division for Diet, Disease Prevention and Toxicology, National Food Institute, Technical University of Denmark, DTU Food, Kemitorvet, building, 202 Kgs. Lyngby, Denmark. [4]Department of Endocrinology, Diabetes and Metabolism, Rigshospitalet, Copenhagen, Denmark. [5]The Danish Diabetes Academy, Odense, Denmark. [6]Vitality - Centre for Good Older Lives, Department of Nutrition, Exercise, and Sports, University of Copenhagen, University of Copenhagen, Rolighedsvej 26, 1958 Frederiksberg C, Denmark.

References

1. Prentice A, Schoenmakers I, Laskey MA, de Bono S, Ginty F, Goldberg GR. Nutrition and bone growth and development. Proc Nutr Soc. 006;65(4):348–60.
2. Lipsky LM, Haynie DL, Liu D, Chaurasia A, Gee B, Li K, et al. Trajectories of eating behaviors in a nationally representative cohort of U.S. adolescents during the transition to young adulthood. Int J Behav Nutr Phys Act. 2015;12:138.
3. Berkey CS, Willett WC, Tamimi RM, Rosner B, Frazier AL, Colditz GA. Vegetable protein and vegetable fat intakes in pre-adolescent and adolescent girls, and risk for benign breast disease in young women. Breast Cancer Res Treat. 2013;141(2):299–306.
4. Wiium N, Breivik K, Wold B. Growth trajectories of health behaviors from adolescence through young adulthood. Int J Environ Res Public Health. 2015;12(11):13711–29.
5. Vereecken CA, Maes L. A Belgian study on the reliability and relative validity of the health behaviour in school-aged children food-frequency questionnaire. Public Health Nutr. 2003;6(6):581–8.
6. Truthmann J, Mensink GB, Richter A. Relative validation of the KiGGS food frequency questionnaire among adolescents in Germany. Nutr J. 2011;10:133.
7. Subar AF. Developing dietary assessment tools. J Am Diet Assoc. 2004;104(5):769–70.
8. Beaton GH. Approaches to analysis of dietary data: relationship between planned analyses and choice of methodology. Am J Clin Nutr. 1994;59(1 Suppl):253s–61s.
9. Willett WC. Nutritional epidemiology. 2nd ed. New York: Oxford University Press; 1998.

10. Tabacchi G, Amodio E, Di Pasquale M, Bianco A, Jemni M, Mammina C. Validation and reproducibility of dietary assessment methods in adolescents: a systematic literature review. Public Health Nutr. 2014;17(12):2700–14.
11. Hong TK, Dibley MJ, Sibbritt D. Validity and reliability of an FFQ for use with adolescents in ho chi Minh City, Vietnam. Public Health Nutr. 2010;13(3):368–75.
12. Overby NC, Johannesen E, Jensen G, Skjaevesland AK, Haugen M. Test-retest reliability and validity of a web-based food-frequency questionnaire for adolescents aged 13-14 to be used in the Norwegian mother and child cohort study (MoBa). Food NutrRes. 2014;58:23956.
13. Rockett HR, Breitenbach M, Frazier AL, Witschi J, Wolf AM, Field AE, et al. Validation of a youth/adolescent food frequency questionnaire. PrevMed. 1997;26(6):808–16.
14. Martinez MF, Philippi ST, Estima C, Leal G. Validity and reproducibility of a food frequency questionnaire to assess food group intake in adolescents. Cadernos de saude publica. 2013;29(9):1795–804.
15. Cade JE, Burley VJ, Warm DL, Thompson RL, Margetts BM. Food-frequency questionnaires: a review of their design, validation and utilisation. Nutr Res Rev. 2004;17(1):5–22.
16. De Moor C, Baranowski T, Cullen KW, Nicklas T. Misclassification associated with measurement error in the assessment of dietary intake. Public Health Nutr. 2003;6(4):393–9.
17. Chambers E, Godwin SL, Vecchio FA. Cognitive strategies for reporting portion sizes using dietary recall procedures. J Am Diet Assoc. 2000;100(8):891–7.
18. Livingstone MB, Robson PJ. Measurement of dietary intake in children. Proc Nutr Soc. 2000;59(2):279–93.
19. Lyng N, Fagt S, Davidsen M, Hoppe C, Holstein B, Tetens I. Reporting accuracy of packed lunch consumption among Danish 11-year-olds differ by gender. Food Nutr Res. 2013;57
20. Olsen SF, Mikkelsen TB, Knudsen VK, Orozova-Bekkevold I, Halldorsson TI, Strom M, et al. Data collected on maternal dietary exposures in the Danish National Birth Cohort. Paediatr Perinat Epidemiol. 2007;21(1):76–86.
21. Zhang C, Hu FB, Olsen SF, Vaag A, Gore-Langton R, Chavarro JE, et al. Rationale, design, and method of the Diabetes & Women's health study–a study of long-term health implications of glucose intolerance in pregnancy and their determinants. Acta Obstet Gynecol Scand. 2014;93(11):1123–30.
22. GUTS. Growning Up Today Study. http://www.gutsweb.org/. Assessed April 2014.
23. Fagt S, Matthiessen J, Trolle E, Lyhne N, Christensen T, Hinsch H-J, et al. 2. Danskernes kostvaner 2000–2001. Udviklingen i danskernes kost - forbrug, indkøb og vaner. Fødevaredirektoratet; 2002. Available from: http://www.food.dtu.dk/publikationer/ernaering-og-kostvaner
24. Fagt S, Christensen T, Groth MV, Biltoft-Jensen A, Matthiessen J, Trolle E. Børn og unges måltidsvaner 2000–2004 (dietary patterns of Danish children and adolescents 2000–2004): Fødevareinstituttet, DTU; 2007. Available from: http://www.food.dtu.dk/publikationer/ernaering-og-kostvaner
25. Bjerregaard AA, Tetens I, Olsen SF, Halldorsson TI. Reproducibility of a web-based FFQ for 13- to 15-year-old Danish adolescents. Journal of nutritional science. 2016;5:e5.
26. Ygil KH. Mål, vægt og portionsstørrelser (Dimensions, Weight and Portion sizes of Foods). Søborg: Fødevareinstituttet, DTU; 2013.
27. Pedersen AN, Christensen T, Matthiessen J, Knudsen VK, Rosenlund-Sørensen M, Biltoft-Jensen A, Hinsch HJ, Ygil KY, Kørup K, Saxholt E, Trolle E, Søndergaard AB, Fagt S. Dietary habits in Denmark 2011–2013. Main results. Report. Søborg. Denmark: National Food Institute; 2015. Available from: http://orbit.dtu.dk/files/110628064/Rapport_Danskernes_Kostvaner_2011_2013.pdf
28. Lauritsen J. Foodcalc v.1.3 http://www.ibt.ku.dk/jesper/foodcalc/ Assessed April 2014.
29. Danish Food Composition Data version www.foodcomp.dk. Assessed May 2015.
30. Cole TJ, Bellizzi MC, Flegal KM, Dietz WH. Establishing a standard definition for child overweight and obesity worldwide: international survey. BMJ. 2000;320(7244):1240–3.
31. Masson LF, McNeill G, Tomany JO, Simpson JA, Peace HS, Wei L, et al. Statistical approaches for assessing the relative validity of a food-frequency questionnaire: use of correlation coefficients and the kappa statistic. Public Health Nutr. 2003;6(3):313–21.
32. Bland JM, Altman DG. Measuring agreement in method comparison studies. Stat Methods Med Res. 1999;8(2):135–60.
33. Xia W, Sun C, Zhang L, Zhang X, Wang J, Wang H, et al. Reproducibility and relative validity of a food frequency questionnaire developed for female adolescents in Suihua, North China. PLoS One. 2011;6(5):e19656.
34. Henn RL, Fuchs SC, Moreira LB, Fuchs FD. Development and validation of a food frequency questionnaire (FFQ-Porto Alegre) for adolescent, adult and elderly populations from southern Brazil. CadSaude Publica. 2010;26(11):2068–79.
35. Viera AJ, Garrett JM. Understanding interobserver agreement: the kappa statistic. Family Med. 2005;37(5):360–3.
36. Rothausen BW, Matthiessen J, Hoppe C, Brockhoff PB, Andersen LF, Tetens I. Differences in Danish children's diet quality on weekdays v. Weekend days. Public Health Nutr. 2012;15(9):1653–60.
37. Andersen R, Biltoft-Jensen A, Christensen T, Andersen EW, Ege M, Thorsen AV, et al. What do Danish children eat, and does the diet meet the recommendations? Baseline data from the OPUS school meal study. J Nutr Sci. 2015;4:e29.
38. Krehbiel CF, DuPaul GJ, Hoffman JA. A validation study of the automated self-administered 24-hour dietary recall for children, 2014 version, at school lunch. J Acad Nutr Diet. 2017;117(5):715–24.
39. Bandini LG, Schoeller DA, Cyr HN, Dietz WH. Validity of reported energy intake in obese and nonobese adolescents. Am J Clin Nutr. 1990;52(3):421–5.
40. Kolodziejczyk JK, Merchant G, Norman GJ. Reliability and validity of child/adolescent food frequency questionnaires that assess foods and/or food groups. J Pediat Gastroenterol Nutr. 2012;55(1):4–13.
41. Johansson I, Hallmans G, Wikman A, Biessy C, Riboli E, Kaaks R. Validation and calibration of food-frequency questionnaire measurements in the northern Sweden health and disease cohort. Public Health Nutr. 2002;5(3):487–96.
42. Haftenberger M, Heuer T, Heidemann C, Kube F, Krems C, Mensink GB. Relative validation of a food frequency questionnaire for national health and nutrition monitoring. Nutr J. 2010;9:36.
43. Lu AS, Baranowski J, Islam N, Baranowski T. How to engage children in self-administered dietary assessment programmes. J Hum Nutr Diet. 2014;27(Suppl 1):5–9.
44. Boushey CJ, Kerr DA, Wright J, Lutes KD, Ebert DS, Delp EJ. Use of technology in children's dietary assessment. Eur J Clin Nutr. 2009;63(Suppl 1):S50–7.
45. Deschamps V, de Lauzon-Guillain B, Lafay L, Borys JM, Charles MA, Romon M. Reproducibility and relative validity of a food-frequency questionnaire among French adults and adolescents. Eur J Clin Nutr. 2009;63(2):282–91.
46. Ma Y, Olendzki BC, Pagoto SL, Hurley TG, Magner RP, Ockene IS, et al. Number of 24-hour diet recalls needed to estimate energy intake. Ann Epidemiol. 2009;19(8):553–9.
47. Casey PH, Goolsby SL, Lensing SY, Perloff BP, Bogle ML. The use of telephone interview methodology to obtain 24-hour dietary recalls. J Am Diet Assoc. 1999;99(11):1406–11.
48. Fox TA, Heimendinger J, Block G. Telephone surveys as a method for obtaining dietary information: a review. J Am Diet Assoc. 1992;92(6):729–32.
49. Serra-Majem L, Pfrimer K, Doreste-Alonso J, Ribas-Barba L, Sanchez-Villegas A, Ortiz-Andrellucchi A, et al. Dietary assessment methods for intakes of iron, calcium, selenium, zinc and iodine. Br J Nutr. 2009;102(Suppl 1):S38–55.
50. Nelson M. The validtaion of dietary assessment. In: Margetts BMN, M., editor. Design concepts in nutritional epidemiology. Second ed. Oxford Scholarship Online 2009.
51. Molgaard C, Dele F, Froberg K, Heitman BL, Holm L, Madsen SA, et al. Forebyggelse af overvægt blandt børn og unge – oplæg til strategi. (*Prevention of Obesity Among Children and Adolescents - Proposal for a* Strategy) Motions- og Ernæringsrådet; 2007. Available from: https://www.sst.dk/publ/MER/2007/FOREBYGGELSE_AF_OVERVAEGT_BLANDT_BOERN_OG_UNGE2007.PDF
52. Sundhedsstyrelsen. Opsporing af overvægt og tidlig indsats for børn og unge i skolealderen. 2014 2014. Copenhagen: Recognition of Overweight and Early Intervention for School-age Children; 2014. Available from: https://www.sst.dk/da/udgivelser/2014/~/media/F7C0D97FB5F840C69CE9388A0BAB4E1B.ashx

Permissions

All chapters in this book were first published in NJ, by BioMed Central; hereby published with permission under the Creative Commons Attribution License or equivalent. Every chapter published in this book has been scrutinized by our experts. Their significance has been extensively debated. The topics covered herein carry significant findings which will fuel the growth of the discipline. They may even be implemented as practical applications or may be referred to as a beginning point for another development.

The contributors of this book come from diverse backgrounds, making this book a truly international effort. This book will bring forth new frontiers with its revolutionizing research information and detailed analysis of the nascent developments around the world.

We would like to thank all the contributing authors for lending their expertise to make the book truly unique. They have played a crucial role in the development of this book. Without their invaluable contributions this book wouldn't have been possible. They have made vital efforts to compile up to date information on the varied aspects of this subject to make this book a valuable addition to the collection of many professionals and students.

This book was conceptualized with the vision of imparting up-to-date information and advanced data in this field. To ensure the same, a matchless editorial board was set up. Every individual on the board went through rigorous rounds of assessment to prove their worth. After which they invested a large part of their time researching and compiling the most relevant data for our readers.

The editorial board has been involved in producing this book since its inception. They have spent rigorous hours researching and exploring the diverse topics which have resulted in the successful publishing of this book. They have passed on their knowledge of decades through this book. To expedite this challenging task, the publisher supported the team at every step. A small team of assistant editors was also appointed to further simplify the editing procedure and attain best results for the readers.

Apart from the editorial board, the designing team has also invested a significant amount of their time in understanding the subject and creating the most relevant covers. They scrutinized every image to scout for the most suitable representation of the subject and create an appropriate cover for the book.

The publishing team has been an ardent support to the editorial, designing and production team. Their endless efforts to recruit the best for this project, has resulted in the accomplishment of this book. They are a veteran in the field of academics and their pool of knowledge is as vast as their experience in printing. Their expertise and guidance has proved useful at every step. Their uncompromising quality standards have made this book an exceptional effort. Their encouragement from time to time has been an inspiration for everyone.

The publisher and the editorial board hope that this book will prove to be a valuable piece of knowledge for researchers, students, practitioners and scholars across the globe.

List of Contributors

Katherine Kent, Simone Lee and Jonathon Mond
Centre for Rural Health, Faculty of Health, University of Tasmania, Launceston, TAS 7250, Australia

Karen E. Charlton
Faculty of Science, Medicine and Health, University of Wollongong, Wollongong, Australia
Illawarra Health and Medical Research Institute, Wollongong, Australia

Joanna Russell
Faculty of Social Sciences, University of Wollongong, Wollongong, Australia

Paul Mitchell
Centre for Vision Research, University of Sydney, Sydney, Australia

Victoria M. Flood
Faculty of Health Sciences, University of Sydney, Sydney, Australia
Western Sydney Local Health District, Sydney, Australia

Ulrike Trautvetter
Department of Nutritional Toxicology, Institute of Nutrition, Friedrich Schiller University Jena, Dornburger Straße 24, 07743 Jena, Germany

Amélia Camarinha-Silva
Institute of Animal Science, University of Hohenheim, Emil-Wolff-Straße. 10, 70599 Stuttgart, Germany

Gerhard Jahreis
Department of Nutritional Physiology, Institute of Nutrition, Friedrich Schiller University Jena, Dornburger Straße 23, 07743 Jena, Germany
Competence Cluster for Nutrition and Cardiovascular Health (nutriCARD) Halle-Jena-Leipzig, Jena, Germany

Stefan Lorkowski
Department of Nutritional Biochemistry and Physiology, Institute of Nutrition, Friedrich Schiller University Jena, Dornburger Straße 25, 07743 Jena, Germany
Competence Cluster for Nutrition and Cardiovascular Health (nutriCARD) Halle-Jena-Leipzig, Jena, Germany

Michael Glei
Department of Nutritional Toxicology, Institute of Nutrition, Friedrich Schiller University Jena, Dornburger Straße 24, 07743 Jena, Germany
Competence Cluster for Nutrition and Cardiovascular Health (nutriCARD) Halle-Jena-Leipzig, Jena, Germany

Adriana Monge
Center for Research on Population Health, National Institute of Public Health, Cuernavaca, Mexico
Escuela de Medicina, Tecnológico de Monterrey, Monterrey, Mexico

Martín Lajous
Center for Research on Population Health, National Institute of Public Health, Cuernavaca, Mexico
Department of Global Health and Population, Harvard T.H. Chan School of Public Health, Boston, USA

Eduardo Ortiz-Panozo and Ruy López-Ridaura
Center for Research on Population Health, National Institute of Public Health, Cuernavaca, Mexico

Beatriz L. Rodríguez
Escuela de Medicina, Tecnológico de Monterrey, Monterrey, Mexico
University of Hawaii at Manoa, Honolulu, HI, USA

José Juan Góngora
Escuela de Medicina, Tecnológico de Monterrey, Monterrey, Mexico

Margaret Raber
Department of Pediatrics Research, University of Texas MD Anderson Cancer Center, Houston, USA

Monika Patterson and Tom Baranowsk
USDA/ARS Children's Nutrition Research Center, Baylor College of Medicine, Houston, USA

Wenyan Jia and Mingui Sun
Department of Neurological Surgery, University of Pittsburg, Pittsburg, USA

Olivia Portolese, Yasmine Chertouk and Jade Leahy
Research Centre, Sainte-Justine University Health Center, Department of Nutrition, Université de Montréal, Montreal, QC H3T 1C5, Canada

Laurence Bertout, Caroline Laverdière, Maja Krajinovic and Daniel Sinnett
Research Centre, Sainte-Justine University Health Center, Department of Pediatrics, Université de Montréal, Montreal, QC H3T 1C5, Canada

Ishor Sharma, Barbara Roebothan, Yun Zhu, Jennifer Woodrow and Peter Peizhong Wang
Division of Community Health and Humanities, Faculty of Medicine, Memorial University of Newfoundland, St. John's, NF, Canada

Patrick S. Parfrey
Clinical Epidemiology Unit, Faculty of Medicine, Memorial University of Newfoundland, St. John's, NF, Canada

John R. Mclaughlin
Public Health Ontario, Toronto, ON, Canada

Matthieu Maillot and Florent Vieux
MS-Nutrition, 27 bld Jean Moulin Faculté de Médecine la Timone, Laboratoire NORT, 13385 Marseille cedex 5, France

Colin D. Rehm
Albert Einstein College of Medicine, Montefiore Medical Center, New York, NY 10467, USA

Chelsea M. Rose and Adam Drewnowski
Center for Public Health Nutrition, University of Washington, Seattle, WA 98195, USA

Zakari Ali and Abdul-Razak Abizari
Department of Nutritional Sciences, School of Allied Health Sciences, University for Development Studies, Tamale, Ghana

Sridharshi Chintha Hewawitharana, Lorrene Ritchie and Karen Lucy Webb
Nutrition Policy Institute, University of California, Agriculture and Natural Resources Division, 2115 Milvia Street, Third floor, Berkeley, CA 94704, USA

Frances Elizabeth Thompson
Risk Factor Assessment Branch, Epidemiology and Genomics Research Program, Division of Cancer Control and Population Sciences, National Cancer Institute, Rm. 4E124, 9609 Medical Center Drive, MSC 9763, Bethesda, MD 20892, USA

Catherine M. Loria
Division of Cardiovascular Sciences, National Heart, Lung, and Blood Institute, 6701 Rockledge Drive, Suite 10018, Bethesda, MD 20892, USA

Warren Strauss and Jyothi Nagaraja
Battelle, 505 King Ave, Columbus, OH 43201, USA

Analí Castellanos-Gutiérrez and Tania G. Sánchez-Pimienta
Center for Nutrition and Health Research, National Institute of Public Health, Mexico. Av. Universidad 655, Col. Santa María Ahuacatitlán. Cerrada los pinos y caminera. C.P, 62100 Cuernavaca, Morelos, Mexico

Alicia Carriquiry
Department of Statistics, Iowa State University, Ames, Iowa 50011, USA

Teresa H. M. da Costa
Department of Nutrition, School of Health Science, University of Brasilia, Brasilia - DF, CEP 70910-900, Brazil

Ana Carolina Ariza
National Council of Science and Technology (CONACYT) - Center for Nutrition and Health Research, National Institute of Public Health, Cuernavaca, Morelos, Mexico

Katherine M. Livingstone and Sarah A. McNaughton
Institute for Physical Activity and Nutrition, School of Exercise and Nutrition Sciences, Deakin University, Melbourne Burwood Campus, 221 Burwood Highway, Geelong, Victoria 3125, Australia

Sandra N. Slagter, Melanie M. van der Klauw, Bruce H. R. Wolffenbuttel and Jana V. van Vliet-Ostaptchouk
Department of Endocrinology, University of Groningen, University Medical Center Groningen, HPC AA31, Groningen, The Netherlands

Eva Corpeleijn and Daan Kromhout
Department of Epidemiology, University of Groningen, University Medical Center Groningen, Groningen, The Netherlands

Anna Sijtsma
Lifelines Cohort Study, University of Groningen, University Medical Center Groningen, Groningen, The Netherlands

Linda G. Swart-Busscher
Department of Paramedical Sciences, University of Groningen, University Medical Center Groningen, Groningen, The Netherlands

Corine W. M. Perenboom, Jeanne H. M. de Vries and Edith J. M. Feskens
Division of Human Nutrition, Wageningen University, 6700, AA, Wageningen, The Netherlands

Anne A. Bjerregaard and Sjurdur F. Olsen
Center for Fetal Programming, Department of Epidemiology Research, Statens Serum Institut, Artillerivej 5, 2300 Copenhagen, Denmark

Thorhallur I. Halldorsson
Center for Fetal Programming, Department of Epidemiology Research, Statens Serum Institut, Artillerivej 5, 2300 Copenhagen, Denmark
The Unit for Nutrition Research, Faculty of Food Science and Nutrition, School of Health Sciences, University of Iceland, Sæmundargata 2, 101 Reykjavík, Iceland

Freja B. Kampmann
Division for Diet, Disease Prevention and Toxicology, National Food Institute, Technical University of Denmark, DTU Food, Kemitorvet, building, 202 Kgs. Lyngby, Denmark
Department of Endocrinology, Diabetes and Metabolism, Rigshospitalet, Copenhagen, Denmark
The Danish Diabetes Academy, Odense, Denmark

Inge Tetens
Vitality - Centre for Good Older Lives, Department of Nutrition, Exercise, and Sports, University of Copenhagen, University of Copenhagen, Rolighedsvej 26, 1958 Frederiksberg C, Denmark

Index

M

N

O

P

R

S

T

W

CPSIA information can be obtained
at www.ICGtesting.com
Printed in the USA
LVHW062019100122
708212LV00002B/329

9 781641 166317